The Neuroanesthesia Handbook

D1135794

The Neuroanesthesia Handbook

DAVID J. STONE, M.D.
Associate Professor of Anesthesiology and Neurological Surgery
University of Virginia Health Sciences Center
Director of Neuroanesthesiology
Virginia Neurological Institute
Charlottesville, Virginia

RICHARD J. SPERRY, M.D., Ph.D.
Associate Professor of Anesthesiology and Neurosurgery
Chief of Neuroanesthesia
University of Utah Health Sciences Center
Salt Lake City, Utah

JOEL O. JOHNSON, M.D., Ph.D.
Assistant Professor of Anesthesiology and Neurosurgery
University of Utah Health Sciences Center
Salt Lake City, Utah

BURKHARD F. SPIEKERMANN, M.D.
Assistant Professor of Anesthesiology
University of Virginia Health Sciences Center
Charlottesville, Virginia

TERRANCE A. YEMEN, M.D.
Assistant Professor of Anesthesiology
University of Virginia Health Sciences Center
Charlottesville, Virginia

*with **94** illustrations*

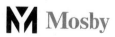

Mosby

St. Louis   Baltimore   Boston
Carlsbad   Chicago   Naples   New York   Philadelphia   Portland
London   Madrid   Mexico City   Singapore   Sydney   Tokyo   Toronto   Wiesbaden

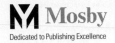

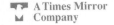

Executive Editor: Susan M. Gay
Developmental Editor: Sandra Clark Brown
Project Manager: Patricia Tannian
Production Editor: Melissa Mraz
Book Design Manager: Gail Morey Hudson
Manufacturing Supervisor: Dave Graybill
Editing and Production: Top Graphics
Cover Designer: Teresa Breckwoldt
Cover Illustration: Courtesy *Journal of
Neurosurgery*

Printed in the United States of America
Composition by Top Graphics
Printing/binding by R.R. Donnelley & Sons Company

Mosby–Year Book, Inc.
11830 Westline Industrial Drive
St. Louis, Missouri 63146

Library of Congress Cataloging in Publication Data

The neuroanesthesia handbook / David J. Stone . . . [et al.].
    p.   cm.
  Rev. ed. of: Manual of neuroanesthesia / Richard J. Sperry, Joseph
A. Stirt, David J. Stone. c1989.
  Includes bibliographical references and index.
  ISBN 0-8151-8145-0
  1. Anesthesia in neurology—Handbooks, manuals, etc.   I. Stone,
David J.   II. Sperry, R.J.   III. Manual of neuroanesthesia.
  [DNLM: 1. Nervous System—drug effects—handbooks.   2. Anesthesia—
handbooks.   3. Nervous System—surgery—handbooks.   WL 39 N4935 1995]
RD87.3.N47N48   1995
617.9'6748—dc20
DNLM/DLC
for Library of Congress   95-34090
                                                                  CIP

95 96 97 98 99 / 9 8 7 6 5 4 3 2 1

CONTRIBUTORS

THOMAS P. BLECK, M.D., F.A.C.P., F.C.C.M.

Associate Professor of Neurology and Neurological Surgery
The John T. and Louise Nerancy Professor of Neurology
Director, Neuroscience Intensive Care Unit
University of Virginia Health Sciences Center
Charlottesville, Virginia

DAVID L. BOGDONOFF, M.D.

Associate Professor of Anesthesiology and Surgery
University of Virginia Health Sciences Center
Charlottesville, Virginia

CHERYLEE W.J. CHANG, M.D.

Fellow, Neuroscience Critical Care
University of Virginia Health Sciences Center
Charlottesville, Virginia

ANDREW G. CHENELLE, M.D.

Resident, Department of Neurological Surgery
University of Virginia Health Sciences Center
Charlottesville, Virginia

COSMO A. DiFAZIO, M.D., Ph.D.

Professor of Anesthesiology
University of Virginia Health Sciences Center
Charlottesville, Virginia

MARCEL E. DURIEUX, M.D.

Assistant Professor of Anesthesiology
University of Virginia Health Sciences Center
Charlottesville, Virginia

STEVEN T. FARNSWORTH, M.D.

Instructor
University of Utah Health Sciences Center
Salt Lake City, Utah

ROBERT S. HOLZMAN, M.D.

Senior Associate in Anesthesia and Director of Extramural
Anesthesia
Children's Hospital
Assistant Professor of Anaesthesia
Harvard Medical School
Boston, Massachusetts

J. MICHAEL JAEGER, M.D., Ph.D.

Assistant Professor of Anesthesiology and Neurological Surgery
University of Virginia Health Sciences Center
Charlottesville, Virginia

JOEL O. JOHNSON, M.D., Ph.D.

Assistant Professor of Anesthesiology and Neurosurgery
University of Utah Health Sciences Center
Salt Lake City, Utah

GEORGE S. LEISURE, M.D.

Assistant Professor of Anesthesiology
University of Virginia Health Sciences Center
Charlottesville, Virginia

LAWRENCE H. PHILLIPS II, M.D.

Associate Professor of Medicine (Neurology)
University of Virginia Health Sciences Center
Charlottesville, Virginia

CHRISTOPHER I. SHAFFREY, M.D.

Fellow, Neurological Surgery
University of Virginia Health Sciences Center
Charlottesville, Virginia

MARK E. SHAFFREY, M.D.

Assistant Professor of Neurological Surgery
University of Virginia Health Sciences Center
Charlottesville, Virginia

RICHARD J. SPERRY, M.D., Ph.D.

Associate Professor of Anesthesiology and Neurosurgery
Chief of Neuroanesthesia
University of Utah Health Sciences Center
Salt Lake City, Utah

BURKHARD F. SPIEKERMANN, M.D.

Assistant Professor of Anesthesiology
University of Virginia Health Sciences Center
Charlottesville, Virginia

DAVID J. STONE, M.D.

Associate Professor of Anesthesiology and Neurological Surgery
University of Virginia Health Sciences Center
Director of Neuroanesthesiology
Virginia Neurological Institute
Charlottesville, Virginia

SCOTT A. THOMPSON, M.D.

Research Fellow in Neuroanesthesiology
University of Virginia Health Sciences Center
Charlottesville, Virginia

TERRANCE A. YEMEN, M.D.

Assistant Professor of Anesthesiology
University of Virginia Health Sciences Center
Charlottesville, Virginia

PREFACE

This handbook is essentially a revision of the *Manual of Neuroanesthesia,* edited by R.J. Sperry, J.A. Stirt, and D.J. Stone and published in 1989. The original editors were gratified to receive positive reviews from our own house staffs, as well as from residents and staff members at other institutions. However, we came to realize that significant changes in neuroanesthesia and neurologic surgery demanded a new edition. Therefore, in conjunction with the staff at Mosby, we decided to produce a fully updated but similar (in style) work in a more portable-sized book. Rather than using the outline form usually expected in a handbook, we have written this book as a mini-textbook. We have not attempted to avoid all repetition or to extract any element of personal style from the individual chapters. Rather, we hope we have provided you with a useful work that is fun and easy to read and fits easily into the back pocket of your scrubs during a rotation on neuroanesthesia or an encounter with a neurosurgical patient under other circumstances.

In addition to updating the content of the *Manual of Neuroanesthesia,* we have made other important new changes in *The Neuroanesthesia Handbook.* We have altered our introductory neurosurgical chapter to be primarily anatomically oriented, including many illustrations that should help you learn about what the neurosurgeon is trying to accomplish. We have also introduced two new chapters: one on craniofacial and craniobasal surgery and another on epilepsy surgery and stereotactic procedures. These additions were necessary because of the continuing advances in neurosurgery. The chapters on pediatric neuroanesthesia, neuroradiology, head trauma, and intensive care have been entirely rewritten by new authors who have brought fresh and interesting approaches to these problems. All the remaining chapters have been thoughtfully and thoroughly updated. We feel confident that *The Neuroanesthesia Handbook* will become an essential piece of equipment in your care of neurosurgical patients.

David J. Stone
Richard J. Sperry
Joel O. Johnson
Burkhard F. Spiekermann
Terrance A. Yemen

CONTENTS

NEUROSURGICAL ANATOMY

1

Andrew G. Chenelle
Mark E. Shaffrey
Christopher I. Shaffrey
David J. Stone

The goal of neuroanesthesia is to provide a safe anesthetic for the patient while improving surgical conditions in keeping with patient safety. To achieve this goal, a basic knowledge of neuroanatomy is important for several reasons. First, a familiarity with the anatomy of the nervous system is part of the database of any well-educated physician. In more practical terms, this knowledge allows the anesthetist to practice more efficient, more directed, and better care of the neurosurgical patient. It also provides for improved communication between surgeon and anesthetist, which is undeniably beneficial for day-to-day and long-term relationships in the neurosurgical operating room and sets the stage for benefits to the patient. Finally, a complete understanding of "what is going on" on the other side of the ether screen makes the whole process of neuroanesthesia more professional and more enjoyable for the resident, the nurse anesthetist, or the attending anesthesiologist involved in the case.

Anesthesia can be achieved by putting the patient to sleep, inserting the appropriate tubes, and keeping the patient from moving until the surgeon has completed the procedure. However, it can also be accomplished by a thoughtful practitioner whose understanding of the medical implications, surgical requirements, and complications of each stage of the procedure contributes to the maintenance and development of the bona fide specialty that neuroanesthesiology has become.

DEFINITIONS

When you encounter any new field of medicine, the first job is to learn the language in order to communicate with the established practitioners. Clinical neurosurgery is no exception to the medical tower of Babel. The following list of terms should assist in your assimilation into this remarkable culture. It is by no means complete but has been selected to include some of the terms used most commonly on a daily basis in the operating room. Other significant terms are found later in this or other chapters.

Most important, if you do not recognize or understand some terminology, ask the surgeon. Rather than exposing yourself as ignorant, this approach will identify you as interested and open up a useful two-way information superhighway on your particular block.

Anterior Circulation—The part of the cerebral circulation, including and emanating from the middle and anterior cerebral arteries, that perfuses the anterior half of the thalamus and the cerebral cortex (except for those areas supplied by the posterior circulation).

Bipolar Needle Electrode—A device used for coagulation in neurosurgery. Unlike the Bovey electrocautery, in which the circuit runs from the coagulator to a distantly placed pad, the bipolar electrode has two (BI-polar) closely positioned tips that contain the flow of heat-producing current to the small area exposed to the tips.

Burr Hole—A small (≤2 cm diameter) hole drilled through the skull to reach the epidural or subdural spaces for emergency evacuation of a hematoma or one drilled completely through the meninges to reach the ventricles for drainage or brain tissue for biopsy. The drilling can be performed with the patient under local anesthesia, supplemented as required by patient discomfort. A bony incision carried out between three (or more) burr holes can be used to create a craniotomy flap (see Fig. 1-1, *F*).

Calvaria—The bones of the cranial vault that, together with the cranial base, make up the skull. They include the frontal, parietal, occipital, sphenoid, and temporal bones (see Fig. 1-1, *A*). To review the anatomy of the cranial base, see Fig. 1-1, *B*.

Camino—The name that surgeons often use to refer to the currently preferred intracranial pressure monitor. Camino is actually the name of the company that manufactures the device (think Xerox). (For further information, see Chapter 4.)

Cavernous Sinuses—Venous sinuses that are situated on either side of the sella turcica and run from the superior orbital fissure anteriorly to the temporal bone posteriorly. Surgery in this area is treacherous because these sinuses contain the third, fourth, sixth, first, and second divisions of the fifth cranial nerve as well as the carotid artery.

Craniectomy—An intracranial operation in which a bone flap is removed and not replaced because it cannot be (severe cerebral edema) or should not be (infection or tumor involvement). In a lobectomy brain tissue is resected, but in a lobotomy brain tissue is merely incised.

Cranioplasty—A procedure in which the craniectomy bone flap is replaced by actual bone or an acrylic substitute to protect the fragile brain tissue. This step is necessary because, unlike the periosteum of long bones, the periosteum of the adult skull is deficient in osteogenic potential.

Craniotomy—An intracranial operation in which a bone flap is removed during surgery and replaced before closure.

Depth Electrodes—Electrodes placed into the brain substance to map an epileptic focus. This type contrasts with grid electrodes, which lie on the brain surface.

Disc—An intervertebral plate that is made up of two parts: a dense outer capsule called the annulus fibrosis and an inner cushion called the nucleus pulposus. Disc herniations occur when a region of annulus fibrosis weakens and allows the nucleus pulposus to extrude.

Dura—Formally, this part of the brain is called the dura mater or "tough mother" (really!). Within the skull, the outer layer of dura forms the inner layer of periosteum. The inner layer of dura makes up the meningeal layers, which divide the intracranial space into several distinct areas:

Falx Cerebri—Fold that divides the cerebral hemispheres in the midline.

Falx Cerebelli—Fold that divides the cerebellar hemispheres in the midline.

Tentorium Cerebelli—Horizontally oriented fold that divides the supratentorial cerebral hemispheres from the infratentorial cerebellum.

Hydrocephalus—Enlargement of the ventricular system and accumulation of cerebrospinal fluid within the brain resulting from failure to reabsorb cerebrospinal fluid (communicating hydrocephalus), obstruction of cerebrospinal fluid flow (noncommunicating hydrocephalus), or overproduction of cerebrospinal fluid by a choroid plexus tumor.

Laminectomy—A spinal operation in which parts of adjacent vertebral laminae are removed to gain access to a herniated disc. This procedure is accomplished with robust instruments such as punches and rongeurs.

Posterior Circulation—The parts of the cerebral circulation that include and emanate from the vertebral, basilar, and posterior cerebral arteries. The areas supplied include the posterior thalamus and the remainder of the brainstem, the cerebellum, the occipital lobes, and the inferior surface of the temporal lobes.

Sella Turcica—Literally "Turkish saddle," this space, located in the cranial base, contains the pituitary gland. It is defined by the cavernous sinuses laterally and anteroposteriorly by the respective clinoid processes. The roof of the sella is formed by a flap of dura known as the diaphragma sellae, which is perforated by the pituitary stalk.

Stereotaxis—The process by which a precise area of brain is identified by an imaging technique and assigned to a three-dimensional coordinate that is fixed by an external head frame. The area of interest can then be identified by the previously defined point in space with reference to the head frame. It is this requirement for precise localization dependent on the position of the head frame that makes neurosurgeons reluctant to move or remove the head frame, for example, for airway management.

Ventriculostomy—Insertion of catheters into the ventricular system by a frontal or parietooccipital approach (see Fig. 1-3, *C*). The catheters can be externalized for drainage and measurement of intracranial pressure or internalized to the peritoneum, pleura, or atrium for more permanent drainage of cerebrospinal fluid.

NEURORADIOLOGY

There have been stunning advances in neuroradiology over the past 20 years, and this section is intended to give only the briefest overview of these developments.

The neuroanesthetist encounters, on a daily basis, different types of clinical findings as they are displayed prominently in the neurosurgical operating room. Therefore it is reasonable to expect the neuroanesthetist to have a basic understanding of what he/she is viewing, especially when implications for anesthetic care are involved. In general, these findings include intracranial masses with edema and shift of midline structures implying increased intracranial pressure (ICP).

Probably the most practical way to gain facility in reading arteriograms, computed tomography (CT) scans, and magnetic resonance imaging (MRI) scans is to review the studies with the surgeons at the beginning of the case, preferably before induction of anesthesia (and not when the patient is present). It is also possible to review studies with the neuroradiologists who may be assigned to cover cases in that area. With practice, the most important lesions usually can be spotted.

CT scanning is the "high-tech" modality that revolutionized neuroimaging about 20 years ago. Although state-of-the-art CT is highly accurate, it has been replaced by MRI as the image of choice for most purposes. However, CT is still employed in emergency situations because it is the preferred means of detecting intracranial hemorrhage and it is less difficult logistically for the acute trauma patient. Contrast myelography with CT is actually more sensitive than MRI in the diagnosis of certain spinal cord lesions, such as small discs that exert pressure on nerve roots. MRI is especially effective in areas such as the posterior fossa and the skull base and is useful in detecting subtle parenchymal lesions, for example, in demyelinating disease. Arteriograms represent a quantal leap in diagnostic difficulty. They are used in the evaluation of aneurysms and arteriovenous malformations (AVMs) but also may be employed in any situation in which hypervascularity represents a potential surgical problem. The vascular blush of an AVM or a vascular tumor is often not extremely difficult to identify and may give a rough idea of the likelihood of excessive bleeding and the need for another IV infusion. The size of the AVM may also suggest the potential for postoperative edema and/or hemorrhage, which is more likely if the AVM is large. *Text continues on p. 27.*

GALLERY OF NEUROANATOMIC ILLUSTRATIONS

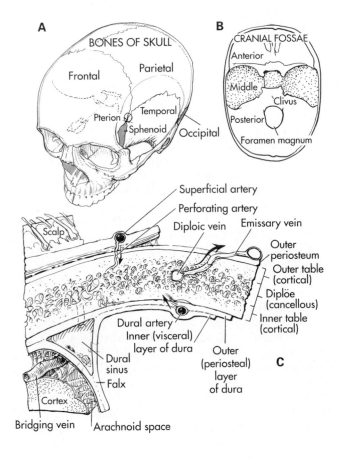

Figs. 1-1 through 1-8 from Shaffrey ME, Shaffrey CI, Chenelle AG, Stone DJ: Central neuroanatomy: an operative approach. In Weinberg GL, editor: *Basic science for anesthesiologists*, New York, 1995, McGraw-Hill.

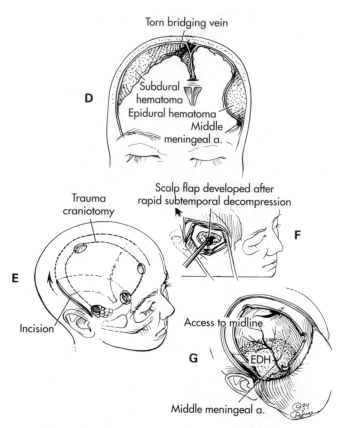

FIG 1-1.

Skull. **A,** Cranial vault or calvaria. Note location of pterion, an important area in neurosurgical access. **B,** Skull base demonstrating three cranial fossae: anterior, middle, and posterior. **C,** Cross section of calvaria. **D,** Coronal section demonstrating epidural (middle meningeal artery) and subdural (torn bridging vein) hematomas. **E,** Large bone flap traditionally raised for exploration in traumatic hemorrhage. **F,** Emergent subtemporal decompression before craniotomy. **G,** Completed craniotomy revealing epidural hemorrhage *(EDH)* and middle meningeal artery, which will need to be coagulated.

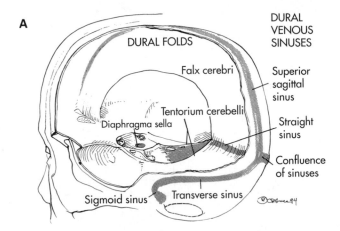

FIG 1-2.
Dural membranes and herniation syndromes. **A,** Cut-away skull section with brain removed demonstrates primary dural partitions and venous sinuses. **B,** Simplified normal coronal section; *SSS,* superior sagittal sinus; *TS,* transverse sinus; *V,* ventricle. **C,** Herniation of uncus of temporal lobe. This type of herniation may result in pressure on oculomotor nerve, posterior cerebral arteries, and cerebral peduncle, producing pupillary abnormalities, contralateral hemiplegia, and, possibly, ipsilateral medial occipital lobe infarction. Extreme pressure on brainstem structures responsible for consciousness (reticular activating system) results in coma. **D,** Subfalcine herniation. This anomaly can directly injure cingulate gyrus and cause ischemia in anterior cerebral artery distribution. Supratentorial masses in midline can cause central herniation syndrome through tentorial hiatus and force brainstem structures down through foramen magnum (known as *coning*). Downward movement of brainstem structures against immobile basilar artery may also result in brainstem hemorrhage. **E,** Tonsillar herniation. Proximity of cerebellum to critical brainstem structures and relatively small size of posterior fossa result in severe problems with lesions that would cause less difficulty if they were supratentorial.

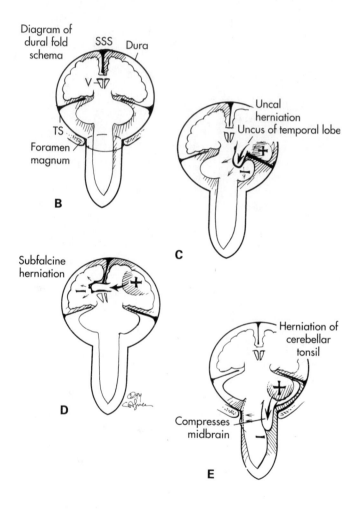

Diagram of dural fold schema

SSS Dura

V

TS

Foramen magnum

B

Uncal herniation
Uncus of temporal lobe

C

Subfalcine herniation

D

Herniation of cerebellar tonsil

Compresses midbrain

E

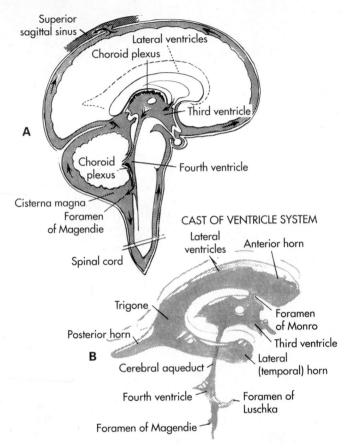

FIG 1-3.
Ventricular System. **A** and **B**, Ventricular anatomy and CSF flow.
CSF is produced in choroid plexus of lateral and fourth ventricles.
It flows from lateral ventricles through foramina of Monro into third
ventricle. CSF then flows from third ventricle via cerebral aqueduct
of Sylvius to rhomboid-shaped fourth ventricle. It exits fourth ventricle via midline foramen of Magendie and lateral foramina of
Luschka and then flows superiorly into cisterns and subarachnoid
space surrounding cerebellum and inferiorly into spinal subarachnoid space. CSF returns to venous system via arachnoid granula-
tions, mainly in superior sagittal sinus.

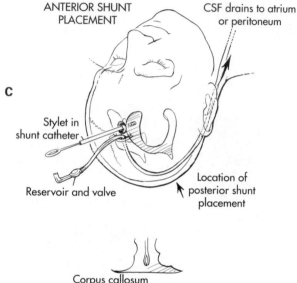

ANTERIOR SHUNT
PLACEMENT

CSF drains to atrium
or peritoneum

C

Stylet in
shunt catheter

Reservoir and valve

Location of
posterior shunt
placement

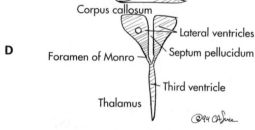

Corpus callosum

Lateral ventricles

D   Foramen of Monro

Septum pellucidum

Third ventricle

Thalamus

FIG 1-3, cont'd.

C, Positions for anterior or posterior shunt placement. For anterior placement, burr hole is located 2 cm anterior to coronal suture in midpupillary line; catheter enters ipsilateral anterior or frontal horn anterior to foramen of Monro. **D,** Simplified cross section with catheter tip situated in lateral ventricle.

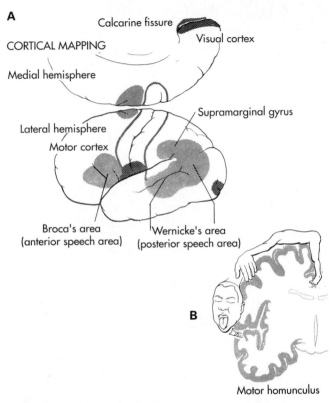

FIG 1-4.
Localization of cortical function. **A,** Cortical localization of vision, motor function (precentral gyrus), and communication. **B,** Motor homunculus representing distribution of brain areas responsible for body movement. Lower extremity is medial, and face is most lateral. Analogous sensory homunculus coexists in postcentral gyrus.

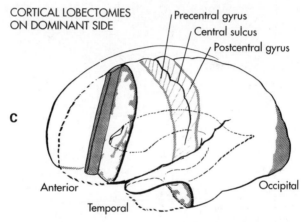

CORTICAL LOBECTOMIES
ON DOMINANT SIDE

Precentral gyrus
Central sulcus
Postcentral gyrus

C

Anterior

Temporal

Occipital

FIG 1-4, cont'd.
C, Cut-away views of frontal and temporal lobectomies. Shaded
area represents potential occipital lobectomy.

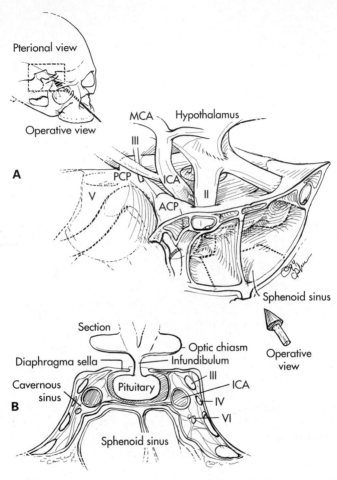

FIG 1-5.
Parasellar anatomy. **A,** Pterional view of parasellar region showing optic nerve (II) and other cranial nerves. *ACP,* Anterior clinoid process; *ICA,* internal carotid artery; *PCP,* posterior clinoid process. **B,** Pituitary gland is situated directly beneath optic chiasm. Coronal section of sella turcica showing surrounding cavernous sinuses, intercavernous cranial nerves, and internal carotid artery (*ICA*).

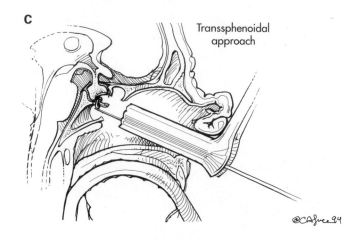

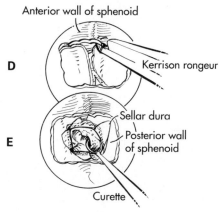

FIG 1-5, cont'd.
C, Sagittal view of completed approach. **D**, Removal of anterior sphenoid sinus wall with Kerrison rongeur. **E**, Removal of tumor with ring curette.

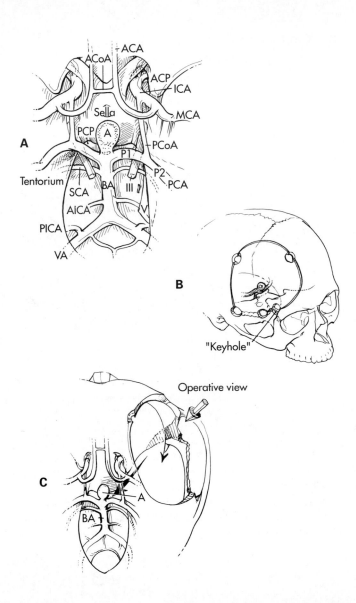

A

ACoA
ACA
ACP
ICA
Sella
MCA
PCP
A
PCoA
P1
Tentorium
P2
PCA
SCA
BA
III
AICA
V
PICA
VA

B

"Keyhole"

Operative view

C

A
BA

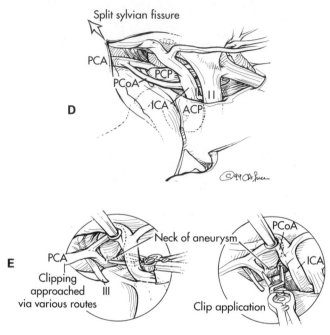

FIG 1-6.

Circle of Willis. **A**, View from above with basilar tip aneurysm present. *A*, Aneurysm; *ACA*, anterior cerebral artery; *ACoA*, anterior communicating artery; *ACP*, anterior clinoid process; *AICA*, anterior inferior cerebellar artery; *BA*, basilar artery; *ICA*, internal carotid artery; *MCA*, middle cerebral artery; *PCA*, posterior cerebral artery; *PCoA*, posterior communicating artery; *PCP*, posterior clinoid process; *PICA*, posterior inferior cerebellar artery; *P1, P2*, first and second segments of posterior cerebral artery; *SCA*, superior cerebellar artery; *VA*, vertebral artery. Circle of Willis is subject to frequent anatomic variations, and "normal" circle is found in only half of population. This structure is critical in providing anastomotic pathways to regions involved with arterial occlusions. **B**, Pterional craniotomy for basilar tip aneurysm demonstrating "keyhole" burr hole in pterion. **C**, Operative view. **D**, View after splitting of sylvian fissure. **E**, Application of aneurysm clip medial *(left)* and lateral *(right)* to internal carotid artery.

A

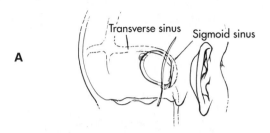

B

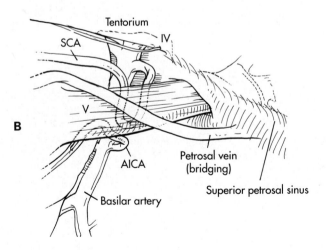

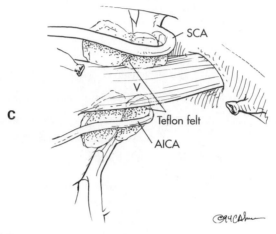

FIG 1-7.

Posterior fossa I: microvascular decompression of trigeminal nerve.
A, View of craniotomy with vascular sinuses exposed. **B**, Trigeminal nerve may be compressed by loops of anterior inferior cerebellar artery *(AICA)* or superior cerebellar artery *(SCA)*. Petrosal vein
drains anterior brainstem and superior cerebellum. This vein runs
close to trigeminal nerve and may need to be divided during approach. Trigeminal nerve originates on lateral surface of pons and
divides into three well-known branches—ophthalmic (V1), maxillary (V2), and mandibular (V3)—that exit skull through superior
orbital fissure, foramen rotundum, and foramen ovale. **C**, Separation of vessels from nerve with Teflon felt.

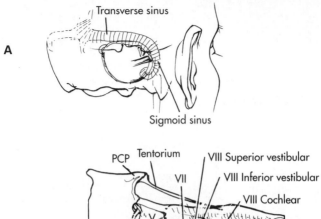

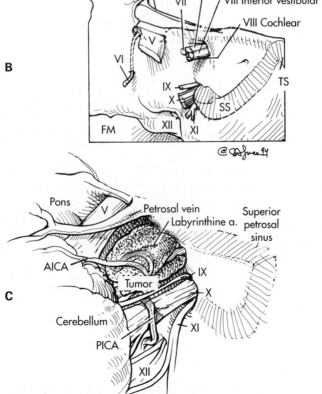

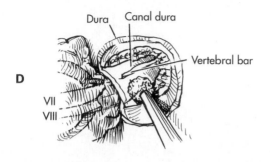

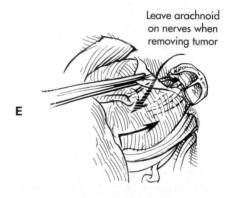

FIG 1-8.

Posterior fossa II: resection of acoustic neuroma. **A**, View of sub-occipital craniotomy. **B**, Region of internal acoustic meatus with brainstem cut away. Note seventh cranial nerve and three branches of eighth cranial nerve entering meatus. *FM*, foramen magnum; *SS*, sigmoid sinus; *TS*, transverse sinus; *PCP*, posterior clinoid process. **C**, Surgical view of tumor. Note close association of anterior inferior cerebellar artery *(AICA)* with tumor and displacement of seventh and eighth cranial nerves. *PICA*, posterior inferior cerebellar artery. **D**, Drilling of internal acoustic meatus. **E**, Separation of tumor from arachnoid plane after internal debulking.

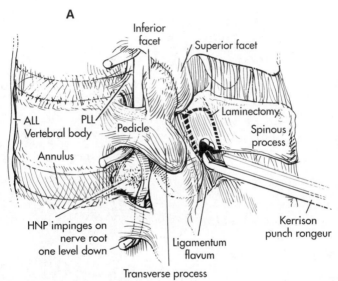

A

Inferior facet

Superior facet

ALL
Vertebral body

PLL

Pedicle

Laminectomy

Spinous process

Annulus

HNP impinges on
nerve root
one level down

Ligamentum
flavum

Kerrison
punch rongeur

Transverse process

FIG 1-9.
Lumbar laminectomy showing vertebral anatomy. **A,** Oblique view of lumbar spine demonstrating anatomic relationships. Anterior longitudinal ligament *(ALL)* and posterior longitudinal ligament *(PLL)* serve as major support structures between vertebral bodies. Often herniated nucleus pulposus *(HNP)* is contained by posterior longitudinal ligament, even though it has ruptured through annulus fibrosis. Nerve roots exit beneath pedicle. Because of anatomy of exiting nerve roots, herniated disc impinges on nerve root named for lower vertebral body (i.e., L4-5 disc impinges on L5 nerve root). Laminectomy is performed by removing approximately half of lamina above and below disc space of interest. Underlying lamina and spinous processes is ligamentum flavum, which also must be removed to gain access to disc space.

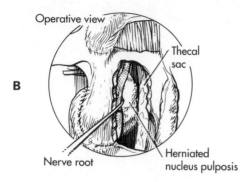

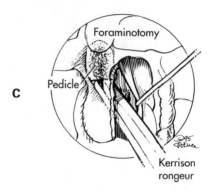

FIG 1-9, cont'd.

B, Once laminectomy has been performed, nerve root can be retracted either medially (more common) or laterally (as illustrated) to
better visualize herniated disc. Disc is then removed with curettes
and rongeurs. **C**, Occasionally pedicles or facets are hypertrophied
and cause compression of nerve root. Foramen can be enlarged by
reaching into foramen and removing hypertrophied bone (foramino-
tomy).

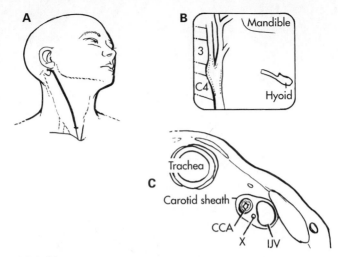

FIG 1-10.

Approach to carotid endarterectomy. **A,** Skin incision for carotid endarterectomy is generous because adequate exposure of distal internal carotid artery is of utmost importance. Incision runs from anterior mastoid process to sternal notch at anterior border of sternocleidomastoid muscle. **B,** Usual carotid bifurcation occurs at level of bodies of C3-C4. **C,** Cross section of neck demonstrating anatomic relationships of important structures in neck. Carotid sheath, containing common carotid artery *(CCA)*, vagus nerve *(X)*, and internal jugular vein *(IJV)*, lies lateral to trachea and slightly underneath sternocleidomastoid muscle. **D,** Once carotid sheath is opened, and patient has received heparin bolus, clamp is placed on common carotid artery *(CCA)*. Common facial vein *(CFV)* and ansa cervicalis are variable in location relative to carotid bifurcation, and occasionally they need to be divided to gain adequate exposure of bifurcation. Hypoglossal nerve *(XII)* is often exposed at superior end of exposure, and great care must be taken not to injure this nerve because tongue paralysis could result. Vagus nerve *(X)* lies posterior to carotid artery and also must be carefully handled. **E,** Before arteriotomy is begun, clamps are placed on external carotid artery *(ECA)*, superior thyroid artery, and internal carotid artery *(ICA)*. Arteriotomy starts at common carotid artery *(CCA)* and extends above plaque on internal carotid artery. Plaque is carefully dissected from intima with use of small spatula.

Continued

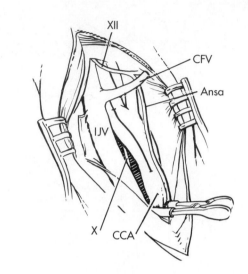

D

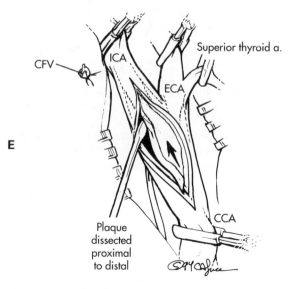

E

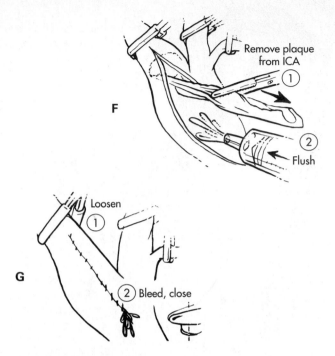

FIG 1-10, cont'd.

F, Once plaque has been freed from wall of vessel, it is removed carefully so that edges on wall of vessel will remain smooth. Intima is washed with heparinized saline. **G,** Arteriotomy is closed with running suture, with particular care taken not to narrow vessel lumen. Before complete closure, internal carotid artery clamp is loosened and internal carotid artery is allowed to back-bleed so that any clot that may have formed during procedure is washed out of internal system. After closure, clamps are removed from common carotid, external carotid, and superior thyroid arteries. Blood is allowed to flow through external system for a few minutes before removal of internal carotid artery clamp, which allows blood to flow in internal carotid system. This method serves to wash debris and clot harmlessly into external system before internal system is opened to blood flow.

CLINICAL CONSIDERATIONS

The specific clinical problems that the anesthesiologist is likely to encounter in a given operation are discussed in the final section of this chapter and throughout the chapters that follow. This section focuses on general problems in neurologic surgery.

One issue that often needs to be pointed out to residents-in-training is the importance of a secure airway in neurosurgical patients. This situation is so because the patient's airway is rarely in the kind of accessible position present in intraabdominal surgery, for instance. Inadvertent extubation with the patient in the head-pinned, prone, 90-degree head-away position and with the brain exposed is a life-threatening emergency. Before the incision is made, care should be taken to establish the unquestionable securement of the endotracheal tube. Taping of the tube should not be rushed in an effort to save 5 minutes in a 5-hour operation. Because the skull cannot be circumvented in intracranial or cervical surgery, beards and mustaches may need to be trimmed or removed to allow an adequate clear area for taping. The patency and security of the airway should be rechecked after the final desired position is achieved to prevent problems that are much more difficult to correct after surgery has begun. If such problems do arise, the patient may need to be placed back in an accessible position, even if this repositioning requires undraping and repinning. If the patient is critically hypoxic, the possibility of postoperative infection is not the primary concern. Finally, the use of the laryngeal mask airway or Combitube should be considered if an endotracheal tube is dislodged and the patient is in a position that makes conventional airway management difficult or impossible.

When intracranial surgery is planned, the skull is frequently placed in head pinions, or, as we say in operating room jargon, the head is "pinned." This step often represents the first major stimulus to the patient following laryngoscopy and intubation. It usually requires amelioration of the hemodynamic response with intravenous agents and increased inhalational agent concentrations, with or without local anesthesia at the pin sites. It is critical for the anesthesiologist to communicate with the patient during all head movements to avoid inadvertent extubation. When applying the head pinions, the surgeon must consider the position he/she wishes to achieve ultimately and avoid placement of pins into areas such as the orbits or the venous sinuses. On removal of the pins, it is important to avoid injury to the patient's eyes. Venous air embolus is a rare but reported complication after removal of head pinions.

When the scalp is "prepped" with cleansing solution, it is essential to avoid drainage of the irritating solution into the eyes. In addition to not using an excessive amount of prep, it is helpful for the patient to wear self-sticking eye goggles during prepping. The lenses of the goggles also serve to protect the eyes from traumatic corneal injuries, for example, from head pins. It is advisable to use eye ointment, and it is essential to tape the eyes completely shut before applying the goggles. With reasonable care, my colleagues and I have cut down drastically on our incidence of corneal abrasion resulting from a slit of eyelid remaining open in a prone patient.

The scalp incision is designed to allow favorable access to the bone flap that is planned and to preserve the vasculature of the scalp and avoid postoperative skin necrosis. The bone flap is planned to provide an avenue to the brain area requiring surgery while avoiding entry to undesirable structures such as the venous sinuses. Inadvertent entry into a venous sinus is a rare but life-threatening emergency that quickly results in the loss of large amounts of blood and is difficult to control surgically. Once any vascular structures are encountered, the possibility of venous air embolism must be considered. This subject is also discussed in Chapter 11 because it occurs most prominently in patients requiring the seated position for supratentorial surgery. However, venous air embolism may occur during any neurosurgical procedure, including lumbar laminectomy, because the operative site is almost always above the heart. Meticulous neurosurgical technique appears to decrease the frequency and magnitude of venous air embolism but cannot eliminate the risk entirely.

Skin incision, raising the bone flap, and incision of the dura represent painful stimuli that should be addressed appropriately by the anesthetist. Once the brain has been entered, there is little to no pain stimulus because the brain tissue has no pain receptors. However, vascular and dural structures appear to sense pain, and compression of certain neural structures may stimulate hemodynamic reflexes. These reflexes can produce a variety of cardiovascular reflexes. The most likely combinations are bradycardia/hypertension (trigeminal nucleus/cerebellar tentorium) and bradycardia/hypotension (brainstem cardiovascular centers/vagal nucleus).

The first-line treatment is to notify the surgeon, who will end stimulation. Second, short-acting drugs should be employed, if necessary, because these changes are usually transient. The physiology of ICP and the intraoperative management of difficulties in brain exposure are discussed in Chapters 2 and 9, respectively. When a mass causing increased ICP is removed, blood pressure may fall because the cardiovascular reflex center no longer senses a need for elevated systemic blood pressures to maintain cerebral perfusion. Decreased blood pressure can also occur when hydrocephalus is relieved. We and others have noticed that severe bradycardia can occur when suction is applied to a supratentorial drainage catheter after closure. The etiology is not clear, but it may represent an upward herniation of brainstem contents or a dural reflex. Whatever the cause, the suction must be discontinued and the situation reevaluated at this point: Reapply suction cautiously to see if there is a real correlation? Apply less suction? Is the brain tight?

During closure, the surgeon generally desires normotension so that bleeding is not masked by low systemic blood pressures. The incidence of postoperative hematoma is about 2% after craniotomy or cerebral biopsy, with almost 90% of these hematomas arising within 6 hours of surgery. The incidence of such hematomas is highest in emergency posterior fossa exploration. Blood pressure must be monitored carefully to avoid excessive increases. The exact definition of an "excessive increase" is situationally dependent and should be discussed with the surgeon. Difficulties in closure may occur in trauma or tumor surgery because of hematoma or edema. The usual steps for ICP control should be implemented, but occasionally the brain may be too swollen to allow replacement of the bone flap. One uncommon problem that should be considered at this time is tension pneumocephalus, especially if the patient underwent surgery in the seated position.

Although it is highly desirable to have a patient who is extubated and awake as soon as the last piece of tape is placed on the head dressing, it is also important not to have the patient awake and in head pins in the prone position with the bed turned away. In general, it is preferable to keep the patient asleep a little longer with volatile anesthetic or short-acting intravenous agents. Unless very large doses of narcotics or barbiturates have been administered, my colleagues and I have found that significantly delayed wake-ups are the result of hypothermia or a neuroanatomic problem such as hematoma, edema, or unintentional loss of perfusion to a key structure (e.g., the reticular activating system). It is critical to notify the surgeon immediately if there is suspicion that wake-up in the recovery room or intensive care unit is taking longer than expected.

SELECTED COMMENTS ON SPECIFIC PROCEDURES

Since the remaining chapters of this book discuss the anesthetic concerns of specific procedures in detail, this section is restricted to anatomic and neurosurgical concerns.

Evacuation of Intracranial Hematoma

A large area of brain must be exposed in this procedure so that the question mark–shaped incision extends from the base of the zygoma to the anterior midline of the scalp (see Fig. 1-1, *E*). Before the craniotomy itself is performed, a temporal burr hole may be used for emergent clot evacuation. During the craniotomy, blood is gently removed from the brain surface by using a combination of irrigation, suctioning, and cup forceps (designed to avoid trauma to the brain surface).

Decompressive Craniotomy

The anatomy of the dural membrane is presented in Fig. 1-2, *A* and *B*. Fig. 1-2, *C* through *E*, shows the classic herniation syndromes, but the lateral displacement of the midline may be the most predictive determinant of the patient's state of consciousness.

When severe generalized edema is present, the surgeon may choose to remove a large portion of the calvarial bone on one side of the skull (hemicraniectomy) or both frontal bones as a single flap (bifrontal craniectomy or Kjellberg procedure). These radical techniques have not been shown to improve outcome.

Cerebrospinal Fluid Diversion

Ideally, a frontal ventriculostomy catheter is placed through a burr hole in the midpupillary line and 1 to 2 cm anterior to the coronal suture. (To review the anatomy of the ventricular system, see Fig. 1-3.) The catheter tip is guided to the junction of the sagittal midline and a coronal line just anterior to the external auditory canal. This approach should place the tip at an area devoid of choroid plexus, which can obstruct the catheter. More acceptable methods of placement of the parietooccipital burr hole may be possible, but most surgeons use landmarks that are several centimeters superior to the transverse sinus and several centimeters lateral to the sagittal sinus. This posterior placement has been reported to result in a lower incidence of subsequent epilepsy.

Cerebral Lobectomy

Localization of function is critical in removing tumors in sensitive areas (e.g., speech, motor) and in epilepsy surgery (see Fig. 1-4). The precentral gyrus contains the primary motor area that gives rise (in part) to the corticospinal tracts. The visual center lies in and around the calcarine fissure in the occipital lobes. It receives visual information from the ipsilateral nasal field and the contralateral temporal field. Speech is located in two main areas: Broca's area in the inferior frontal lobe, which controls expression of communication, and Wernicke's area in the temporoparietal cortex, which is involved in the interpretation of language. Language localization is found in the left hemisphere in 96% of the population, including some people who would identify themselves as left-handed.

For frontal lobectomy, a modified transcoronal skin incision is made to allow a large bone flap that begins near the skull base and extends to 1 cm from the midline. In general, 7 cm of lobe may be removed from the nondominant hemisphere, whereas only 5 cm can be safely resected from the dominant side while avoiding injury to Broca's area. Temporal lobectomy involves a small bone flap based on a burr hole in the zygoma. In the nondominant hemisphere, about 6 cm of tissue can be resected, but in the dominant hemisphere only 5 cm is generally removed to avoid causing language deficits. However, the language area can extend more anteriorly, and some surgeons perform temporal lobectomy in the conscious sedated patient in order to mark out the speech area precisely for that individual. The intention is to maximize resection of pathologic tissue while minimizing irreversible neurologic injury to speech, motor, and visual areas.

Transsphenoidal Hypophysectomy

This ingenious approach to the pituitary was developed by Harvey Cushing, the father of American neurosurgery, and has been further refined and popularized in the era of the operating microscope. The initial incision may be made in the nasal mucosa or the upper gingival mucosa. The dissection is carried back to the anterior wall of the sphenoid sinus, which looks like a boat keel (see Fig. 1-5, *D*). Then the sinus is entered. After radiographic confirmation of the location, the sella is entered via its anterior wall. It is critical to stay in the midline to avoid the carotid arteries, which are a dangerous, though uncommon, source of bleeding. It is also important not to open the dural entrance into the sella too far superiorly or a cerebrospinal fluid (CSF) leak may result (see Fig. 1-5, *E*). If a leak is detected, the sella is packed with fat from the patient's thigh or abdomen. The tumor (macroadenoma) is then resected with care to preserve the normal pituitary gland, if possible. For large tumors, a lumbar drain may be used to introduce 5 to 10 cc of air that can be seen outlining the tumor on x-ray film and pushing the suprasellar tumor down into the sella. Care must be taken to avoid damage to the optic nerves, which lie above the sella. The precise preoperative localization of microadenomas by MRI or selective venous sampling helps to minimize damage to the remaining normal gland.

Basilar Artery Aneurysm

Half of all posterior circulation aneurysms occur at the basilar artery tip or apex. Such aneurysms are particularly difficult to deal with technically because of the proximity of other essential vascular and neural structures. Aneurysms at or just above the posterior clinoid process are approached by a pterional exposure (see Fig. 1-6, *B*), whereas those below this point are approached by a subtemporal or subtemporal-transtentorial route. Exposure of the former type of aneurysm is improved by drilling off the sphenoid ridge and separating the sylvian fissure (see Fig. 1-6, *D*). The identification of the P1 segments, the contralateral superior cerebellar artery, and the oculomotor nerve are keys to successful clipping (see Fig. 1-6, *A*). It is essential to attempt to avoid occlusion of the many small perforating vessels that arise from P1 and supply critical brainstem structures. Exposure of the less common aneurysm arising below the sella includes elevation of the temporal lobe, possibly with division of the tentorium. The temporal elevation may compromise the inferior anastomotic vein (of Labbé) as it traverses from the posterioinferior temporal lobe to the junction of the transverse and sigmoid sinuses. This interference with venous outflow can cause a venous infarction (analogous to a compartment syndrome) or edema. Injury to the fourth cranial nerve is another specific risk of this approach.

Microvascular Decompression

The observation that vascular compression in the posterior fossa could cause trigeminal neuralgia was made by Walter Dandy in the

1920s, but the operative technique currently used was devised in the 1970s. The superior and anterior inferior cerebellar arteries often have significant loops in their course and run proximally to the trigeminal nerve. It is thought that the vascular pulsations of these arteries cause the severe, lancinating pain of trigeminal neuralgia in these instances. Care taken to avoid major venous sinuses is important for this (and any) procedure. Fig. 1-7, *A,* demonstrates the bone flap employed for this procedure. If the mastoid air cells are entered, they must be packed with muscle and bone wax to avoid postoperative CSF leak. Once the dura is opened, the trigeminal nerve is located by looking for the junction of the tentorium and the petrous dura. The cerebellum is carefully retracted, and auditory evoked potentials may be used to detect injury to the trigeminal nerve. Once the source of the vascular compression is identified, the blood vessel is carefully separated from the nerve and a small piece of Gelfoam, muscle, or Teflon pad is inserted between the vessel and the nerve.

Acoustic Neuroma

Acoustic neuromas are tumors that arise from the vestibular nerve. They may compress the facial and cochlear nerves, but they rarely arise from these nerves. With modern microscopic operative techniques and facial nerve and brainstem auditory evoked potential monitoring, the preservation of facial nerve function is usually possible and that of hearing is sometimes possible. The three traditional approaches to acoustic neuromas are the suboccipital, translabyrinthine, and middle fossa.

The suboccipital approach is chosen when the tumor is >2.5 cm in diameter or when preservation of hearing is possible. The patient may be supine with the head turned away, in the "park bench" position (halfway between lateral and prone), or seated. After the dura is opened, an exposure similar to that shown in Fig. 1-8, *C*, is achieved. The close juxtaposition of many critical cranial nerves is demonstrated in Fig. 1-8, *B*. In addition to direct damage, neural function can be impaired by injuring the blood vessels supplying those nerves. The tumor is carefully removed, with care taken to avoid damage to nerves and blood vessels. Drilling out the internal acoustic meatus, as shown in Fig. 1-8, *D*, may help in identification of nerves and safe removal of the tumor.

The translabyrinthine approach may be preferred when the tumor is small and particularly when useful hearing has already been lost on the same side. This approach avoids cerebellar retraction and allows for identification of the facial nerve during the dissection.

The middle fossa approach is limited to small intracanalicular acoustic neuromas that allow preservation of hearing.

Lumbar Hemilaminectomy and Discectomy

This operation begins with a vertical incision over the spinous process of the vertebral level of interest, usually L4-5 or L5-S1. The incision is carried down to the paraspinal musculature, which is dissected off the spinous process and lamina in subperiosteal fashion. After the interlaminar ligament and ligamentum flavum are opened, an intraoperative x-ray film (with a radiopaque object in place) is used to confirm the operative level. A Kerrison punch rongeur is then used to remove about half of the lamina above and below the level of interest, and the hemilaminectomies are carried laterally to the facet joint. After removal of laminae and ligamentum flavum, the dura is exposed and bleeding from the epidural veins is controlled. The lateral recess of the spinal canal is then explored for the herniated disc. For lumbar discs, the location is usually in the "shoulder" of the nerve root. For cervical discs, it is most often the "axilla" of the nerve root. If there is a "free fragment" dorsal to the posterior longitudinal ligament, the disc fragment can be removed without opening this ligament. More often the ligament must be incised to reach and remove as much nucleus pulposus as possible. Before closure, a piece of subcutaneous fat is placed over the hemilaminectomy site to prevent scar formation over the nerve root.

Carotid Endarterectomy

For a review of the anatomy involved in this procedure, see Fig. 1-10. The length and direction of the neck incision employed for this operation is variable. The underlying platysma muscle is opened in the same direction as the skin and undermined to obtain greater retraction. The sternocleidomastoid (SCM) muscle is identified, and care is taken to preserve its thin fascia. With blunt dissection of the anterior border of the SCM, the carotid sheath is identified after division of the omohyoid muscle and, often, the ansa cervicalis nerve branches from C1-3 that can be divided without subsequent neurologic deficit. Care must be taken to avoid damage to the hypoglossal nerve, which passes underneath the digastric muscle at the superior part of the incision.

The carotid sheath is a fascial condensation containing the carotid arteries, the internal jugular vein, and the vagus nerve. The sheath is opened anteriorly to expose the vital area of the end-arterectomy. The dissection must be carried superiorly 3 to 4 cm up the internal carotid artery so that exposure created beyond the plaque facilitates closure. The superior thyroid artery, the first branch of the external carotid artery, is always exposed during the operation. At our institution the nerve to the carotid sinus is divided and the sinus itself is cauterized to reduce subsequent hemodynamic changes. After the exposure of the vessels is adequate, heparin is administered and clips are placed on the superior thyroid artery, the common carotid artery, the internal carotid artery distal to the plaque, and the external carotid artery. The arteriotomy is begun 1 cm below the bifurcation and is extended up the internal carotid artery as far as possible. A plane is developed between the athero-sclerosed intima and media, and the plaque is removed. After careful inspection of the area, the arteriotomy is closed, with back-bleeding from the internal carotid artery allowed just before final closure. The internal carotid artery clip remains in place while a few minutes of common carotid to external carotid artery flow is permitted to allow debris to flow into the less vulnerable external system. The skin and the platysma muscle are then closed with running sutures.

NEUROPHYSIOLOGY 2

Steven T. Farnsworth
Richard J. Sperry

CEREBRAL METABOLISM
CEREBRAL BLOOD FLOW
    CONTROL
    METABOLIC REGULATION
    AUTOREGULATION
    BLOOD GASES
    DRUGS AND CEREBRAL BLOOD FLOW
CEREBRAL ISCHEMIA AND BRAIN PROTECTION
CEREBROSPINAL FLUID

It is important to understand the many aspects of central nervous system (CNS) physiology in order to provide optimal anesthetic management for surgery of the CNS. This chapter focuses on the salient features of cerebral metabolism and blood flow, which are integral to neuroanesthesia and neurologic intensive care.

CEREBRAL METABOLISM

Brain tissue has a very high energy requirement. For adults the cerebral metabolic rate of oxygen consumption ($CMRO_2$) is approximately 3.5 ml O_2/100 g [brain tissue]/min. This rate equals 50 ml/min for the typical 1400 g brain, or roughly 20% of the whole body O_2 consumption. The $CMRO_2$ is higher in children: 5.2 ml O_2/100 g/min. Glucose is the main substrate for energy production in the brain. With adequate O_2, glucose is metabolized via the glycolytic pathway. Then citric acid cycles to generate adenosine triphosphate (ATP) and reduced nicotinamide adenine dinucleotide (NADH) from adenosine diphosphate (ADP) and nicotinamide adenine dinucleotide (NAD), respectively. In an awake young adult man, the cerebral metabolic rate of glucose consumption (CMRG) is 31 μm (5 mg)/100 g brain tissue/min. In the absence of adequate O_2, the glucose is metabolized via glycolysis to pyruvate and then to lactate. This process generates only two molecules of ATP per molecule of glucose, producing insufficient ATP for the brain's needs and leading to lactic acidosis.

Although the global resting metabolic rate of the brain is fairly constant, there is a heterogeneity in brain metabolism. This heterogeneity reflects a different basal metabolic rate for different brain structures. Since neural activity results in an increased metabolic rate, patient stimulation causes a variable pattern of neuronal activation that enhances this heterogeneity.

Brain O_2 consumption supports two major functions: (1) basic cellular maintenance (45% of total) and (2) nerve impulse generation and transmission (55% of total) (see Box 2-1). A basic assumption in this model is that a neuron will cease to propagate impulses in favor of cellular integrity. Hence, when energy substrate delivery falls, a loss of function occurs but cell viability is preserved. When substrate delivery falls further, cell viability is threatened.

CEREBRAL BLOOD FLOW

Normal cerebral blood flow (CBF) is approximately 50 ml/100 g/min, or about 15% of cardiac output. Because most cell metabolism occurs in the cell body, gray matter has a greater average blood flow (75 to 80 ml/100 g/min) than does white matter (20 to 30 ml/100 g/min). In infants and children, global CBF is higher than in adults: 65 ml/100 g/min.

Several techniques for measuring CBF exist, but only a few are applicable to humans. Measurements of CBF are virtually never made in the clinical practice of anesthesiology. However, it is critical for anesthesiologists to understand how these measurements are obtained because the information from these measurements is used daily in clinical care.

BOX 2-1.
Cellular Energy Requirements

Maintenance of transmembrane electrical potential and other ion pumping
Cellular metabolism
Molecular transport within cells

The most common method in humans involves the use of a diffusable indicator and the Fick principle. This technique, described by Kety and Schmidt in 1945, requires a 10- to 15-minute period of breathing an inert gas such as krypton (^{85}Kr), xenon (^{133}Xe), or nitrous oxide (N_2O) and a collection of arterial and venous blood samples. This method yields a global value for CBF.

The method most applicable to the operating room is a modification of the Kety-Schmidt technique that uses scintillation detectors to monitor the washout of ^{133}Xe. The washout curves of the inert gas can be related to blood flow. If a series of small focused scintillation counters is employed, blood flow to discrete areas of the brain (regional CBF) can be determined. However, it is important to realize that this technique measures blood flow only in the outer layer of the cerebral cortex.

Another technique that can be used with humans is positron emission tomography (PET) scanning. PET is an important and powerful method for investigating cerebral physiology. It can noninvasively measure CBF, cerebral metabolic rate (CMR), cerebral blood volume, the blood-brain barrier, and drug pharmacokinetics. PET has great promise for the future, but it is very expensive and PET scanners are not widely available at this time.

^{133}Xe-enhanced computed tomography (CT) uses nonradioactive ^{133}Xe to alter the radiodensity of CT brain images. The concentration at any given location in the brain is dependent on CBF, allowing derivation of a quantitative measure of CBF. However, the validity of these measurements has been challenged because ^{133}Xe itself has been reported to increase CBF.

Recently, a technique involving proton magnetic resonance imaging (MRI) has been described to measure cerebral perfusion. Proton MRI was used to measure CBF in a rat model using water as a freely diffusable tracer. The inflowing water proton spins in the arterial blood are labeled by inverting them at the neck region and observing the effects on brain MRI intensity. This technique allows regional perfusion rates to be measured from an image with spin inversion, a control image, and a T_1-weighted image by solving modified Bloch equations.

Other techniques are commonly used in experimental animals and are reported in the literature of many disciplines. They include autoradiography, radioactive microspheres, hydrogen clearance, direct observation of pial vessels, and measurement of cerebral arterial inflow or venous outflow.

Each technique for measuring CBF has certain advantages and disadvantages. In the intact animal and human, values for global CBF represent an average of all brain structures, and values for regional blood flow represent only a sample of values from several distinct areas of thin outer cerebral cortex. True regional blood flow, or flow to all substructures of the brain, is not measured in humans. Because CBF can vary dramatically among different structures of the brain, a variance that can be greatly altered under pathologic conditions, it is important to remember the average nature of CBF measurements.

Control

Multiple factors integrate to regulate CBF. Brain metabolism, blood pressure, arterial O_2 and CO_2 tension, and drugs all interact to produce the overall value of CBF in a given region of the brain. A pathologic state within the CNS can also affect the global or regional value of CBF. Although the various mechanisms of CBF control are presented independently, all these mechanisms may interact to produce a very complex picture of CBF. A good approach to patient care, however, is to dissect the control of CBF into its various parts and devise a treatment plan based on that dissection.

Metabolic Regulation

The normally functioning brain has a fairly constant global metabolic rate and a rather stable value of global CBF. This global constancy, however, can be very misleading since regional metabolism and blood flow are not homogeneous. The heterogeneity of cerebral metabolism and blood flow is the result of two factors. First, various substructures within the brain have different basal metabolic rates. Second, a given substructure of the brain has a variable pattern of neuronal activation, depending on the activities of a patient; that is, more neuronal work requires greater O_2 and glucose delivery.

Blood flow and metabolism are tightly coupled in the normal brain. For example, during voluntary movement of the hand, CBF and $CMRo_2$ rapidly increase in the contralateral cortical area representing the hand. Pain, anxiety, and seizure activity can also cause a significant increase in brain metabolism and blood flow. The brain is a very dynamic organ, with metabolism regulating an ever-changing CBF pattern.

The exact mechanisms of metabolic regulation have not yet been determined. It has been proposed that the extracellular fluid concentrations of ions such as hydrogen, potassium, and calcium and of metabolic products such as adenosine, thromboxane, and prostaglandins may act as local vasoregulators that couple local blood flow to local metabolism and may be responsible for neural adjustment of flow to function.

Autoregulation

Autoregulation maintains CBF at a constant value over a wide range of cerebral perfusion pressure (Fig. 2-1). Cerebral perfusion pressure is defined as the difference between mean arterial pressure (MAP) and intracranial pressure (ICP) (or central venous pressure [CVP] if it is higher than ICP).

Autoregulation is accomplished by active arteriolar constriction when the distending pressure increases and by arteriolar dilation when the distending pressure decreases. Autoregulatory adjustments may take up to 2 minutes to become effective. Autoregulation has both lower and upper limits. The lower limit for autoregulation is approximately 50 mm Hg MAP. Below this limit, CBF decreases linearly with decreasing perfusion pressure. The upper limit for autoregulation is 130 to 150 mm Hg. At the upper autoregulatory limit,

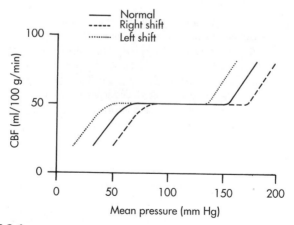

FIG 2-1.
Normal autoregulatory curve with right shift and left shift depicted.

arteriolar constriction is maximal, and a greater pressure cannot be contained. This situation results in forced dilation of brain arterioles, allowing blood flow to increase and pressure to be transmitted to the more fragile downstream vessels. The blood-brain barrier may subsequently be disrupted, leading to focal plasma leakage, hemorrhage, and cerebral edema.

The limits of autoregulation are not well defined in children. Autoregulatory limits for spinal cord blood flow are roughly the same as for CBF.

The mechanism by which autoregulation occurs is uncertain. A myogenic hypothesis states that autoregulation is an intrinsic property of the smooth muscle cells in the arteriolar wall, as seen in isolated vessels. A stretching of the smooth muscle cell by increased arterial pressure leads to active constriction; decreased distending pressure causes smooth muscle relaxation.

A metabolic hypothesis states that arteriolar dilation is regulated by tissue O_2 and glucose requirements. A decrease in perfusion pressure decreases CBF and O_2 delivery to a value lower than that required for tissue demands. This decrease in substrate delivery leads to a reflex arteriolar dilation.

The autoregulatory curve may be shifted in either direction. A shift to the right, increasing the lower and upper limits of autoregulation, occurs with chronic hypertension and sympathetic activation (e.g., shock or stress). With chronic hypertension, this shift is caused by hypertrophy of the vessel walls and is established over about 4 to 8 weeks. A right-shifted curve means that a greater perfusion pressure is necessary to maintain CBF, but it also allows for a greater perfusion pressure to be contained before autoregulatory breakthrough and disruption of the blood-brain barrier occur. A left-shifted autoregulatory curve is produced by hypoxia, hypercarbia, and vasodilators. A left-shifted curve allows CBF to be maintained at a lower than normal perfusion pressure.

It is key to understand that pressure containment protects the chronically hypertensive patient from disruption of the blood-brain barrier. However, the chronically hypertensive patient will suffer a dangerous decrease in CBF at a greater arterial blood pressure than would a normotensive patient. A gentle and sustained blood pressure reduction in a chronically hypertensive patient may shift the autoregulatory curve back toward normal.

It is also important to understand that, because hypovolemic hypotension is associated with sympathetic activation and a right-shifted autoregulatory curve, CBF will be better maintained with pharmacologic (rather than with hypovolemic) hypotension.

Autoregulation is affected by many cerebral disease processes, and it is easily impaired. Trauma, hypoxia, and some anesthetic drugs can abolish autoregulation.

Blood Gases

Alterations in arterial oxygen partial pressure (Pa_{O_2}) and arterial carbon dioxide partial pressure (Pa_{CO_2}) can have a profound effect on CBF (Fig. 2-2).

OXYGEN

CBF changes with arterial O_2 content to maintain the appropriate tissue O_2 tension for cerebral metabolism. The precise chemical mediator for this response to O_2 is not known. However, a metabolic product, adenosine, is thought to play an important role in this response. CBF is not affected until the Pa_{O_2} decreases below 50 mm Hg. At this point, cerebral vasodilation begins and CBF increases. At a Pa_{O_2} of 35 mm Hg, CBF is increased 32%; at 15 mm Hg, it is

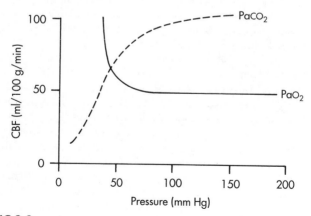

FIG 2-2.
Relationship between oxygen and carbon dioxide tension and CBF.

four times normal. This increase in CBF is contingent on a normal blood pressure. At very high PaO_2 levels (>300 mm Hg) CBF may undergo modest decreases.

Neonatal circulation responds to smaller changes in PaO_2. This response may reflect the lower hemoglobin molecule 50% saturated (P_{50}) value of fetal hemoglobin. The exact age at which this increased responsiveness changes is unknown.

CARBON DIOXIDE

The relationship of CBF to $PaCO_2$ is linear between a $PaCO_2$ of 25 mm Hg and 75 mm Hg. Increased $PaCO_2$ causes increased CBF, and decreased $PaCO_2$ causes decreased CBF. CBF changes 4% (2 ml/100 g/min) for each 1 mm Hg change in $PaCO_2$. A useful approximation is that a $PaCO_2$ of two times normal (80 mm Hg) will double CBF, and a $PaCO_2$ of one half normal (20 mm Hg) will decrease CBF by one half.

The effects of CO_2 on CBF are mediated by the pH of cerebrospinal fluid (CSF). As the arterial $PaCO_2$ increases, more CO_2 diffuses freely across the blood-brain barrier into the CSF. Bicarbonate ion, the major buffer in the CSF, does not cross the blood-brain barrier. Thus, as CO_2 enters or leaves the CSF, the pH will change in a manner predictable by the Henderson-Hasselbalch equation. An increase in CO_2 will decrease the pH, and a decrease in CO_2 will increase the pH. Eventually the bicarbonate ion concentration is equilibrated, and the pH returns to normal (normal CSF pH is 7.32). This adjustment has a half-life of approximately 6 hours.

The effect of CO_2 on the magnitude of blood flow change in the spinal cord is approximately one half the effect on CBF. The response of the vasculature takes 20 to 30 seconds.

The maximal increase in CBF from hypercapnia and hypoxemia is the same. At submaximal levels of change, the effects of hypercapnia and hypoxemia are additive. Hence, a poorly ventilated and marginally oxygenated patient will have a dramatic increase in CBF.

Hypocapnia data from normal subjects suggest that brain ischemia will not occur with a $PaCO_2$ >20 mm Hg. Metabolic abnormalities have been seen, however, with extreme hypocapnia to $PaCO_2$ <15 mm Hg.

Drugs and Cerebral Blood Flow

The CBF-drug connection can be confusing. Historically, in most clinical situations and laboratory studies, the measured variable has been CBF. Many anesthetic agents cause an increase in CBF (Table 2-1). A superficial reading of these studies may lead one to conclude that an increase in CBF is harmful in patients with intracranial pathology. It is not the increase in CBF per se that is harmful but rather the increase in cerebral blood volume (CBV) that may follow an increase in CBF. An increase in CBV can cause an increase in ICP and subsequent ischemia and brain tissue shifts (herniation).

To the extent that CBV and CBF track together in both direction and magnitude, it makes sense to focus on the most conveniently measured variable, CBF. Measurements of CBV are technically more difficult to perform. However, making assumptions about CBV from CBF can be misleading. For example, high concentrations of any volatile anesthetic will significantly increase both CBF and CBV at normal blood pressure. Because the volatile anesthetic agents blunt autoregulation, CBF will fall if blood pressure is reduced. Therefore the CBF value could be reduced to normal, or even subnormal, by lowering the blood pressure. However, CBV would not be expected to decrease much, if at all, as the blood pressure is reduced. In this possible clinical situation, CBF and CBV would lie in opposite directions from their baseline values.

In addition, many drugs have different effects on capacitance and resistance vessels in the peripheral circulation. It is reasonable to

TABLE 2-1. Effects of Anesthetic Drugs on CBF and CMR_{O_2}

Anesthetic	CBF	CMR_{O_2}
Halothane	↑↑↑	↓
Enflurane	↑↑	↓
Isoflurane	↑	↓↓
Desflurane	↑	↓↓
Sevoflurane	↑	↓↓
Nitrous oxide	↑	↑
Thiopental	↓↓↓	↓↓↓
Etomidate	↓↓↓	↓↓↓
Propofol	↓↓	↓↓
Midazolam	↓↓	↓↓
Ketamine	↑↑	↑
Fentanyl	↓	↓
Sufentanil	Uncertain	Uncertain
Alfentanil	Uncertain	Uncertain

NOTE: Increases are indicated as slight (↑), significant (↑↑), or marked (↑↑↑). Decreases are indicated as slight (↓), significant (↓↓), or marked (↓↓↓). No significant change (—).

presume that this situation is also true for the cerebral circulation. Thus, alterations in CBF and CBV should not be conceived as being interchangeable values. Table 2-1 shows the usual changes in CBF accompanying the administration of various anesthetic drugs. Although CBF data have been generated for the indicated drugs, CBV and ICP data have not been published for most of the drugs. A further discussion can be found in Chapter 3.

PATHOLOGIC STATES

Blood flow in and around areas of tumor, infarction, and trauma may be abnormal. Vasomotor paralysis, in which blood vessels have lost the ability to control their own resistance actively, occurs in these areas with subsequent loss of blood pressure autoregulation and response to CO_2. In this state of vasomotor paralysis, CBF becomes pressure-dependent, rendering this area of brain more susceptible to ischemia at lower blood pressures and more likely to sustain injury at higher pressures.

Also, as the $Paco_2$ increases and normal blood vessels dilate, blood is shunted away from the abnormal areas of brain that do not respond to CO_2. This phenomenon is called *steal*. An *inverse steal* (or *Robin Hood phenomenon*) occurs when the $Paco_2$ is reduced and the normal areas of brain vasoconstrict, shunting blood to the abnormal brain, which does not vasoconstrict. This inverse steal phenomenon can also occur when drugs that cause cerebral vasoconstriction (e.g., barbiturates) are administered.

• • •

As demonstrated by Fig. 2-3, ICP, $Paco_2$, Pao_2, and arterial pressure are the clinically important variables that control CBF. With the exception of the $Paco_2$ curve, all these curves change at a pressure of about 50 mm Hg. Also, the average normal CBF is 50 ml/100 g/min, and the normal total brain O_2 consumption is 50 ml/min. The number 50 is a useful one to keep in mind.

CEREBRAL ISCHEMIA AND BRAIN PROTECTION

Cerebral perfusion pressure (CPP) is the driving force for substrate (O_2, glucose) delivery to the brain. Cerebral perfusion pressure is defined as MAP minus ICP. Both MAP and ICP should be measured at the level of the brain. A good external landmark for the circle of Willis is the external auditory meatus.

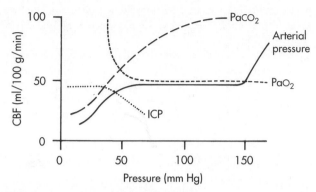

FIG 2-3.
Summary of CBF control.

CBF can be used to calculate O_2 delivery to the brain. A standard formula is used:

$$Do_2 = Cao_2 \times CBF$$

where:

Do_2 = Delivered oxygen
Cao_2 = Arterial oxygen content
CBF = Cerebral blood flow

Normal Cao_2 is 16 to 20 ml O_2/100 ml arterial blood. Cao_2 is dependent on hemoglobin content and Pao_2. Normal Do_2 is (16 to 20 ml O_2/100 ml) $\times$ 50 ml/100 g/min = 8 to 10 ml O_2/100 g/min. Since normal O_2 consumption (Vo_2) is 3.5 to 5 ml O_2/100 g/min, there is a safety factor of 1.5 to 2 Do_2 to Vo_2. These figures are a global average, and it is vital to keep in mind that the brain is a very heterogenous organ. Local areas of the brain may have a different ratio of Do_2 to Vo_2 secondary to a pathologic CBF or an altered metabolic rate.

Brain ischemic symptoms are seen when CBF falls to about 20 ml/100 g/min ($Do_2 = 4$ ml O_2/100 g/min). Electroencephalographic silence occurs at a CBF of 15 ml/100 g/min ($Do_2 = 3$ ml O_2/100 g/min; CPP 30 to 40 mm Hg). Cellular ion leakage and eventual cell death occurs at a CBF of 8 to 12 ml/100 g/min ($Do_2 = 2$ ml O_2/100 g/min). Although the effects on cerebral function and the electroencephalogram (EEG) occur rather rapidly and reversibly, the irreversible effects on cell viability occur as a function of time and the level of Do_2 (Fig. 2-4).

Of all the body's organs, the brain is the most sensitive to ischemia. When blood supply to the brain is decreased below a critical level, ischemic damage occurs. The mechanisms leading to neuronal damage are likely similar, and calcium is central in the pathophysiology. Ischemia leads to excessive release of neurotransmitters, which cause increased calcium influx. Ischemic injury is characterized by a decrease in O_2 delivery and by a decrease in the supply of glucose and other metabolites. One of the earliest manifestations of

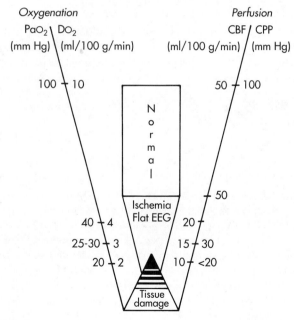

FIG 2-4.
Representation of brain function related to two measures of oxygenation (arterial oxygen partial pressure *[Pao$_2$]* and delivered oxygen *[Do$_2$]*) and two measures of perfusion (cerebral blood flow *[CBF]* and cerebral perfusion pressure *[CPP]*).

cerebral ischemia is an abrupt reduction in the concentrations of energy metabolites and, eventually, ATP. When tissue ATP is depleted, the Na^+-K^+ ATPase-dependent ion pumps fail, leading to Na^+ influx, K^+ efflux, and membrane depolarization. Membrane depolarization results in an uncontrolled influx of Ca^{++}, which leads to disruption of mitochondrial and cell membranes and the release of free fatty acids, including arachidonic acid. Since ATP is necessary to clear the calcium from the cytosol, increased cytosolic calcium levels occur. Calcium activates many intracellular enzymes, and the increased levels of calcium result in enzymatic breakdown of membranes with subsequent fatty acid (including arachidonic acid) and chemically reactive free radical production. These molecules and their biochemical products contribute to the vasodilation, vasoconstriction, and membrane permeability alterations associated with the evolution of ischemic neuronal injury.

Incomplete ischemia differs from complete ischemia in that there is a continuing supply of glucose despite tissue hypoxia. This supply of glucose sustains anaerobic metabolism, increasing the brain lactic acid level. Above a certain threshold, lactic acid damages neurons. This effect is the basis for the concern that increased preischemic serum glucose levels may increase or hasten the ischemic tissue damage.

Ischemia leads instantly to brain edema. Edema can worsen ischemia, and the cycle can quickly spiral into brain death.

At the tissue level, hypoxia can be defined as a reduction in O_2 availability to a level insufficient for tissue demands. Tissue hypoxia can be caused by either hypoxemia (low Pa_{O_2}) or ischemia (low CBF). The effects of these two insults are not equivalent. Hypoxemia with a Pa_{O_2} of 50 mm Hg causes an increased brain lactate. Hypoxemia with a Pa_{O_2} of 35 mm Hg also causes a decrease in phosphocreatine. However, if arterial pressure does not drop significantly, brain ATP stores are not decreased. Therefore neuronal survival is not threatened until the Pa_{O_2} is <25 mm Hg. This defense of ATP levels occurs because hypoxemia induces a compensatory increase in CBF and a sixfold increase in cerebral glucose metabolism.

Pure hypoxemic injuries to the human brain rarely occur. The reason is because severe hypoxemia is required before neuronal death occurs and also because one of the earliest effects of hypoxemia is cardiac dysfunction and resultant ischemia. Anesthesiologists have a significant opportunity to cause hypoxemic brain injury if they render a patient hypoxemic and then artificially support the patient's blood pressure.

Ischemia can be global or focal, complete or incomplete. With complete global ischemia, the EEG becomes isoelectric in 15 to 25 seconds, the brain phosphocreatine concentration approaches 0 in approximately 1 minute, and the tissue high-energy phosphate concentration approaches 0 in 5 to 7 minutes.

Brain protection addresses the preservation of neuronal integrity during periods of hypoxemia and ischemia. Brain protection and brain resuscitation are fundamentally different. Protection is instituted before an insult; resuscitation is administered following an insult. This discussion addresses only the issue of protection.

To prevent neuronal death from ischemia or hypoxemia, two basic strategies can be employed: prevention of tissue hypoxia primarily or modification of the events that lead to cell injury and death subsequent to energy failure. The prevention of tissue hypoxia can be divided into two general categories: decreasing tissue O_2 demand and increasing O_2 supply. There are not many techniques to decrease true tissue O_2 demand—that is, the level of Po_2 required for neuronal survival. Hypothermia decreases the cellular O_2 requirement for both synaptic transmission and cellular maintenance. A temperature reduction from 38°C to 28°C decreases $CMRo_2$ to 45% of the normothermic value. A temperature of 18°C lowers the $CMRo_2$ to 20% of the normothermic value. A canine study showed that cooling to 22°C produced EEG burst suppression, though cooling further to 14°C increased periods of suppression but did not eliminate burst activity. It has been proposed that the ischemia protection of hypothermia is caused by a reduction in release of glutamate and dopamine.

Short of hypothermia, the major way we affect tissue hypoxia is by increasing O_2 supply. Keeping a normal blood hemoglobin, Pao_2, cardiac output, and tissue blood flow all serve the function of maintaining O_2 delivery. However, tissue O_2 tension can also be significantly affected by the use of drugs, frequently anesthetics.

Some semantic confusion exists regarding the O_2 supply-demand balance effects of anesthetic agents. Both isoflurane and barbiturates decrease $CMRo_2$ by a maximum of 55%. This $CMRo_2$ suppression comes from abolishing neuronal synaptic transmission. However, the amount of O_2 required for the maintenance of cellular integrity is not decreased. (The maintenance of cellular integrity consumes about 45% of $CMRO_2$.) Hence the lower limit of acceptable local hypoxia is not altered as it is with hypothermia. This situation is the basis for the semantic confusion. The reduced VO_2 by the brain with high doses of isoflurane or barbiturates essentially increases the supply of O_2 to the distal watershed areas of the capillary bed. The earliest sites of tissue hypoxia will be those areas of the microcirculation farthest from blood inflow, that is, at the venous end of the capillaries. By retarding synaptic transmission, and hence VO_2 by the upstream neurons, anesthetics decrease the amount of tissue at risk during ischemic periods by increasing the supply of O_2 to the most vulnerable areas of the capillary bed.

In addition to decreasing $CMRO_2$, the barbiturates may have several actions that provide brain protection. Barbiturates decrease ICP and cerebral edema, which improves CBF. They may also increase the supply of O_2 to areas of regional ischemia by the inverse steal phenomenon. Overall, however, drugs cannot provide the extent of protection offered by hypothermia because decreasing temperature decreases the $CMRO_2$ necessary for both neural activity and cellular maintenance.

CEREBROSPINAL FLUID

The adult human has approximately 150 ml of CSF within the cranium and the spinal space. The CSF is formed primarily by the choroid plexus, although transependymal diffusion makes a small contribution. CSF is formed (and reabsorbed) at a rate of 18 to 25 ml/hour, providing a replacement of the entire CSF volume 3 to 4 times/day. The extracellular milleu provided by the CSF must be maintained within strict limits because of the sensitivity of neurons. The composition of the CSF is generally similar to that of extracellular fluid elsewhere in the body (Table 2-2), although most ions are present in CSF in slightly lower concentrations and there is very little protein in normal CSF. In addition to providing a critical extracellular environment for neurons, the CSF cushions the brain and is adjusted to compensate for changes in ICP. Acute intracranial hypertension is compensated for by decreased blood flow, whereas chronic compensation is accomplished through decreased CSF volume. Most of the commonly used general anesthetic agents influence CSF secretion and absorption (Table 2-3).

TABLE 2-2. Composition of CSF and Serum

Component	CSF	Serum
Sodium (mEq/L)	138.0	140.0
Potassium (mEq/L)	2.8	4.0
Calcium (mEq/L)	2.4	4.6
Magnesium (mEq/L)	2.7	1.8
Chloride (mEq/L)	124.0	99.0
Glucose (mg/dl)	60.0	99.0
Protein (g/dl)	0.05	7.08

TABLE 2-3. Anesthetics and CSF Secretion and Absorption

Anesthetic	Secretion	Absorption
Halothane	↓	↓
Enflurane	↑	↓
Isoflurane	—	↑
Fentanyl	—	↑
Ketamine	—	↓
Nitrous oxide	—	—

CSF flows from the lateral ventricles down through the third and fourth ventricles and cisterna magna. It then circulates about the brain and spinal cord in the subarachnoid space before being reabsorbed into venous sinuses via arachnoid villi. Reabsorption is passive because, in normal conditions, the CSF is under higher pressure than the venous sinuses and the arachnoid villi have unidirectional valves for flow.

The brain's capillary endothelial cells have tight junctions that prevent substances from passing through them. In addition, these capillary endothelial cells are separated from neurons by processes extending from astrocyte glial cells. These processes make up the blood-brain barrier. Lipid-soluble molecules pass through the blood-brain barrier much more quickly and efficiently than do hydrophilic compounds. The brain is required to transport many essential substances in a carrier-mediated fashion, often requiring energy to do so. The blood-CSF barrier is very similar, but it is formed by tight junctions in the choroid plexus epithelial cells. These choroid epithelial cells surround the fenestrated choroid capillaries that produce the CSF. The blood-brain barrier is disrupted by many pathologic conditions, including ischemia, acute hypertension, tumor, trauma, and irradiation.

Suggested Readings

Algotsson L, Messeter K, Nordstrom CH, et al: Cerebral blood flow and oxygen consumption during isoflurane and halothane anesthesia in man, *Acta Anaesthesiol Scand* 32:15, 1988.

Artru AA, Katz RA, Colley PS: Autoregulation of cerebral blood flow during normocapnia and hypocapnia in dogs, *Anesthesiology* 70:288, 1989.

Busto R, Dietrich WD, Globus MYT: Small differences in intra-ischemic brain temperature critically determine the extent of ischemic neuronal injury, *J Cereb Blood Flow Metab* 7:729, 1987.

Cucchiara RF, Theye RA, Michenfelder JD: The effects of isoflurane on cerebral metabolism and blood flow, *Anesthesiology* 40:571, 1974.

Drummond JC, Moore SS: The influence of dextrose administration on neurologic outcome after temporary spinal cord ischemia in the rabbit, *Anesthesiology* 70:64, 1989.

Ellinggen I, Hauge A, Nocolaysen G, et al: Changes in human cerebral blood flow due to step changes in Pao_2 and $Paco_2$, *Acta Physiol Scand* 129:157, 1987.

Gisvold SE, Steen PA: Drug therapy in brain ischemia, *Br J Anaesth* 57:96, 1985.

Graham DI: The pathology of brain ischemia and possibilities for therapeutic intervention, *Br J Anaesth* 57:3, 1985.

Grubb RL, Raichle ME, Eichling JO, et al: The effects of changes in $Paco_2$ on cerebral blood volume, blood flow, and vascular mean transit time, *Stroke* 5:630, 1974.

Heiss WD: Flow thresholds of functional and morphological damage of brain tissue, *Stroke* 14:329, 1983.

Kelly BJ, Luce JM: Current concepts in cerebral protection, *Chest* 103:1246, 1993.

Kety SS, Schmidt CF: The determination of cerebral blood flow in man by the use of nitrous oxide in low concentrations, *Am J Physiol* 143:53, 1945.

Lanier WL, Stangland KJ, Scheithauer BW: The effects of dextrose infusion and head position on neurologic outcome after complete cerebral ischemia in primates: examination of a model, *Anesthesiology* 66:39, 1987.

Lassen NA, Christensen MS: Physiology of cerebral blood flow, *Br J Anaesth* 48:719, 1976.

Messick JM, Milde LN: Brain protection, *Adv Anesthesia* 4:47, 1987.

Michenfelder JD: The interdependency of cerebral function and metabolic effects following massive doses of thiopental in the dog, *Anesthesiology* 41:231, 1974.

Michenfelder JD, Milde JH: The relationship among canine brain temperature, metabolism, and function during hypothermia, *Anesthesiology* 75:130, 1991.

Milde LN: Cerebral protection. In Cucchiara RF, Michenfelder JD, editors: *Clinical anesthesia,* New York, 1990, Churchill Livingstone.

Olesen J: Contralateral local increase in cerebral blood flow in man during arm work, *Brain* 94:635, 1971.

Plum F, Posner JB, Zee D: The relationship of cerebral blood flow to CO_2 tension in the blood and pH in the CSF, respectively, *Scand J Clin Lab Invest Suppl* 102:8F, 1968.

Rogers MC, Nugent SK, Traystman RJ: Control of cerebral circulation in the neonate and infant, *Crit Care Med* 8:570, 1980.

Siesjo BK: Cerebral circulation and metabolism, *J Neurosurg* 60:883, 1984.

Siesjo BK, Bengtsson F: Calcium fluxes, calcium antagonists, and calcium-related pathology in brain ischemia, hypoglycemia, and spreading depression: a unifying hypothesis, *J Cereb Blood Flow Metab* 9:127, 1989.

Smith AL, Wollman H: Cerebral blood flow and metabolism: effects of anesthetic drugs and techniques, *Anesthesiology* 36:378, 1972.

Spetzler RF, Hadley MN: Protection against cerebral ischemia: the role of barbiturates, *Cerebrovasc Brain Metab Rev* 1:212, 1989.

Strandgaard S, Olesen J: Autoregulation of brain circulation in severe arterial hypertension, *Br Med J* 1:507, 1973.

Symon L: Flow thresholds in brain ischemia and the effects of drugs, *Br J Anaesth* 57:34, 1985.

PHARMACOLOGY *3*

Steven T. Farnsworth
Joel O. Johnson

Patients who are taken to the operating room for neurosurgical procedures often have a very tenuous neurophysiologic status. The pharmacologic agents used by the anesthesiologist significantly impact this often fragile state. This chapter discusses the neurophysiologic effects of sedative-hypnotic, analgesic, inhalation, and neuromuscular blocking drugs.

SEDATIVE-HYPNOTIC AGENTS

Barbiturates

Barbiturates are intravenous anesthetic agents that are commonly used in neuroanesthesia because they possess a number of favorable neurophysiologic features. By reducing neuronal activity, they decrease the cerebral metabolic rate of oxygen consumption ($CMRO_2$). This reduction causes a concomitant reduction in cerebral blood flow (CBF) and thus intracranial pressure (ICP). The reduced CBF is secondary to cerebral vasoconstriction. This vasoconstriction occurs only in areas of normal brain tissue while areas of injury or ischemia fail to react and remain maximally dilated. The result is the physiologically favorable shunting of blood from normal to ischemic areas (*inverse steal* or *Robin Hood phenomenon*). Barbiturates can maximally lower $CMRO_2$ to approximately 50% of normal, the electroencephalographic point of isoelectricity. Higher doses will not lower $CMRO_2$ further (because the other approximately 50% of $CMRO_2$ is required for maintenance of cellular integrity and membrane function). Cerebrospinal fluid (CSF) dynamics are not significantly affected.

Barbiturates produce their pharmacologic effects by enhancing the inhibitory synaptic transmissions and blocking the excitatory ones via interaction with the gamma-aminobutyric acid (GABA) receptor complex. The binding site for barbiturates is different from that of benzodiazepines. The duration of GABA occupancy is prolonged by barbiturates, thus extending the duration of its inhibitory activity. Nonselective depression of transmission occurs at higher doses. In addition, barbiturates decrease the free radical activity in the central nervous system (CNS), which may prevent further neuronal injury and ameliorate postischemia cytotoxic cerebral edema.

Barbiturates are also potent anticonvulsants. Small doses of these agents increase electroencephalogram (EEG)-recorded beta activity, whereas larger doses lead to burst-suppression and isoelectricity. A typical induction dose will temporarily produce burst-suppression. Larger doses will increase latency and decrease, but not abolish, the amplitude of somatosensory-evoked potentials (SSEPs), even when the EEG is "flat."

Negative side effects associated with the use of barbiturates include dose-dependent cardiovascular and respiratory depression and peripheral vasodilation via lowered sympathetic tone. This cardiovascular depression can decrease blood pressure to the point of decreasing cerebral perfusion pressure (CPP). Respiratory depression can lead to hypoxia and hypercarbia with accompanying increases in CBF and ICP. In addition, tolerance may develop with chronic barbiturate administration.

Barbiturates easily penetrate the blood-brain barrier and enter the CNS. The properties of a drug that determine its entry into the CNS are lipid solubility, ionization, plasma concentration, and protein binding. Barbiturates are largely nonionized weak acids at physiologic pH and are very lipid soluble. Since barbiturates are highly protein bound, their free plasma concentration may be increased by low-protein states or other drugs that displace them from carrier proteins.

Plasma concentration depends on dose and speed of administration. An induction dose of barbiturate produces brain uptake in <30 seconds with peak levels at 45 seconds (approximately one circulation time). Termination of the barbiturate's induction effects occurs by redistribution from vessel-rich to vessel-lean tissues. Peak uptake in fat tissue occurs at 2.5 hours.

Thiopental is the most frequently used barbiturate in neuroanesthesia. It is capable of inducing anesthesia smoothly within one circulation time (about 45 to 60 seconds). Recovery from an induction dose results from redistribution. The metabolism of thiopental is hepatic. Dose-dependent cardiac depression does occur. If thiopental is used as an infusion to maintain burst-suppression of the EEG, it is common to use concurrent inotropic blood pressure support once a total dose of 2 to 4 g or more has been given.

Thiamylal has most of the same properties as thiopental and therefore will not be discussed separately.

Methohexital is commonly used for sedation and induction of anesthesia for brief procedures (i.e., electroconvulsive therapy). The metabolism of methohexital is hepatic, but it occurs more rapidly than that of thiopental. Of significant interest in the neurosurgical population is the fact that methohexital enhances epileptogenic activity in patients with focal seizure. Also, excitatory phenomena are common with methohexital, and induction is not as smooth as with thiopental. An advantage of methohexital is that it is effective when given rectally, a useful property of induction/sedation in the pediatric population.

Thiopental is the barbiturate most commonly used in neuroanesthesia, but methohexital and thiamylal are also used. Although these agents share a great many pharmacologic properties, they have some important differences. Table 3-1 presents a comparative summary of these three barbiturates.

Propofol

Propofol is an intravenous agent used for both induction and maintenance of anesthesia (Table 3-2). Like the barbiturates, it pos-

TABLE 3-1. Pharmacology and Use of Barbiturates

Factor	Thiopental	Thiamylal	Methohexital
Induction dose (mg/kg)	4-5	4-5	1-2 IV (25-30 PR)
Time to awakening (min)	5-10	5-10	3-8
Respiratory effects	Minimum depression with hypnotic dose progressing to apnea with high doses Laryngeal/cough reflexes intact Vasodilation, myocardial depression	Similar to thiopental	Similar to thiopental with shorter duration
Hemodynamic effects	Blood pressure decreases markedly if hypovolemia present Reflex increase in heart rate Small amount of histamine release	Similar to thiopental	Similar to thiopental
CNS effects	↓ CBF, CMR_{O_2}, ICP Flat EEG with induction dose	Similar to thiopental	Similar to thiopental Increased excitatory phenomena Seizures common after withdrawal of high dose infusion Increased seizure activity
Complications (%)			
Cough/hiccup	5	5	25
Pain/phlebitis	9/1	9/1	12/8
Movements	7	7	35

Modified from Stoelting RK: Barbiturates. In *Pharmacology and physiology in anesthetic practice*, Philadelphia, 1987, JB Lippincott, pp 102-116, and Corssen G et al: Barbiturates. In *Intravenous anesthesia and analgesia*, Philadelphia, 1988, Lea & Febiger, p 85.

sesses many favorable properties for the treatment of neurosurgical patients. Propofol lowers CBF, $CMRo_2$, and ICP. Also like barbiturates, propofol causes dose-dependent cardiovascular and respiratory depression and can decrease CPP. The cardiac depression caused by propofol is slightly greater than that of thiopental. Propofol can be a highly effective agent for maintenance of anesthesia as long as blood pressure is maintained. Recent reports indicate that a propofol-based anesthetic for neurosurgical procedures compares favorably to inhalation and nitrous oxide/narcotic techniques in terms of cost, intensive care unit stay, and side effects. Propofol blunts the response to laryngoscopy and intubation more effectively than thiopental or etomidate does.

Propofol causes EEG shifts from alpha to delta waves, and burst-suppression is possible with higher doses. No epileptiform activity is seen on EEG. Recovery is rapid, and emergence from anesthesia is smooth, with little nausea or vomiting. A rapid, smooth recovery is very important to most surgeons since they prefer to assess the patient's neurologic status immediately following a neurosurgical procedure. SSEPs show increased latency and decreased amplitude with propofol.

Etomidate

Etomidate is an agent with remarkable hemodynamic stability and many useful neuropharmacologic properties (Table 3-3). It is a cerebral vasoconstrictor that reduces CBF and ICP without decreasing CPP. With administration of etomidate, $CMRo_2$ is reduced by 50%, although in a less uniform way than the global reduction produced by thiopental. Reductions in the cortical regions are greater than the brainstem reductions associated with etomidate. Cardiac index, blood pressure, afterload, and preload all show minimal changes with etomidate. Etomidate causes no histamine re-

TABLE 3-2. Clinical Use of Propofol

Use	Dose (mg/kg)	Onset	Duration (min)
Induction	2-3	Rapid	5-10
Maintenance	50-150 µg/kg/min	—	5-10 after stopped

TABLE 3-3. Clinical Use of Etomidate

Use	Dose (mg/kg)	Onset	Duration (min)
Induction	0.2-0.4	Immediate	5-10
Infusion	100 μg/kg/min × 10 min then 10 μg/kg/min	2 min	10 after discontinued

lease. It is metabolized almost exclusively in the liver and undergoes renal excretion.

Etomidate produces an EEG pattern of delta waves followed by burst-suppression after an induction dose. Myoclonic movement is associated with the delta-wave stage. Etomidate confers cerebral protection and improved outcomes following ischemia. Its effects on SSEPs include significantly increased amplitude and smaller increases in latency, but the SSEP is unchanged at the spinal cord level.

Negative effects of etomidate include the possible precipitation of seizure in patients with a history of a seizure disorder (although this drug has been used successfully to treat status epilepticus). Etomidate also suppresses the adrenocortical axis. Adrenal suppression is probably a clinical concern only when etomidate is used for chronic infusion rather than as an induction agent. Nausea and vomiting, and pain on injection are side effects seen with etomidate (Box 3-1).

Benzodiazepines

Benzodiazepines are sedative-hypnotic agents that act via the CNS to facilitate the inhibitory neurotransmitter action of GABA. These drugs also act as amnestics, anticonvulsants, and anxiolytics (Table 3-4).

The benzodiazepines provide a degree of cerebral protection by producing dose-dependent decreases in $CMRo_2$ and, subsequently, CBF and ICP. They cause an EEG shift from alpha to low-voltage beta and then theta waves. These agents are excellent anticonvulsants. SSEPs at the spinal cord are not significantly affected. The

BOX 3-1.

Complications of Etomidate Use

Adrenocortical suppression
  Via 11-beta hydroxylase
  Decreases cortisol—persists for several hours after induction dose
Myoclonic movements
  Occur in up to 80% of patients
  Not associated with seizure activity on EEG
  Use of muscle relaxants often required
Nausea and vomiting
  Occurs in 30%-40% of patients
  Largest source of complaints
Pain on injection
  Due to high osmolarity of formulation
  High incidence of thrombophlebitis
  Decreased with use of larger veins

TABLE 3-4. Benzodiazepine Uses

	Anesthesia Induction Agent	Anesthesia Premedicant	Night Hypnotic	Anxio- lytic	Anticon- vulsant
Chlordiaz- epoxide		X	X	X	
Clonazepam					X
Diazepam	X	X	X	X	X
Flurazepam			X		
Lorazepam		X	X	X	
Midazolam	X	X			X
Triazolam			X	X	

barbiturates provide a greater degree of cerebral protection than do the benzodiazepines.

The benzodiazepines comprise a class of drugs with a wide variety of half-lives and active metabolites. They are highly protein-bound drugs. Metabolism occurs primarily in the liver, often with production of active metabolites. A comparison of the commonly used benzodiazepines, together with dosages and routes of administration, is presented in Table 3-5.

TABLE 3-5. Comparison of Commonly Used Benzodiazepines

Drug	Dose	Comments
Midazolam	0.5-0.1 mg/kg IM premed 0.5-2.5 mg to 0.1 mg/kg IV sedation 0.2-0.4 mg/kg IV induction 4-6 mg/hr IV infusion	Shortest duration* 20 min of hypnosis after induction
Diazepam	0.1-0.2 mg/kg PO premed 0.3-0.6 mg/kg IV induction	Postoperative sedation may last for several hours
Triazolam	0.25-0.5 mg PO premed	Shorter duration than diazepam with less postoperative sedation and greater amnesia
Lorazepam	0.5-4 mg (max 0.05 mg/kg) PO premed 2-4 mg IM	Prolonged postoperative sedation Amnesia at higher doses for 6-8 hr

*Duration of benzodiazepines is variable; sedation lasts much longer than hypnosis.

Historically, *diazepam* has been considered the standard benzodiazepine. It is now most commonly used as an oral premedicant. This drug possesses excellent sedation and anticonvulsant activity, and it remains the treatment of choice for status epilepticus. Diazepam is highly protein-bound and is metabolized by the liver to active metabolites. The use of diazepam in the neurosurgical population is limited because its elimination half-life is >24 hours. This factor can delay awakening and evaluation of some patients, even following a lengthy surgical procedure. Diazepam is not highly water soluble, and as an intravenous preparation it is a painful venous irritant.

Midazolam is a water-soluble drug with excellent anterograde amnestic properties. It is supplied in an ionized water-soluble form at an acidic pH. Once midazolam is in the plasma, the higher physiologic pH causes it to become nonionized and highly lipid soluble. This drug is 3 to 4 times as potent as diazepam, and it has a much faster onset and recovery. Midazolam is an excellent anticonvulsant because of its rapid CNS penetration and potency. Its shorter duration of activity makes midazolam an ideal premedicant because it does not prolong awakening. Midazolam is metabolized by the liver to inactive metabolites.

Lorazepam is another benzodiazepine commonly used for premedication. It is 5 to 10 times as potent as diazepam, and it can be given either orally or parenterally. Like diazepam, lorazepam is less attractive as a neuroanesthetic premedicant because its long elimination half-life can lead to prolonged postoperative sedation.

Flumazenil is a relatively new drug that acts as a CNS benzodiazepine receptor antagonist to reverse the sedation and amnesia caused by benzodiazepines. Flumazenil is given intravenously in 0.1 to 0.2 mg doses every 60 seconds until adequate reversal is achieved. However, just as naloxone needs repeat dosing because its half-life is shorter than that of certain opioids, flumazenil may necessitate repeat dosing every 45 to 60 minutes if it is used to reverse the effects of a long-acting benzodiazepine.

Ketamine

Ketamine is a dissociative anesthetic agent with limited application in the neurosurgical patient (Table 3-6). It increases ICP by multiple mechanisms. Ketamine increases blood pressure and causes cerebrovasodilation, this increasing CBF and CPP. This agent also increases resistance to CSF reabsorption. $CMRO_2$ does not change significantly with administration of ketamine, although it may increase slightly.

Ketamine is lipid soluble and penetrates the CNS effectively. It is metabolized by the liver, with renal elimination. Delirium with hallucinations and agitation may be seen on emergence, although these effects are greatly lessened by concomitant administration of benzodiazepines. Ketamine noncompetitively antagonizes the excitatory amino acid glutamate, particularly in the limbic areas. A state of dissociation occurs with ketamine because the brain becomes un-

TABLE 3-6. Clinical Use of Ketamine

Use	Dose (mg/kg)	Onset	Duration (min)*
Induction			
IV	1-2	Immediate	6-10
IM	5-10	2-3 min	10-25
Repeat doses (IV)	½ of initial dose†	Immediate	8-15
Infusion	1-2 mg/kg/hr†		

*May be markedly prolonged if used with volatile anesthetics.
†Much lower if used with N_2O or narcotic.

able to properly analyze sensory information. Ketamine is a potent somatic analgesic.

Muscle tone and purposeless movements are enhanced by ketamine. In epileptic patients, cortical and subcortical seizures have been reported with the use of ketamine. However, no epileptiform activity is seen on EEG analysis. In fact, ketamine suppresses such EEG activity. With unresponsiveness, the EEG changes to theta waves, followed by high-amplitude delta waves. Burst-suppression is not seen.

Ketamine is a sympathetic nervous system stimulator that causes increases in heart rate, blood pressure, and cardiac output. If a patient is already in a chronic state of high sympathetic outflow (i.e., congestive heart failure), ketamine can decrease cardiac output and blood pressure via direct cardiac depression. It is also a vasodilator, both systemically and intracranially.

Respiratory depression is less marked with ketamine than with barbiturates and propofol. This effect, combined with ketamine's marked somatic analgesic properties, makes it a good choice for very brief but painful procedures. Since apnea can be induced by administration of ketamine, its use warrants the same vigilant attention to airway maintenance that would be given to any other potent sedative agent. Ketamine decreases elevated airway pressures but increases respiratory secretions. The increase in secretions can be blunted by administration of anticholinergic drugs.

Droperidol

Although droperidol was formerly used as a neuroleptic anesthetic agent in combination with fentanyl, it is now used mainly as an antiemetic. Droperidol has a rapid distribution but a slow half-life. Its side effects include dyskinesia, akathisia, hallucinations, agitation, and dysphoria. This agent may cause confusion during the postoperative period, even in moderate doses. Droperidol is also an alpha-adrenergic blocking agent and produces mild decreases in blood pressure. It is a vasoconstrictor that decreases CBF, and possibly ICP, without significantly changing $CMRO_2$. These effects could threaten ischemic brain tissue.

Droperidol is a useful drug for neuroleptic sedation for awake procedures such as fiberoptic endotracheal intubation. However, if used in moderate or high doses, it may cause postoperative sedation and dysphoria without providing analgesia.

ANALGESICS

Opioids

The opioids are a group of drugs that bind to any of several types of opioid receptors. Drugs in this class have slightly different affinities for mutiple receptor subtypes. In general, opioids trigger presynaptic events, at a CNS level, that result in decreased neurotransmitter release. Specifically, the neurotransmitters norepinephrine, substance P, acetylcholine, and dopamine are most affected.

Opioids are profound analgesics and produce sedation. They do not, however, produce amnesia reliably. They cause dose-dependent slowing of the EEG, with a shift from alpha to delta activity. They do not produce burst-suppression or a flat EEG. $CMRo_2$ is submaximally reduced, with preservation of the concomitant decrease in CBF. Overall, opioids decrease ICP, although alfentanil, fentanyl, and sufentanil may increase ICP in patients with head injury if hypotension occurs concomitantly.

In general, the opioids allow a great deal of cardiac stability and preserve myocardial contractility. The principal cardiac effect is bradycardia caused by central vagotonic action and direct sinoatrial (SA) and atrioventricular (AV) nodal depression. Infrequently, tachycardia can be seen compensating for vasodilation produced by histamine release when large doses of morphine are given rapidly. Decreases in blood pressure can occur, most likely secondary to a blunting of central sympathetic outflow.

Two potential side effects of opioids that are of special significance in neurosurgical patients are respiratory depression and muscle rigidity. Opioids cause a dose-dependent depression of central respiratory centers, producing decreased respiratory rate, CO_2 response, and minute and tidal volumes. If untreated, the resultant hypercapnia will lead to increased CBF and ICP.

The incidence of muscle rigidity is related to the dose and speed of intravenous administration of opioids. Rigidity can make ventilation difficult, leading to hypercapnia and its consequences. In addition, the muscular rigidity can increase central venous pressure (CVP) and reduce venous drainage from the brain, thereby increasing cerebral blood volume (CBV) and ICP. If large doses of opioids are given for induction of anesthesia, neuromuscular blocking agents must be immediately available to be administered concurrently or at the first signs of rigidity.

Additional side effects seen with opioids are nausea and vomiting, decreased gastrointestinal motility, increased gastric volume, and urinary retention and urgency. Many of these effects predispose the patient to aspiration, especially when the sedative effects of opioids are considered. Therefore, although opioids are excellent anesthetic agents, their safe use requires a thorough understanding of their systemic pharmacologic effects. Relevant doses of opioids are outlined in Table 3-7.

Morphine is relatively lipid insoluble and has poor CNS penetration. Plasma levels change more rapidly than CNS levels do, and therefore the onset and duration of the drug's central effects correlate poorly with plasma levels. Morphine exhibits first-order kinetics, with metabolism done primarily by the liver and, to a lesser amount, by the kidneys. Renal elimination accounts for 80% of the metabolite excretion, with the remainder eliminated via the biliary system.

A significant systemic effect of morphine is hypotension, produced by a combination of diminished sympathetic tone with vasodilation, slowed heart rate, and histamine release. Prior administration of histamine-blocking agents can attenuate the histamine-related blood pressure effects.

Meperidine is unique because it possesses structural similarity to atropine. Therefore it can cause an increase in heart rate. Unlike other opioids, meperidine is a negative inotrope that may cause hypotension secondary to decreased cardiac output. This atropine-like effect may also prevent the miosis noted with other opioids.

TABLE 3-7. Clinical Doses of Opioids

Drug	IV Dose	Onset (min)	Approximate Duration
Morphine	0.05-0.3 mg/kg	5-10	3-5 hr
Meperidine	0.5-1.0 mg/kg	5-10	2-3 hr
Fentanyl	1-5 μg/kg	2	45 min-2 hr
	5-10 μg/kg*		1-3 hr
Sufentanil	0.5-2 μg/kg	<1	2 hr
Alfentanil	10-40 μg/kg	<1	<30 min
	30-80 μg/kg*		<60 min
	0.5-3.0 μg/kg/min		Discontinue 10-15 min before end of case

*Larger doses will result in increased duration.

Meperidine has one tenth the potency of morphine. Its metabolism is primarily hepatic, with a small amount excreted unchanged by the kidneys. Normeperidine, an active metabolite, causes central nervous system (CNS) excitation and seizures if levels accumulate. Its accumulation is a concern in patients with renal insufficiency. Meperidine is generally not used in neurosurgery patients.

Fentanyl is 100 times more potent than morphine and has a rapid onset and shorter duration of effect. Fentanyl possesses many favorable properties for use in the neurosurgical population. It slightly lowers ICP, decreases the resistance to CSF absorption, reduces CBV, and maintains CPP better than sufentanil or alfentanil (Fig. 3-1).

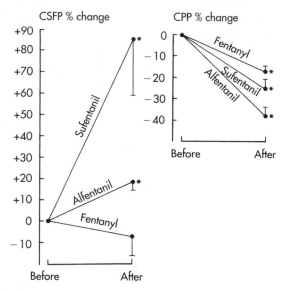

FIG 3-1.

Peak changes in cerebrospinal fluid pressure and CPP before and 10 minutes after administration of fentanyl, sufentanil, or alfentanil during N_2O-O_2-vecuronium anesthesia, expressed as percent change from control. All values: mean ± SE. Asterisks indicate $P < 0.05$ vs. control values. (From Marx W et al: Sufentanil, alfentanil, and fentanyl: impact on *CSF* pressure in patients with brain tumors, *Anesthesiology* 69:A627, 1988.)

Fentanyl is highly lipid soluble and has a large volume of distribution. It is metabolized to inactive metabolites in the liver. At lower doses, its short duration is the result of redistribution rather than metabolism.

Like other opioids, fentanyl causes dose-dependent respiratory depression, which closely follows plasma decay. It also causes bradycardia via depression of SA and AV nodes and central vagal tone enhancement. Anticholinergic agents are given to prevent this bradycardia. Unlike morphine, fentanyl does not cause histamine release.

Sufentanil is a very potent lipid-soluble opioid. It enters the CNS rapidly (peak onset about 5 minutes), with a lower volume of distribution and a higher percentage that is protein bound than fentanyl. Sufentanil is metabolized by the liver with elimination occurring via both the kidneys and the biliary system.

Sufentanil is five to ten times more potent than fentanyl when given intravenously (possibly only two to three times as potent when given intrathecally). It has the highest therapeutic index of the clinically used opiates and affords excellent hemodynamic stability. However, sufentanil may increase ICP via cerebral vasodilation. Also, like fentanyl, it can cause bradycardia when given without anticholinergic agents.

Alfentanil has a rapid onset and shorter duration than other opioids. It has a small volume of distribution and is highly protein bound. It is approximately one tenth as potent as fentanyl. When used in high doses for induction, alfentanil can slightly increase ICP, lower blood pressure, and cause rigidity. Because of its rapid onset and short duration, it is a useful drug for preventing potentially harmful responses to painful stimuli such as skin incision and stereotactic head-frame pin placement.

Naloxone is an opioid drug that binds receptors and antagonizes other opioids. It is the most commonly used perioperative antagonist. Doses should be small and titrated (in 40 μg increments) to prevent hypertension, tachycardia, severe pain, and pulmonary edema. If this agent is administered to reverse opioid-induced respiratory depression, it must be remembered that the duration of action of intravenous naloxone is <45 minutes, and repeat doses may be necessary to prevent "renarcotization."

Nonsteroidal Antiinflammatory Agents

Indomethacin has been investigated regarding its role as an inhibitor of the arachidonic acid metabolic pathways. It has not been found to be effective as a treatment for cerebral edema, probably because brain edema is linked to the production of leukotrienes and not prostaglandins.

Although *ketorolac* is used for postoperative pain control in nonneurosurgical cases, it is avoided after craniotomy because of concern about its inhibitory effect on platelet aggregation.

A summary of comparative pharmacology of the commonly used intravenous anesthetic agents can be found in Tables 3-8 and 3-9.

INHALATION AGENTS

The CNS effects of inhalation anesthetic agents assume an integral role in the management of neurosurgical patients. The inhalational agents produce dose-dependent CNS depression with progressive slowing of the EEG. They reduce $CMRo_2$ from 40% to 50% if given in high enough concentrations to produce an isoelectric EEG. Unlike the previously mentioned anesthetic drugs, inhalational agents uncouple the relationship of CBF to $CMRo_2$. Cerebral autoregulation is affected in a dose-related manner (Fig. 3-2). The ratio of CBF to $CMRo_2$ is 14 to 18:1 in the awake brain. Although other anesthetic drugs that decrease CBF have a concurrent fall in $CMRo_2$, the inhalational agents produce an increase in CBF with a decrease in $CMRo_2$.

The inhalational agents produce cerebral vasodilation, which increases CBF. They also reduce $CMRo_2$ in a dose-dependent fashion, which somewhat blunts, but does not prevent, the increase in CBF. CBF also responds to changes in $Paco_2$, although to varying degrees depending on the volatile agent. All volatile anesthetics produce an initial increase in CBV of about 10%, which falls to preanesthetic levels after about 3 hours. This change in CBV occurs early and is responsible for increases in ICP.

An important determinant of ICP that is significantly affected by inhalation agents is cerebrospinal fluid (CSF). CSF volume depends on its rate of formation and rate of absorption (affected by resistance to absorption). The normal rate of formation of CSF is

TABLE 3-8. Pharmacokinetic Values for Intravenous Anesthetics

Drug	$t_{1/2\alpha}$ (min)	$t_{1/2\beta}$ (hr)	VD_{ss} (L/kg)	Clearance (ml/kg/min)	Protein Bound (%)	pk_a	Unionized at pH 7.4 (%)
Barbiturates							
Thiopental	2-4	10-12	2-3	3-4	75	7.45	50
Methohexital	5-6	3-5	1.5-3	7-13	75	7.9	75
Benzodiazepines							
Diazepam	10-15	20-40	1.9	0.4	98	3.4	>90
Midazolam	7-15	2-4	1.7	7	95	6.2	90
Lorazepam	3-10	10-20	1.3	1.2	95	1.5 and 11.5	?
Ketamine	11-17	2-3	1-3	17	Low	7.5	50
Etomidate	2-4	2-5	4.5	14	75	4.2	>90
Propofol	2-4	1-3	5-20	20-30	98	11	<10
Narcotics							
Morphine	10-20	2-4	3-5	15	30	8.0	25
Fentanyl	5-20	2-4	3-5	11.5	85	8.4	<10
Sufentanil	5-15	2-3	2.5	10	93	8.0	20
Alfentanil	5-20	1-2	0.5-1.0	6.4	93	6.5	90

Modified from Youngberg JA: Intravenous induction agents. In Attia RR et al, editors: *Practical anesthetic pharmacology.* Norwalk, Conn, 1986, Appleton & Lange, pp 42-43.

TABLE 3-9. Comparative Pharmacology of Intravenous Induction Agents

Agent	Induction	Cardiovascular	Respiratory	Analgesia	Amnesia	Emergence
Thiopental	Smooth/rapid	Depression	Transient depression	None	Minimal	Smooth/rapid
Ketamine	Excitatory/rapid	Stimulation	Minimal	Yes	Minimal	Stormy/intermediate
Etomidate	Smooth/rapid	None	Transient depression	None	Minimal	Smooth/rapid
Propofol	Smooth/rapid/pain	Depression	Depression	None	Minimal	Smooth/rapid
Diazepam	Smooth/slow/pain	Minimal	Depression	None	Yes	Smooth/prolonged
Midazolam	Smooth/intermediate	Vasodilation	Depression	None	Yes	Smooth/intermediate
Alfentanil	Smooth/rapid/rigidity	Depression	Depression	Yes	Minimal	Smooth/rapid
Sufentanil	Smooth/rapid/rigidity	Minimal	Depression	Yes	Minimal	Smooth/intermediate

Modified from White PF: Clinical use of newer intravenous induction drugs, Cleveland, 1988, *IARS review course lectures*, pp 102-112.

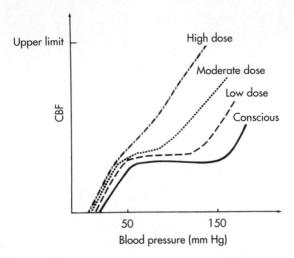

FIG 3-2.
Schematic representation of effect of progressively increased dose of typical volatile anesthetic agent on CBF autoregulation. Both upper and lower thresholds are shifted to left. (From Shapiro HM: Anesthesia effects upon cerebral blood flow, cerebral metabolism, electroencephalogram, and evoked potentials. In Miller RD, editor: *Anesthesia,* ed 2, vol 2, New York, 1986, Churchill Livingstone, p 1263.)

about 25 ml/hour. Anesthetic drugs of all kinds do, however, have varying effects on these factors related to CSF volume (Table 3-10).

Evoked potentials are affected by inhalational anesthetics. All but nitrous oxide increase latency and decrease amplitude. Doses of <0.75 to 1 minimum alveolar concentration (MAC) are clinically acceptable for allowing reliable monitoring of evoked potentials. Keeping the doses of enflurane and isoflurane <0.5 MAC is preferable if SSEPs are being monitored.

Inhalational anesthetic agents have profound cardiopulmonary effects. They all cause hemodynamic depression via varying degrees of direct cardiac depression or vasodilation. They produce depression of spontaneous respiration, with decreases in tidal volume greater than increases in the respiratory rate. Resting arterial carbon dioxide partial pressure ($Paco_2$) increases, and the ventilatory

TABLE 3-10. Effects of Anesthetics on Cerebral Physiology

Drug	CBF	CMRo$_2$	CBF/ CMRo$_2$	CBV	CSF Formation (V$_f$)	CSF Resistance to Absorption (R$_a$)	CPP*
Inhalational							
N$_2$O	↑	0†	↑	0	0	0	↓
Halothane	↑	↓	↑	↑	↓	↑	↓
Isoflurane	↑	↓	↑	↑	0	↓	↓
Enflurane	↑	↓	↑	↑	↑	↑	↓
Desflurane	↑	↓	↑	↑	↑	0	↓
Sevoflurane	↑	↓	↑	↑	?	?	↓
Intravenous							
Barbiturates	↓	↓	0	↓	↓	↓	0
Etomidate	↓	↓	0	↓	↓	↓	0
Propofol	↓	↓	0	↓	?	?	↓
Ketamine	↑	0	↑	↑	0	↑	↓
Midazolam	↓	↓	0	?	↓‡	?	0
Morphine	0	0	0	?	?	↓	↓
Fentanyl	0	0	0	↓	0	?	0
Alfentanil	0	0	0	?	?	?	↓
Sufentanil	↑(?)	0	0	?	?	?	↓

Modified from Michenfelder JD: *Anesthesia and the brain*, New York, 1988, Churchill Livingstone, p 41, and Artru AA: New concepts concerning anesthetic effects on intracranial dynamics: CSF and CBV, *ASA annual refresher course lectures*, no. 133, 1987.
*Depends on ICP and blood pressure.
†No effect.
‡At very high doses.

response to CO_2 is blunted. Even low doses of inhalation agents abolish the ventilatory response to hypoxia. Specific cardiopulmonary effects are discussed for each individual agent.

Halogenated Agents

Halothane markedly impairs cerebral vascular autoregulation and increases CBF more than the other volatile anesthetics do. The increase in ICP can be prevented by initiation of hyperventilation before administration of halothane. With halothane, the resistance to reabsorption of CSF is increased more than the production of CSF is decreased.

Halothane does lower the $CMRO_2$, but less so than the other volatile agents do. A concentration of 4.5% is required to produce an isoelectric EEG and its associated 50% decrease in $CMRO_2$. The problem is that concentrations of halothane >2% cause significant cardiac depression and interruption of normal mitochondrial function.

Cerebral ischemia is less well tolerated with halothane than with enflurane or isoflurane. The critical CBF value (minimum CBF below which EEG changes are seen with unilateral carotid artery occlusion) for halothane is 20 ml/100 g/min, while values for enflurane and isoflurane are 15 ml/100 g/min and 10 to 12 ml/100 g/min, respectively.

Decreased blood pressure with halothane is primarily caused by depressed cardiac contractility rather than peripheral vasodilation. Halothane also sensitizes the myocardium to catecholamine-induced arrhythmias more than does isoflurane.

Enflurane lowers $CMRO_2$ more than halothane does but less than isoflurane. At >1 MAC, a drop of 30% to 50% is attainable. One significant disadvantage to enflurane is its potential to cause EEG seizure activity at doses of 1.5 to 2 MAC, especially if the patient is hypocapnic. This seizure activity increases $CMRO_2$ several hundred percent and leads to increased CBF.

Enflurane causes increased formation of CSF and increased resistance to reabsorption of CSF. Cerebral ischemia protection is intermediate, better than that of halothane but less than that of isoflurane. Decreases in blood pressure are caused by both cardiac depression and peripheral vasodilation.

Isoflurane is the volatile anesthetic agent of choice in neuroanesthesia for a number of reasons. It produces a 50% reduction in $CMRO_2$, with the attainment of an isoelectric EEG at approximately 2 MAC. Ischemic protection is potentially greater than that with either halothane or enflurane. However, isoflurane does not produce protection from global ischemia severe enough to produce a flat EEG. It is less protective than thiopental for regional ischemia.

Isoflurane is a cerebral vasodilator, but increases in CBF can be prevented by concomitant hyperventilation to produce a decreased $Paco_2$. Autoregulation is impaired but does remain functional, up to 1.5 MAC. Isoflurane increases CBV but decreases resistance to CSF absorption. As long as hyperventilation is maintained, increased ICP can be avoided with isoflurane.

Cardiac output is maintained with isoflurane because the vasodilation is compensated for by increased heart rate. Since isoflurane is a potent vasodilator, decreased blood pressure is the result of decreased systemic vascular resistance. The cerebral vasodilation also makes the phenomenon of "steal" a potential problem in the brain, as it is in the heart. "Steal" is the shunting of blood from already maximally vasodilated ischemic regions to nonischemic areas vasodilated by isoflurane.

Desflurane, with its very low solubility, has rapid uptake and elimination. It is quite pungent, however, which precludes inhalation induction and may cause unwanted coughing on emergence from anesthesia in the neurosurgical patient. However, the potential for rapid awakening at the conclusion of surgery is desirable. Desflurane is less potent than the other volatile agents, and its MAC is 6%.

Desflurane, like isoflurane, increases heart rate. It depresses myocardial contractility, but less so than halothane. Like isoflurane, desflurane maintains cardiac output. Sensitivity to catecholamines is not increased. Animal studies show desflurane to decrease $CMRO_2$, with a dose-dependent cerebrovasodilation. Cerebral vascular response to $Paco_2$ appears to be preserved, although less so than with isoflurane. Desflurane depresses the EEG in a dose-related fashion without causing seizure activity. Conflicting reports indicate that desflurane may increase or have no effect on lumbar CSF pressure in patients with supratentorial tumors. The increase in pressure is possibly caused by increased production of CSF with no change in the rate of resorption.

The effects of *sevoflurane* are similar to those of isoflurane. This agent has the associated advantages of lower solubility than isoflurane and is not pungent. Sevoflurane causes dose-related EEG depression. No increase in heart rate is seen with sevoflurane, although it is a peripheral and cerebral vasodilator. Sensitivity to catecholamines is not increased with administration of sevoflurane.

Approximately 2% of absorbed sevoflurane is metabolized, with the production of two toxic metabolites: inorganic fluoride and hexafluoroisopropanol. Toxic metabolites have not been seen to be of any significant negative clinical effect, although the longevity of many neurosurgical procedures makes these metabolites of more concern than they would be for many other types of surgery.

Nitrous Oxide

Nitrous oxide (N_2O) is a controversial inhaled anesthetic agent that is used in neuroanesthesia. It differs significantly from the volatile anesthetics because it has little effect on, or slightly increases, $CMRo_2$. N_2O is a cerebral vasodilator, even at doses of 0.5 MAC. The increase in CBF caused by N_2O is attenuated by barbiturates, opioids, and hypocapnia. N_2O has no significant effect on CBV or CSF dynamics. Although N_2O does not induce EEG slowing, it does not cause seizures.

Because N_2O will diffuse into an air-filled space approximately 30 times as rapidly as nitrogen diffuses out of the space, its use in sitting craniotomies and other surgical procedures with the potential for air embolism requires careful consideration. However, no change in patient outcome has been shown in cases of air embolism, whether or not the patient was receiving N_2O. If an air embolism is suspected, N_2O should be stopped immediately. N_2O allows for lower doses of intravenous and volatile agents to be used, with the possibility of a more rapid awakening for postoperative evaluation.

NEUROMUSCULAR BLOCKING AGENTS

This section reviews depolarizing and nondepolarizing neuromuscular blocking drugs as they pertain to neuroanesthesia. Muscle relaxants are used for facilitating endotracheal tube placement, providing relaxation necessary for surgery, and preventing patient movement. Specific effects that require careful consideration are the drug's side effects, duration of action, metabolism, and elimination.

Depolarizing Agents

The only depolarizing neuromuscular blocker in common clinical use today is succinylcholine. Succinylcholine is an acetylcholine dimer that competes for acetylcholine receptor sites. It serves as an agonist at those sites, initiating a depolarization of the muscle membrane endplate. This binding is more prolonged than that of acetyl-choline because succinylcholine is more slowly degraded by plasma cholinesterase. Succinylcholine acts postsynaptically and causes visible muscle fasciculations followed by profound relaxation. The muscle fasciculations can be blunted reliably by pretreatment with a small dose of a nondepolarizing agent. Monitoring reveals decreased twitch height, without fade of tetanus or train-of-four, and no posttetanic facilitation.

Phase II block can be produced by succinylcholine, especially at higher doses or after repeat doses. Infusion to a total dose as low as 2 mg/kg can cause a phase II block. Onset of this phenomenon is preceded by tachyphylaxis and the development of monitoring characteristics of nondepolarizing drugs (e.g., fade in train-of-four). Attempting pharmacologic reversal of a phase II block may paradoxically prolong recovery, perhaps through inhibition of plasma cholinesterase necessary for degradation of succinylcholine. Allowing spontaneous recovery from a phase II block is the recommended course. The duration of action of succinylcholine is normally <10 minutes. However, patients with atypical plasma cholinesterase or those taking certain drugs (i.e., aminoglycoside and polymixin antibiotics) can experience a very prolonged duration of neuromuscular blockade.

Other systemic effects of succinylcholine primarily relate to its property of being an agonist at nicotinic ganglionic receptors and cardiac muscarinic receptors. The cardiac effects can cause a significant bradycardia, particularly in children under age 1 year or after a second dose that shortly follows the first. Pretreatment with atropine can effectively blunt this bradycardiac response.

Several aspects of succinylcholine use have a profound impact on neurosurgical patients. Succinylcholine has no significant effects on CSF dynamics, but it may increase ICP through increased CBF via activation of gamma afferent nerve fibers. A defasciculating dose of metocurine attenuates this increased ICP (Fig. 3-3). Succinylcholine may also cause a hyperkalemic, life-threatening arrhythmia in patients with diffuse muscular injury, whether it is caused by denervation, burn, sepsis, or crush injury (Fig. 3-4). In normal patients, intubation doses of succinylcholine will increase the serum potassium level by about 0.5 mEq/L. In patients with neuromuscular disease, the proliferation of extrajunctional acetylcholine receptors will allow a large potassium flux. Pretreatment with a defasciculating dose will not reliably prevent this hyperkalemic response. Although a period of at least 24 to 48 hours following the inciting event ap-

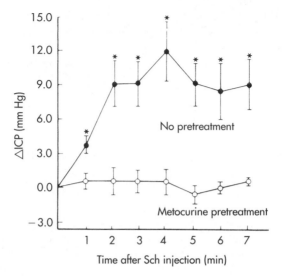

FIG 3-3.
Changes (mean ±SEM) in ICP after administration of succinylcholine *(Sch)* 1 mg/kg to anesthetized patients with malignant brain tumors. Open circles indicate values after administration of metocurine 0.03 mg/kg and Sch (group 1); solid circles indicate values after administration of saline and Sch (group II). Baseline values before Sch administration were similar; after Sch, ICP increased significantly in group II and remained elevated. Asterisks indicate *P* ≤0.5 compared to baseline value before Sch injection. (From Stirt JA et al: "Defasciculation" with metocurine prevents succinylcholine-induced increases in intracranial pressure, *Anesthesiology* 67:50-53, 1987.)

pears necessary before a hyperkalemic response will occur, it is most prudent to avoid giving succinylcholine to any patient who fits the at-risk criteria. In addition, succinylcholine is believed to be a triggering agent for masseter muscle spasm and malignant hyperthermia. Its use should also be avoided in patients considered to be at increased risk for malignant hyperthermia. Neurosurgical patients with upper motor neuron injury or intracerebral compromise are at risk for the development of hyperkalemia after succinylcholine administration. The presence of blood in the CNS, closed head injury,

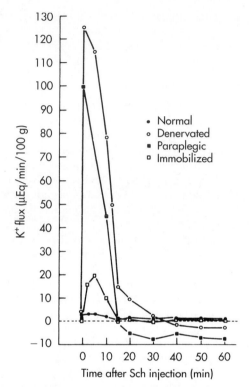

FIG 3-4.
Potassium ion fluxes of normal, immobilized, paraplegic, and denervated canine skeletal muscle after injection of succinylcholine (Sch) 0.25 mg/kg. (From Thiagarajah S: Anesthetic management of spinal surgery. In Frost EM, editor: Practical neuroanesthesia, *Anesthesiol Clin North Am* 5:593, 1987.)

and encephalitis are associated with increases in serum potassium, possibly through disuse atrophy of the affected musculature in some patients (Table 3-11). In contrast, brain lesions such as those of ischemic brain disease and tumors have a low incidence of hyperkalemia after administration of succinylcholine but are associated with decreased compliance and increased ICP.

Although succinylcholine has some significant side effects, it is valuable for use in rapidly securing the airway. Careful patient evaluation for side effect risk factors needs to be done, and appropriate premedication must be carried out (Table 3-12). However, when used appropriately, succinylcholine is a very rapid, potent, and effective neuromuscular blocking agent.

Nondepolarizing Agents

The nondepolarizing neuromuscular blocking drugs act as competitive antagonists of neuromuscular junction acetylcholine receptors, both presynaptically and postsynaptically. These agents show fade with train-of-four and sustained tetanus and exhibit posttetanic potentiation. It is the presynaptic action of these drugs, decreasing acetylcholine release, that is believed to be responsible for the fade and posttetanic facilitation. Nondepolarizing drugs vary greatly as to their cardiovascular and CPP effects, metabolism, and duration of action (Tables 3-13 and 3-14). They tend to be very large quaternary molecules that cross the placenta poorly. The nondepolarizing relaxants, like succinylcholine, are affected by preexisting neurologic disorders (see Table 3-11).

Atracurium has an intermediate duration of action and is metabolized by ester hydrolysis and Hofmann elimination. The latter produces the metabolite laudanosine, which can cause CNS excitation, although not at the concentrations obtained with normal clinical use. The metabolism of atracurium is not affected by either liver or renal dysfunction (or plasma cholinesterase), and it is a good choice for patients with disease of the liver or the kidneys. The duration of action is about 40 minutes following an induction dose.

Atracurium has no effect on ICP, but it does elicit mild release of histamine. Thus blood pressure may drop slightly following the rapid administration of large doses. Otherwise, cardiovascular stability is maintained.

The drug *d-tubocurarine* is a long-acting and cumulative agent that elicits a large histamine release with intravenous administration. It exhibits marked ganglionic and presynaptic blockade. Not significantly metabolized, it is excreted unchanged primarily by the kidneys and, to a small extent, via the biliary system. Curare does not directly affect CBF or $CMRo_2$, but it can raise ICP in at-risk patients. Although pretreatment with H_1- and H_2-blocking drugs can attenuate the histamine effects, use of large doses of curare is best avoided in patients in whom ICP is a concern. Today, curare is primarily used in small doses as a defasciculating agent before the administration of succinylcholine.

TABLE 3-11. Response to Muscle Relaxants in Neuromuscular Disorders

Disorder	Nondepolarizers	Succinylcholine
Intracranial lesions		
Hemiplegia	Decreased	Hyperkalemia
Parkinsonism	Normal	Normal
Multiple sclerosis	Normal	Hyperkalemia
Diffuse head injury	?	Hyperkalemia
Encephalitis	?	Hyperkalemia
Ruptured cerebral aneurysm	?	Hyperkalemia
Tetanus	Normal	Hyperkalemia
Spinal cord lesions		
Paraplegia/quadriplegia	Increased	Hyperkalemia
Amyotrophic lateral sclerosis	Increased	Contracture
Poliomyelitis	Increased	?
Acute anterior horn disease	?	Hyperkalemia
Peripheral nerve lesions		
Neurofibromatosis	Increased	Resistance
Peripheral neuropathies	Decreased	?
Muscular denervation	Normal	Contracture/ hyperkalemia
Neuromuscular junction lesions		
Myasthenia gravis		
Active	Increased	Resistance (early phase II block)
Remission	Normal	?
Muscular lesions		
Myasthenic syndrome	Increased	Increased
Myotonia	Normal/increased	Unpredictable Malignant hyperthermia association
Muscular dystrophy	Normal/increased	Hyperkalemia Malignant hyperthermia (Duchenne)
Ocular muscular dystrophy	Increased	?

Modified from Azar I: The response of patients with neuromuscular disorders to muscle relaxants: a review, *Anesthesiology* 61:173-187, 1984.

TABLE 3-12. Contraindications to Succinylcholine Use

Absolute	Relative
History of malignant hyperthermia	Increased ICP*
Severe burns ≤6 mo of age	Open eye injury
Severe trauma	Severe glaucoma
Upper motor neuron lesions	Hyperkalemia
Denervation	History of masseter spasm
Neuromuscular disorders	

*Attenuated or prevented by pretreatment.

TABLE 3-13. Effects of Muscle Relaxants on Hemodynamics and ICP

Drug	Mean Arterial Pressure	Heart Rate	ICP
Succinylcholine	—	↓	↑
Atracurium	↓	↑	—
Vecuronium	—	—	—
Pancuronium	↑	↑↑	—
Metocurine	↓	↑	—
d-Tubocurarine	↓↓	↓ or ↑*	↑†
Gallamine	↑	↑↑↑	— to ↑
Pipecuronium	—	—	?
Doxacurium	—	—	?
Mivacurium	↓	↑	?
Rocuronium	—	—	?

NOTE: Arrows indicate increase (↑) or decrease (↓). Number of arrows signifies magnitude of change. No effect (—). Unknown (?).
*Initially increased because of histamine release; as this dissipates, the ganglionic blockade predominates.
†Caused by histamine release.

Doxacurium is a very potent, long-acting benzylisoquinolinium that is devoid of significant cardiovascular side effects. No significant negative cerebral effects have been described. Doxacurium is minimally metabolized by plasma cholinesterase and is excreted essentially unchanged by the kidneys. Recovery to 25% of twitch height after an intubation dose takes about 2 to 3 hours. Because of its lack of side effects and long duration of action, doxacurium is an excellent choice for many neurosurgical procedures.

Gallamine is a long-acting drug with significant cardiovascular side effects. It produces a strong block of muscarinic cardiac recep-

TABLE 3-14. Autonomic and Histamine Effects of Muscle Relaxants

Drug	Cardiac Muscarine Receptor	Autonomic Ganglia	Histamine Release
Succinylcholine	Stimulates	Stimulates	Slight
Atracurium	—	—	Slight
Vecuronium	—	—	—
Pancuronium	Moderate block	—	—
Metocurine	—	Weak block	Slight
d-Tubocurarine	—	Moderate block	Moderate
Gallamine	Strong block	—	—
Pipecuronium	—	—	—
Doxacurium	—	—	—
Mivacurium	—	—	Slight
Rocuronium	—	—	—

Modified from Miller RD: The rational approach to the choice of a muscle relaxant, *ASA refresher course no. 52,* 1986.

tors, with a resultant tachycardia. Excretion occurs with the drug unchanged by the kidneys. Gallamine is not commonly used in today's clinical arena, although it is effective in defasciculation before succinylcholine administration.

Metocurine is a long-acting drug that has few cardiovascular side effects and minor ganglionic blockade action. It does liberate a significant amount of histamine if given rapidly. Metocurine is primarily excreted unchanged via the kidneys. ICP is not directly affected by metocurine, but the histamine effects must be taken into account. Metocurine is principally used as a defasciculating agent or in combination with pancuronium for long-acting blockade.

Mivacurium is a short-acting benzylisoquinolinium that undergoes rapid hydrolysis by plasma cholinesterase to inactive metabolites at a rate about 80% of succinylcholine. As with succinylcholine, duration of blockade is significantly prolonged in patients with atypical cholinesterase. The drug's rapid hydrolysis makes it an attractive agent for infusion. Some histamine release occurs with mivacurium, especially with intubating doses given rapidly.

Pancuronium is a long-acting drug that may increase ICP via tachycardia-induced increases in CBF. It is a vagolytic that produces tachycardia via altered SA and AV nodal conduction. Such changes can be beneficial in young children. Metabolism of pancuronium occurs via the liver with significant excretion through the kidneys.

Pipecuronium is a steroidal drug that is long-acting and devoid of significant cardiovascular side effects. It is primarily excreted unchanged from the kidneys. No significant negative cerebral effects have been described. It is very similar to vecuronium, although significantly longer acting—a benefit in many craniotomy surgeries.

Rocuronium is an intermediate-acting steroidal drug. Its pharmacokinetic and dynamic patterns are similar to those of vecuronium, with the important exception that the onset of rocuronium is more rapid. This characteristic makes rocuronium an extremely attractive agent for intubation in patients at risk for succinylcholine side effects. Hemodynamic stability is very well maintained at intubation doses of rocuronium. Rocuronium is not metabolized. It is excreted unchanged by the kidneys and especially via the biliary system.

Vecuronium is a steroidal drug that does not alter ICP or CSF dynamics. Cardiovascular side effects are almost nonexistent, even with very high doses. This situation allows vecuronium to be used for intubation with maintenance of stable hemodynamics. Bradycardia has been noted when vecuronium is used in combination with high doses of opioids because of the unopposed vagotonic effect of the opioids. Overall, the neuromuscular blocking properties are well separated from autonomic nervous system effects. Recovery from its effects occurs as a result of both hepatic metabolism and redistribution. The metabolites, one of which has some neuromuscular blocking activity, are excreted through the biliary system.

Tables 3-15 and 3-16 summarize the doses and duration of action of commonly used muscle relaxants.

ANTICHOLINESTERASES

Reversal of neuromuscular blockade is achieved by competitive inhibition of acetylcholinesterase (AChE) at the neuromuscular junction. The normal breakdown of acetylcholine (ACh) is inhibited, resulting in displacement of the neuromuscular blocking agents from the ACh receptor. Train-of-four measurement or evaluation of tetanic fade is commonly used as an endpoint for determination of the effectiveness of reversal of blockade at the nicotinic receptor. Dose, onset, and duration of the anticholinesterases are outlined in Table 3-17.

The nonspecific inhibition of AChE results in significant increases in ACh at the muscarinic receptor, causing bradycardia, salivation, increased gut motility, and other minor cholinergic side effects. Coad-

TABLE 3-15. Guidelines for Clinical Use of Muscle Relaxants

Drug	Normal Intubating Dose (mg/kg)	Onset to 100% block (min)	Duration (min)
Succinylcholine	1.0	0.5-1.0	5-10
Atracurium	0.5	2.5	30-45
Vecuronium	0.1	2.5	45-60
Pancuronium	0.1	3	120
Metocurine	0.4	4	150
d-Tubocurarine	0.5	4	150
Pipecuronium	0.1	4	120-150
Doxacurium	0.05	4	100-120
Mivacurium	0.2	1.5-2	≤30
Rocuronium	0.6	1.0-1.5	45-60

Modified from Miller RD: The rational approach to the choice of a muscle relaxant, *ASA refresher course no. 52,* 1986.

TABLE 3-16. Rapid Sequence Induction with Muscle Relaxants (Intubation within 90 sec)

Drug	Priming Dose (mg/kg)	Intubation Dose (mg/kg)	Duration* (min)
Succinylcholine	—	1 (1.5 mg/kg with pretreatment)	5-10
Atracurium	0.07	0.6-1.0	45-60
Vecuronium	0.01	0.2-0.3	60-90
Mivacurium	0.03	0.25	15
Rocuronium	0.07	0.6	45-60

From Savarese JJ: *The newer muscle relaxants,* no. 142, American Society of Anesthesiologists, 1986.
*Minimum to 25% twitch recovery.

ministration of an anticholinergic agent such as atropine or glycopyrrolate prevents excessive muscarinic stimulation. Atropine readily crosses the blood-brain barrier and may be associated with CNS effects. Appropriate doses and effects are summarized in Table 3-18.

Reversal of profound neuromuscular blockade is best accomplished with neostigmine combined with glycopyrrolate. The inability to reverse a neurosurgical patient's muscle relaxation adequately should result in continued ventilation to avoid hypercarbia and increases in blood pressure. A second dose of reversal agent

TABLE 3-17. Clinical Use of Anticholinesterases

Anti-AchE	Dose (mg/kg)	Onset (min)	Duration (min)
Edrophonium	0.5-1.0	1-2	60
Neostigmine	0.04-0.07	7-10	70
Pyridostigmine	0.2-0.35	12-16	120

TABLE 3-18. Pharmacology of Anticholinergics

	Atropine	Glycopyrrolate
Dose		
With edrophonium	7 μg/kg-10 μg/kg	0.01*
With neostigmine	15 μg/kg	0.01
With pyridostigmine	15 μg/kg†	0.01
Duration	15-30 min	2-4 hr
Effect on CNS	Mild sedation	None
Secretions	↓↓	↓↓↓
Smooth muscle tone	↓↓	↓↓↓
Heart rate	↑↑↑	↑↑

*Give several minutes before edrophonium because of differences in onset.
†Not recommended because of differences in onset.

may be attempted when electrolyte disturbances, acidosis, and drug interactions have been considered and the nerve stimulation indicates that reversal is probable (1 to 2 twitches).

Suggested Readings

Michenfelder JD: *Anesthesia and the brain*, New York, 1988, Churchill Livingstone.

Partridge BL: Advances in the use of muscle relaxants, *Anesth Clin Am* 11(2):205, 1993.

Stoelting RK: *Pharmacology and physiology in anesthetic practice,* ed 2, Philadelphia, 1991, JB Lippincott.

Vandesteene A, Trempont V, Engelman E, et al: Effect of propofol on cerebral blood flow and metabolism in man, *Anaesthesia* 43(suppl):42, 1988.

MONITORING *4*

Joel O. Johnson

MONITORING OF ADEQUACY OF CEREBRAL BLOOD FLOW
CEREBRAL BLOOD FLOW MONITORING
INTRACRANIAL PRESSURE MONITORING
CEREBRAL METABOLISM MONITORING
ELECTROPHYSIOLOGIC MONITORING
ELECTROENCEPHALOGRAPHY
EVOKED POTENTIALS
ELECTROMYOGRAPHY

The patient who is to undergo neurosurgery requires the usual physiologic monitors outlined by the American Society of Anesthesiologists, including the continued presence of qualified anesthesia personnel (see Box 4-1). This chapter focuses on other types of monitoring that may be used to make clinical decisions about the course of a neurosurgical anesthetic. Monitoring of specific neurosurgical procedures, such as carotid endarterectomy, sitting-position craniotomy, supratentorial surgery, and aneurysm clipping, is covered in other chapters.

The goal of most neuroanesthesia monitoring is to assess the adequacy of oxygenated blood flow to the central nervous system (CNS) or to monitor the functional integrity of neural structures at risk. This goal is accomplished by directly measuring blood flow or by using a secondary measure, either functional or physical, to make assumptions about the presence of ischemia or damage. The monitoring methods that are currently available or under study are outlined in Table 4-1.

MONITORING OF ADEQUACY OF CEREBRAL BLOOD FLOW

The anatomy and physiology of the brain is reviewed in Chapters 1 and 2, respectively. The cerebral metabolic and neurodynamic effects of different anesthetic therapies are discussed in Chapter 3. Brain monitoring devices cannot independently improve outcome,

---

BOX 4-1.
American Society of Anesthesiologists Standards for Basic Anesthetic Monitoring

---

Standard I

Qualified anesthesia personnel must be present in the room throughout the conduct of all general anesthetics, regional anesthetics, and monitored anesthesia care.

Standard II

The patient's oxygenation, ventilation, circulation, and temperature must be continuously evaluated.
  Oxygenation
    Oxygen analyzer with a low-limit alarm
    Pulse oximetry or observation of patient color
  Ventilation
    Observation: chest rise, breathing bag excursion
    Auscultation: via esophageal or precordial stethoscope
    Measurement: $ETco_2$ monitoring encouraged
    Intubation: clinical assessment mandatory and $ETco_2$ analysis after placement recommended
  Circulation
    Continuous electrocardiogram (ECG)
    Blood pressure every 5 minutes
    Pulse detection via palpation, auscultation, intraarterial blood pressure monitors, pulse oximetry, or plethysmography
  Temperature
    Available for continuous monitoring

Modified from American Society of Anesthesiologists: *ASA standards, guidelines, and statements,* Chicago, 1994, The Society.

---

and no single monitoring method can define the degree to which ischemia is present. This situation is a result of the marked nonhomogeneity of the brain and cerebral blood flow (CBF). CBF ranges from 20 ml/100 g/min to 80 ml/100 g/min in white and gray matter, respectively. Autoregulation maintains a constant CBF in normal adults by arteriolar adjustment to mean arterial blood pressure, arterial carbon dioxide partial pressure ($Paco_2$), and arterial oxygen partial pressure (Pao_2) (Fig. 4-1). CO_2 may alter flow by as much as 1.75 ml/100 g/min for each 1 mm Hg change in $Paco_2$, and CBF increases if Pao_2 falls below 50 mm Hg.

The optimal delivery of O_2 to the various portions of the brain is a function of arterial O_2 content (Cao_2) and regional CBF, which is

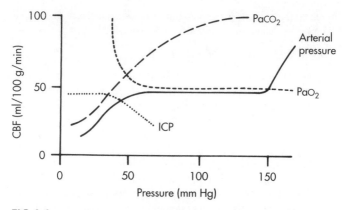

FIG 4-1.
Summary of CBF control. *ICP* represents intracranial pressure.

TABLE 4-1. Monitoring Methods of CNS Used in Neuroanesthesia

Measurement	Method/Device
Adequacy of cerebral blood flow (CBF)	[133]Xenon: quantitative measurement of CBF
	Cerebral blood flow velocity (CBFV)
	Stump pressure
Intracranial pressure monitors	Epidural
	Subdural bolt
	Intraventricular catheter
	Intraparenchymal device
Cerebral metabolism	Oxygen extraction: direct measurement
	Continuous jugular venous oxygen saturation ($Sjvo_2$)
	Transcranial oxygen saturation
Electrophysiologic monitoring	Electroencephalogram (EEG)
	Evoked potentials (EPs)
	Somatosensory evoked potentials (SSEPs)
	Brainstem auditory evoked potentials (BAEPs)
	Visual evoked potentials (VEPs)
	Motor evoked potentials (MEPs)
	Electromyography (EMG)

autoregulated by the metabolic demand, or cerebral metabolic rate of oxygen consumption ($CMRO_2$). In general, brain monitors directly or indirectly assess blood flow, O_2 content (through arterial oxygen saturation, Sao_2), or metabolism. Electrophysiologic devices monitor the functional characteristics of nervous tissue, indicating damage by detection of deviation from baseline values.

Cerebral Blood Flow Monitoring

Quantitative measurement of CBF in man was described by Kety and Schmidt in 1945. Originally calculated with nitrous oxide (N_2O), the technique now uses radioactive [133]xenon (^{133}Xe) clearance to calculate CBF. [133]Xe is inhaled or injected, and scintillation counters positioned over various regions of the scalp record the clearance of radioactive counts. The calculated CBF is the "gold standard" as it relates to blood flow, and it has been shown to have a good prognostic value in patients with head injury. However, the disadvantages of the method preclude its general use as a CBF monitor in the operating room. These include the need to use a radioactive agent, the technical difficulty in measurement, and the lack of specificity for ischemia. However, this method remains a valuable research tool.

Cerebral blood flow velocity (CBFV) (cm/sec) is measured with a transcranial Doppler device by insonation of the middle cerebral artery, as shown in Fig. 4-2. The measurement is both a function of CBF and the diameter of the artery. It has proven useful for the detection of vasospasm after subarachnoid hemorrhage, as a monitor during carotid endarterectomy (CEA), and for the diagnosis of brain death. In addition, it can detect emboli during CEA or cardiopulmonary bypass surgery and assess changes in ICP during shunt malfunction in children. As a brain monitor, CBFV is used intermittently or continuously. This method is noninvasive and relatively easy to use with commercially available equipment. It is not useful as a monitor of regional CBF or during the intraoperative period. The angle of insonation (δ) is critical for accuracy of measurement. Difficulties arise because of variation in CBFV among individual patients and its relation to CBF as measured by [133]Xe.

Stump pressure measurement during CEA is used to assess the adequacy of CBF originating from the contralateral internal carotid artery. Pressure is transduced distal to the operative site, and a critical value of <50 mm Hg indicates risk for ischemia. A lack of correlation with regional CBF has led to decreased use of stump pressure as a reliable monitor.

Nasal plethysmography and conjunctival partial pressure of O_2 (PO_2) have been investigated as indirect monitors of CBF because of their blood supplies from the anterior ethmoidal and ophthalmic ar-

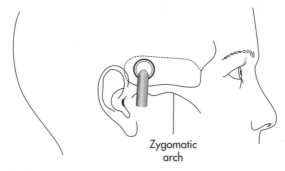

Zygomatic
arch

FIG 4-2.
Diagram of area *(dotted line),* above zygomatic arch, where Doppler signals from intracranial arteries can be obtained. Most likely location to obtain signals is shown by position of probe. (From Aaslid R, Markwalder TM, Nornes H: Noninvasive transcranial Doppler ultrasound recording of flow velocity in basal cerebral arteries, *J Neurosurg* 57:769, 1982.)

teries, respectively. However, there is no correlation between these measures and CBF.

Intracranial Pressure Monitoring

Intracranial pressure (ICP) monitoring devices are used to define the adequacy of CBF by the relationship of mean arterial blood pressure (MAP) to cerebral perfusion pressure (CPP):

$$CPP = MAP - ICP \text{ (or CVP if higher)}$$

Normal CPP in a normal adult is 100 mm Hg. The lower limit of acceptable CPP in a healthy normotensive patient with intact autoregulation is about 50 mm Hg.

Craniotomy patients require continuous monitoring of estimated CPP. This monitoring is routinely accomplished by placing an indwelling arterial catheter before induction of anesthesia. The transducer is placed at the level of the external auditory meatus, allowing an accurate estimate of CPP if ICP is normal (5 to 15 mm Hg). In addition, an arterial catheter allows for intermittent measurement of blood gas tensions to assess the difference between end-tidal CO_2 ($ETCO_2$) and $PaCO_2$ and make appropriate adjustments in ventilation. Although ICP monitoring is an accepted part of management in patients with head injury, it is not routinely used in other neurosurgical procedures. Therefore in patients with an apparently normal ICP, an estimate of CPP based on arterial blood pressure is acceptable.

Intracranial hypertension is defined as a sustained elevation of ICP >15 mm Hg in the supine position. Indications for the placement of an invasive ICP monitor include a midline shift of >5 mm on computed tomography (CT) of the head, papilledema, severe vomiting, headache, or transient blindness. There are four cranium-based methods of monitoring ICP, as illustrated in Fig. 4-3, and lumbar cerebrospinal fluid pressure (CSFP) monitoring.

Lumbar CSFP is measured via a catheter placed below the L2-3 interspace and advanced in a cephalad direction. Under normal circumstances, free communication takes place between the spinal and intracranial spaces, allowing measurement of the ICP. Advantages include the remote nature of the monitoring site and the ability to adjust and sample CSF. The risk of infection requires the use of strict aseptic technique. In patients with noncommunicating hydrocephalus, herniation may develop through the foramen magnum if large pressure changes occur; also, injury to the spinal cord during or after catheter insertion has been reported.

Epidural ICP is monitored through the use of a pressure sensor or transducer placed directly in contact with the surface of the dura. Although this method preserves the parenchyma of the brain and is associated with a low incidence of infection, there are several disadvantages. Recalibration of the system after placement is impossible, the system overestimates pressure (by 5 to 30 mm Hg as compared to intraventricular pressure), and there is significant variance over a 24-hour period. Since the epidural space cannot be transduced with a fluid column attached to a transducer, pressure is monitored with a strain gauge, a pneumatic pressure–sensing device, or a fiberoptic transducer operating on a pneumatic compensating system.

Subdural ICP is monitored through a threaded bolt, as shown in Fig. 4-3. The parenchyma of the brain is again spared damage, and placement complications are rare if the venous sinuses and the proposed surgical site are avoided. Brain tissue may plug the hollow bolt, and therapeutic maneuvers such as drainage of cerebrospinal fluid (CSF) are impossible. The measurements obtained are not as reliable as those taken from an intraventricular catheter.

Intraventricular ICP catheters are placed through the brain into the lateral ventricle contralateral to the side of the lesion. A burr

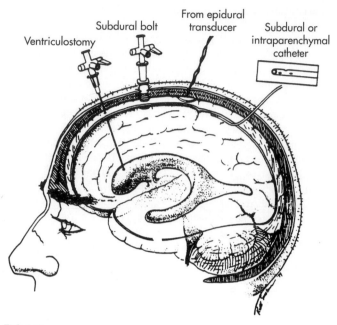

FIG 4-3.
Commonly employed techniques and sites for ICP measurement.
(From Shapiro HM. Neurosurgical anesthesia and intracranial hypertension. In Miller RD, editor: *Anesthesia,* ed 2, vol 2, New York, 1986, Churchill Livingstone, p 1577.)

hole near the coronal suture is used to gain entry to the cranial vault
and the lateral horn of the ventricle. The zero position for the transducer is at the level of the external auditory meatus. Such a system,
which allows for accurate measurement of CSFP and therapeutic
removal of CSF, is considered the "gold standard" for ICP monitoring. Noncommunication of the lateral ventricle with other intracranial compartments invalidates the measurement. Disadvantages include destruction of viable brain tissue, difficult placement,
possible acute decreases in CSFP, intraventricular bleeding, and significant risk of infection. Although 10% of patients with intraventricular catheters have positive CSF cultures, only 1% of these
results are clinically significant. The risk of infection increases sig-

nificantly after 3 days, and prophylactic antibiotics have little or no beneficial effect.

Intraparenchymal ICP monitors are used routinely at our institution for patients at risk for intracranial hypertension. The fiberoptic catheter is placed through a burr hole into the parenchyma of the brain. Pressure is sensed through detection of the movement of a light-reflecting membrane at the tip of the catheter. Calibration (zeroing) of the system is done before insertion, and the output can be displayed in an analog or digital form. Although expensive, the system is easy to use and resistant to artifacts. It accurately reflects ICP changes in an electronically storable format. Disadvantages include the destruction of viable neural tissue, cost, and possible damage to the fiberoptic cable.

ICP waveforms, initially described by Lundberg, may be related to specific outcomes necessitating prompt treatment:

A Waves—Sustained pressure waves (60 to 80 mm Hg) occurring every 5 to 20 minutes. A waves are life-threatening and represent cerebral vasodilation in response to decreased CPP.

B Waves—Small, brief waves (10 to 20 mm Hg) occurring every 30 to 120 seconds. B waves are seen in patients with decreased intracerebral compliance and are caused by fluctuations in cerebral blood volume.

C Waves—Small oscillations (0 to 10 mm Hg) in patients with decreased compliance reflecting changes in systemic arterial pressure.

Cerebral Metabolism Monitoring

Cerebral metabolism is measured by estimating the extraction of O_2 by the brain through the following equation:

$$CMRo_2 = CBF \times (Cao_2 - Cvo_2)$$

in which CvO_2 is the venous O_2 content measured at the jugular venous bulb. This relationship becomes more clinically meaningful if the equation is rearranged to reflect measurable values on the left side of the equation:

$$Cao_2 - Cvo_2 = CMRo_2/CBF$$

As long as the coupling of CBF and $CMRo_2$ remains intact, measurement of the difference between arterial and venous O_2 content

(AVD$_{O_2}$) or more simply, following the O_2 saturation at the jugular bulb (Sjv$_{O_2}$) reveals a constant value. This relationship between demand for O_2 and CBF is disrupted in certain pathologic states, including head injury and brain infarction/ischemia.

O_2 extraction is measured directly by retrograde placement of a jugular venous catheter with any of the commercially available products. Ca$_{O_2}$ is assumed to be the same at the radial artery sampling site and the internal carotid artery. A normal value of Ca$_{O_2}$ − Cv$_{O_2}$ for adults is 7 ml O_2/dl. If the difference is significantly smaller (4 ml O_2/dl), the supply of O_2 exceeds the demand. In contrast, if the difference is significantly larger (>9 ml O_2/dl), the patient is at risk for ischemia. Careful titration of hyperventilation to optimize ICP management while monitoring O_2 extraction should decrease the possibility of hyperventilation-mediated regional ischemia.

Continuous Sjv$_{O_2}$ monitoring is a commercially available simplification of O_2 extraction. Because of the relationship between O_2 content and O_2 saturation, Sjv$_{O_2}$ is used to predict situations in which the supply of O_2 is not meeting the demand. Normal Sjv$_{O_2}$ is 60% to 70%. A decrease to 54% indicates compensated cerebral hypoperfusion, and lower values are associated with electroencephalographic (EEG) changes consistent with ischemia. A value of 40% or less precipitates ischemia in patients with head injury. Although not a proven technique in terms of outcome, this type of monitoring is relatively easy to use and similar to the use of continuous mixed venous oxygenation in the systemic circulation. The effluent blood represents various brain regions and thus cannot predict regional blood flow disturbances. As a consequence, although a decreased Sjv$_{O_2}$ indicates cerebral ischemia, normal or elevated values do not always indicate adequate perfusion in all areas of the brain.

Regional transcranial O_2 saturation is a noninvasive technique that uses near-infrared spectroscopy to estimate O_2 saturation over a chosen region of the brain. A light source directs a shallow beam (transversing scalp and cranium) and a deep beam (scalp, cranium, and cerebral cortex), which are detected simultaneously. Changes in wavelength proportional to the relative concentrations of oxygenated and deoxygenated blood in the cerebral cortex are quantified. This method awaits clinical validation, but it has significant merit as a noninvasive measure for monitoring "at risk" areas of the cerebral cortex.

ELECTROPHYSIOLOGIC MONITORING

The functional integrity of the nervous system may be monitored through various neurophysiologic techniques. There are three criteria that should be met:

1. The nervous system component at risk is amenable to monitoring.
2. A monitoring device and experienced personnel are available to detect abnormalities in the electrophysiologic signal.
3. Therapeutic intervention is possible if an abnormality is detected.

Several techniques meet these criteria, including EEG, evoked potentials (EPs), electromyography (EMG), and motor evoked potentials (MEPs).

Electroencephalography

BASIC PRINCIPLES

EEG waves are the summation of excitatory and inhibitory synaptic potentials spontaneously generated by the pyramidal cells of the cerebral cortex and influenced by rhythmic discharges from the thalamus. Electrical activity is linked to metabolic activity, and the EEG, being a measure of electrical activity, is therefore affected by anything influencing metabolic activity, such as O_2 uptake or cortical blood flow.

Within any individual's EEG, variations are very small. This characteristic makes the EEG a useful parameter for monitoring because any change from a stable baseline indicates a significant change in the brain's metabolic activity. During surgery any transient EEG abnormality that is immediately recognized and corrected usually results in a normal recovery. In contrast, when a major EEG abnormality persists from the time of the insult to the end of the surgery, there is a significantly higher chance of permanent neurologic injury.

TECHNICAL ASPECTS

Fig. 4-4 shows the standard reference point for electrode placement with use of the International 10-20 Electrode System. Placement of electrodes is calculated by using a percentage of the patient's head circumference and the interaural and nasion-inion distance. The designation 10-20 refers to the fact that the percentages are 10% or 20% of the overall distances. By convention, the left side of the skull is given odd numbers; the right side, even. The code used is as follows:

F_p	Frontal pole
F	Frontal
C	Central
T	Temporal
A	Auricular
P	Parietal
O	Occipital
Z	Midline

In the operating room all available channels usually are not used. The placement of the electrodes is subject to variations in surgical incisions, and since most intraoperative recording involves a comparison of the two sides of the brain, symmetry of placement is critical.

In general, all channels of the EEG use two active electrodes and a reference electrode (monopolar montage, Fig. 4-5). The technique illustrated is called common mode rejection and is also used in electrocardiography.

Fig. 4-6 shows the difference between bipolar and common reference montage. With a common reference montage, five channels

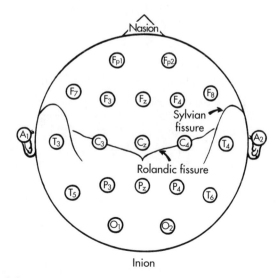

FIG 4-4.
Position for EEG electrodes according to International 10-20 Electrode System.

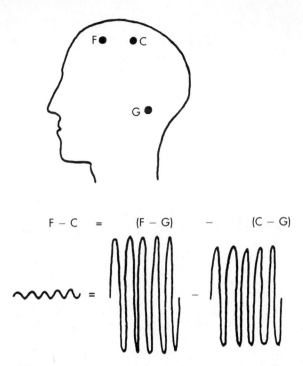

FIG 4-5.
Elimination of artifact by difference amplification. To obtain signal between *F* and *C*, reference point *G* is selected. Since electrical artifact appears to be of equal amplitude for *F-G* and *C-G*, subtracting these two electronically produces *F-C*, desired signal, free from electrical interference.

are available, with differences between adjacent electrodes being measured with the reference electrode at A_1. The advantage of this set-up is that the amplitude of the tracings is high, which is significant in the electrically hostile operating room. The main disadvantage is that if there is any technical difficulty with A_1, all five channels become inoperable. The bipolar montage on the right side of the diagram records four channels. Even if one electrode fails in this configuration, some information remains.

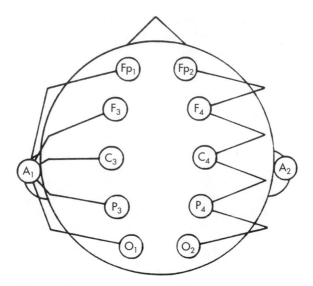

FIG 4-6.

Bipolar and common reference montages. Left parasagittal electrodes are connected in common reference montage with left earlobe (A_1) used as common reference electrode. Five channels are recorded, each between parasagittal electrode and ear electrode. Differences among these channels represent differences in cerebral activity among various parasagittal electrodes because each channel is recorded as difference between activity at parasagittal electrode and at ear electrode. For comparison, right parasagittal electrodes have been connected in bipolar chain. In this configuration, only four channels of EEG data are recorded. Each channel of data represents electrical difference between two adjacent electrodes. (From Levy WJ: Monitoring. In Kaplan, editor: *Cardiac anesthesia,* ed 2, Orlando, Fla, 1987, Grune & Stratton, p 323.)

ELECTRODE POSITIONS (MONTAGE)

Since the EEG signal is normally symmetrical, lead placement is also symmetrical. Asymmetry in the face of a previously symmetrical pattern is suggestive of a catastrophic occurrence.

Electrode placement depends on what information is sought. The gold standard remains the classic 16-channel EEG. For detection of global ischemia, for the patient with therapeutically induced barbiturate coma, or for monitoring of anesthetic depth, a simple two-channel lead placement, as shown in Fig. 4-7, *A,* can be used because most changes that may result from the typical responses to surgery and anesthesia in the operating room can be monitored without a complex montage.

A basic principle is that the EEG recorded at an electrode represents the electrical activity generated in a 2.5 cm radius. The closer an electrode is to an area that becomes ischemic, the better are the chances of seeing a change. However, widely spaced scalp electrodes are also sensitive to cortical events in areas greater than the area of cortex directly beneath the electrode (global ischemia). Therefore some have advocated use of the simple montage (Fig. 4-7, *A*).

Placement of electrodes in a frontomastoid configuration alone might be adequate for assessing global ischemia, but this approach is probably inadequate for monitoring middle cerebral artery ischemia. Thus, when less than a 16-channel montage is used, electrodes ideally should be located so that the middle cerebral artery watershed area is being monitored. Fig. 4-7, *B,* shows a montage that accomplishes this goal.

Many types of electrodes have been developed to make application easy and efficient. The scalp is typically cleansed and degreased with alcohol. Electrolyte conductive paste is placed between the silver disc electrode and the scalp and attached with collodion. Simple pregelled adhesive patches are used on hairless areas. Impedance testing of all electrode sites should reveal values <5000 ohms. Stainless steel needle electrodes can be rapidly applied into the skin, and in the properly premedicated patient they will produce only minimal discomfort. However, the presence of infection, hematoma, or anticoagulation in cardiac surgery are contraindications to needle placement.

INTERPRETATION AND NORMAL FINDINGS

The EEG signal generated in the cerebral cortex is of low energy, around 2 to 200 μV as compared with the 500 to 1000 μV for the ECG. Interpretation of the EEG involves measuring frequency and amplitude as well as evaluating the morphology of the waveform.

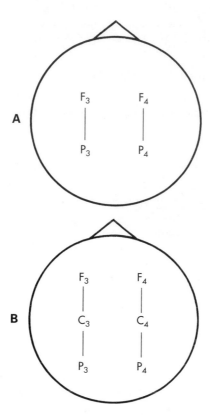

FIG 4-7.
A, Two-channel and, **B,** four-channel lead placement.

Frequency.   The electrical waveform of the EEG is subdivided into sine waves of specific frequencies (cycles/sec or Hertz [Hz]) as follows (Fig. 4-8):

Delta (δ) 0 Hz to 4 Hz—These are high-amplitude, low-frequency waves consistent with stage 4 "deep sleep," deep anesthesia, or neuropathologic states such as cerebral ischemia or infarction.

Theta (θ) 4 Hz to 7 Hz—Theta waves are high-amplitude slow waves seen predominantly in premature infants, in healthy children during sleep, and during hyperventilation. They are also prominent during moderate to deep anesthesia.

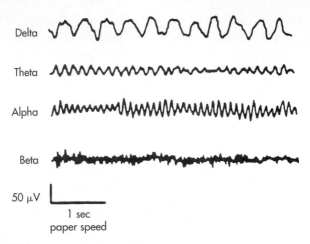

FIG 4-8.
Four basic EEG waveforms.

Alpha (α) 8 Hz to 13 Hz—Alpha waves are typically seen in a person who is relaxed, alert, and with eyes closed. Alpha waves originate primarily from the parietooccipital regions. The typical alpha range averages approximately 10 to 11 Hz, with this baseline slowing with advancing age. In children the mean frequency is within the low 8 Hz range, advancing to higher frequencies of 10 to 11 Hz during adulthood. Light anesthesia is characterized by a dominance of 10 to 14 Hz frequencies.

Beta (β) 14 Hz to 30 Hz—Beta rythmn is characterized by low-voltage fast activity typically seen in the awake, alert individual. It also occurs with low-dose anesthesia produced by barbiturates and 50% N_2O.

An isoelectric (flat line) EEG signifies electrical inactivity and is consistent with ischemia, hypothermia, barbiturate coma, >2 MAC (minimum alveolar concentration) isoflurane anesthesia, or brain death.

Amplitude.   Amplitude refers to the height of the waveform and is expressed in microvolts:

    Low amplitude: <20 μV
    Medium amplitude: 20 to 50 μV
    High amplitude: >50 μV

Symmetry.   Normal brain activity demonstrates symmetry. Acute asymmetry signifies a potentially devastating event. However, an asymmetrical pattern during a neurovascular procedure such as CEA, in which the watershed area of the middle cerebral artery is affected, is at times seen with slowing of the EEG relative to the contralateral side without change in outcome.

ANESTHETIC EFFECTS

When general anesthesia is induced, variability of the EEG among individuals decreases, and the regional differences in frequency and amplitude become minimal. The EEG varies according to the type of anesthetic agent being given, but since most anesthesiologists employ a combination of drugs, this variation is of little practical importance. The changes typically seen with increasing depth of anesthesia are primarily dose dependent rather than agent specific. It is important to realize that the patterns of change caused by increasing doses of anesthetics are similar to those seen with ischemia.

Induction.   Initial fast waves in the EEG are replaced by spindle-shaped bursts with a frequency of 5 to 12 Hz superimposed on the fast activity. As the patient loses consciousness, the EEG develops high-amplitude slow waves of 1 to 3 Hz, at which time skin incision may be made.

Sub-MAC Anesthetic Concentrations.   As the alpha rhythm gives way to increased beta activity, a widespread anterior rhythmic pattern is seen in the low beta and alpha frequencies. As anesthesia deepens, the excitement phase disappears, and a progressive slowing in frequency occurs.

Supra-MAC Anesthetic Concentrations.   Large doses of anesthetics shift the EEG from theta to delta, with increased slowing and finally a decrease in amplitude with burst-suppression and ultimately an isoelectric EEG. Table 4-2 shows the effects of various physiologic and anesthetic conditions on the EEG.

Ischemic Changes.   The EEG begins to show ischemic changes when CBF falls to about 50% of normal in awake individuals (25 ml/min/100 g), or when the PaO_2 falls below 35 mm Hg. In general, critical levels of perfusion and oxygenation decrease with the increasing anesthetic state of the individual. Recognizable ischemic EEG changes precede somatosensory evoked potential or brainstem auditory evoked potential changes. Frontal alpha waves ap-

TABLE 4-2. Factors Affecting EEG

Factor	Effect
Increasing frequency	Hyperoxia
	Hypercarbia
	Hypoxia
	Seizures
	Low-dose barbiturates
	Low-dose benzodiazepines
	N_2O 30%-70%
	Inhalational agents <1 MAC
	Ketamine
Low frequency, low amplitude	Hypoxia
	Hypercarbia
	Barbiturates
	Hypoglycemia
Low frequency, high amplitude	Hypoxia
	Hypocarbia
	Hypothermia
	Barbiturates
	Etomidate
	Narcotics
	Inhalational agents >1 MAC
Isoelectric	Brain death
	Hypoxia (Pao_2 <25 mm Hg)
	Hypothermia (<17°C)
	Barbiturate coma
	Isoflurane 2 MAC

pear, then delta waves, followed by burst-suppression and electrical silence.

PROCESSING

The raw EEG records the changes of voltage over time, which may be stored on strip chart (hard copy) or computer disk. Computerized analysis converts these complex data through the use of fast Fourier transformation into power (amplitude squared) versus frequency. Fourier analysis uses a complex mathematical manipulation to reduce the complex EEG waveform into its component harmonically related sine waves. Displays of the unprocessed EEG signal are still very important and give the observer the chance to assess the validity of the processed data. Thus the 16-channel EEG monitored by an experienced electroencephalographer remains the gold standard.

Cerebral Function Monitor. The cerebral function monitor is a simplified version of the EEG in which the amplitude of the sine waves is measured and displayed as the average peak voltage on a strip chart recorder. This modality traces the product of power and frequency. The trace of the upper border represents amplitude at its highest point, whereas the lower border represents the lowest point of the amplitude. The percentage of total voltage in any particular frequency range is reported. The monitor was originally designed to follow EEG activity in the intensive care setting. It remains a fairly good monitor for global ischemia, but it is inadequate in detecting focal ischemia and is a poor choice for the measurement of depth of anesthesia.

Power-Spectrum Analysis. Power-spectrum analysis breaks the EEG down and digitizes it using fast Fourier transformation. To simplify the data, a one-dimensional (univariate) descriptor of the power spectra may be determined. As the waveform is simplified into these univariate descriptors, much of the information inherent in the waveform is deleted and can be misleading. The advantages of this technique are its ease of use and reliability as an indicator of global ischemia. It is quite sensitive to artifact and baseline drift.

Compressed Spectral Array. Compressed spectral array (CSA) is a three-dimensional display of frequency and power over time. Frequency is described on the X-axis, power on the Z-axis, and time on the Y-axis. Time and amplitude are then rotated onto the same axes. This graphic display of information is presented with clarity on a two-dimensional screen (Fig. 4-9). One of the concerns with this type of display is that high-amplitude activity tends to obscure concurrent low-amplitude activity at the same frequency.

Density-Modulated Spectral Array. In order to avoid the loss of data behind the peaks within the CSA display, density-modulated spectral array (DSA) uses light intensity or density of a dot matrix to represent the power at any frequency. Both CSA and DSA can be coupled with spectral edge frequency, which is the frequency below which 97% of the power is found. Spectral edge frequency may be of some benefit in estimating depth of anesthesia.

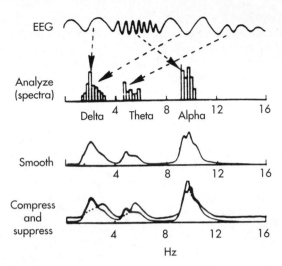

FIG 4-9.
Steps in generation of compressed spectral array from segments of raw EEG data.

Evoked Potentials
PRINCIPLES OF EVOKED POTENTIALS

The EEG measures the surface summation of random spontaneous electrical cortical activity. An EP is the response of the nervous system to an externally applied stimulus. As such, normal sensory evoked potentials (SEPs) reflect the integrity of the pathway being studied. These pathways are ascending sensory tracts that usually involve a peripheral or cranial nerve.

Typically, EPs tend to get buried in the EEG signal because of their low amplitude (1 to 5 μV). Signal averaging helps to amplify the EP, and extraneous random EEG activity and other "noise" is filtered out electronically. However, when a large portion (25%) of any EP waveform is eliminated, the waveform generated may be misleading.

Various factors, such as electrical noise, hypothermia, ischemia, changes in $Paco_2$, anesthesia, age, gender, stimulus characteristics, and electrode placement, can affect EPs. Fig. 4-10 is a typical example of somatosensory evoked potentials (SSEPs).

CLASSIFICATION AND TERMINOLOGY

Latency.   Latency is the elapsed time between application of the stimulus and its recording. It is measured in milliseconds and increases with hypothermia, anesthesia, and ischemia.

Amplitude.   The amplitude of the EP is approximately an order of magnitude less than the EEG (EPs are approximately 1 to 5 μV in amplitude compared to the EEG, which runs approximately 10 to 200 μV in amplitude). The amplitude may also be affected by anesthesia, ischemia, hypothermia, and the strength and site of the application of the neural stimulus.

Near-Field Potentials and Far-Field Potentials.   The characteristics of these potentials are outlined in Table 4-3. Near-field potentials are stimuli that are recorded by electrodes close to the neurogenerative source (e.g., the sensory cortex). Far-field potentials arise from subcortical neurogenerative sources that are relatively far away anatomically from the scalp electrode (e.g., the brainstem).

TYPES OF EVOKED POTENTIALS

Somatosensory Evoked Potentials.   The method used by most electrophysiologists is to monitor two channels, with electrodes placed over the anatomic pathways to be studied. Sites are chosen so that pathways below and above the proposed surgical site are monitored. For scoliosis or aortic surgery, typically the median nerve (above) and the posterior tibial nerve (below) are stimulated, respectively, along with corresponding cortical sites (Fig. 4-11). If there is a thoracic- or lumbar-level insult, a change may be seen on the posterior tibial trace. Interruption of the conduction pathway at any point between the site of stimulation and the cerebral cortex can alter the cortical SSEPs. This effect may occur secondary to ischemia, retraction, or direct surgical disruption. Surgical treatment of scoliosis is associated with 1% to 3% risk of spinal cord damage, depending on the technique used in the application of Harrington or Luque fixation.

Increasing concentrations of all volatile anesthetics prolong the latency and decrease the amplitude of SSEPs. Monitoring must be done at stable concentrations of <0.5 MAC. The use of N_2O will cause similar changes and may be avoided by changing to a propofol infusion as a supplement in a balanced technique. Barbiturates and benzodiazepines decrease SSEPs, whereas narcotics have little effect.

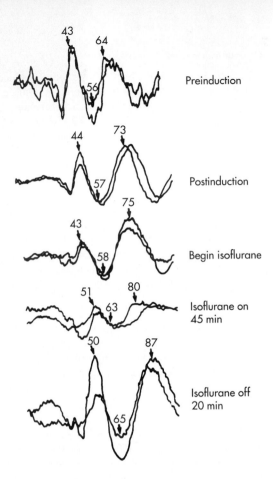

FIG 4-10.
Cortical SSEPs for awake and anesthetized patient. Posterior tibial nerve of patient was stimulated 1024 times with 5.1 stimuli/sec. All cortical responses were averaged. To suppress extraneous signals, filter was used to eliminate all frequencies <30 Hz and >250 Hz. Numbers attached to positive and negative potentials represent time (in milliseconds) that elapsed after stimulation (latency). Thus all recorded potentials arose with latency of <100 msec. Such potentials are called near-field potentials. These are assumed to arise in nervous tissue near scalp electrode, in cortex of patient's brain. Figure shows how isoflurane increases latency and decreases amplitude of near-field SSEP. (From Gravenstein JS, Paulus DA, editors: *Clinical monitoring practice,* Philadelphia, 1987, JB Lippincott, p 265.)

TABLE 4-3. Characteristics of Near-Field and Far-Field Evoked Potentials

Near-Field	Far-Field
Cortical neurogenerator	Brainstem neurogenerator
Longer latency (<100 msec)	Short latency (<45 msec)
Shorter distances	Longer distances
High amplitude (higher voltage)	Lower amplitude (lower voltage)
Less amplification required	Requires more amplification
Fewer individual responses required (50–200)	Requires more rapid rates of stimulation (1000s)
More sensitive to anesthetic/ physiologic effects	Less sensitive to anesthetic/ physiologic effects

Traditionally a "wake-up" test is performed to see if, after instrumentation and before closure, the patient can voluntarily move his/her legs. Depending on the results, the patient is either reanesthetized and possible corrections are instituted or closure of the incision is completed. Although SSEP monitoring is a valuable tool for the diagnosis of spinal cord ischemia, false-negative results have been reported. The wake-up test provides proof of intact function; however, it does so only at a single point in time. SSEPs enhance surveillance by offering an acceptably reliable continuum in the measurement of sensory pathway integrity. Depending on the institution, a wake-up test may be performed before closure in all patients undergoing scoliosis repair, or it may be done immediately intraoperatively only in those with changes in the SSEP.

In the event of a deterioration in the electrophysiologic signal, therapeutic maneuvers consist of both physical and hemodynamic alterations. Retractors may be removed or repositioned, and the spinal column may be repositioned to eliminate pressure on neural structures. Optimization of blood flow and O_2 delivery by increasing arterial pressure, hematocrit, and volume are effective therapies. A transient but reversible loss of SSEPs should preserve postoperative function, but an irreversible loss of SSEPs usually implies a loss of function in the monitored pathway.

Brainstem Auditory Evoked Potentials. Brainstorm auditory evoked potentials (BAEPs) are generated by an audible click delivered to each ear in sequential fashion to stimulate the eighth cranial nerve and associated brainstem pathways. The signal is then recorded by scalp electrodes. At present, BAEP monitoring is used

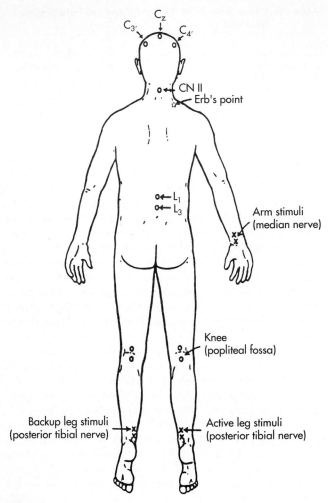

FIG 4-11.
Median nerve and posterior tibial nerve of patient are stimulated. Electrode locations for both stimulating and sensing are shown (patient is prone). $C_{3'}$ is located contralateral to site of stimulation and 3 cm posterior to C_3. $C_{4'}$ is ipsilateral to stimulation and 3 cm posterior to C_4. (From Gravenstein JS, Paulus DA, editors: *Clinical monitoring practice,* Philadelphia, 1987, JB Lippincott, p 270.)

during surgery involving the eighth cranial nerve, such as for acoustic neuromas, or with surgery in the posterior fossa, in which the brainstem may be at risk.

BAEPs are short-latency potentials that may be affected by surgical retraction of the eighth cranial nerve or by any of the other variables previously described. Loss or alteration of waveform may be reversible if the intervention occurs in a timely fashion. No patient with preserved BAEPs has been reported to incur permanent hearing loss; therefore loss of the BAEP waveform may be a highly specific prognostic indicator of unilateral deafness.

Visual Evoked Potentials. Visual evoked potentials (VEPs) are generated by flashes of light presented monocularly through the closed eyelid. The eyes are protected in the usual fashion with ointment and clear plastic tape. Intraoperative monitoring with VEP has been performed during surgery for pituitary lesions and resection of lesions in the anterior cranial fossa. VEPs are highly variable and are very sensitive to metabolic changes and anesthetics. At this time VEP is considered unreliable and of little value in the operating room.

Motor Evoked Potentials. The motor cortex is stimulated by electrodes placed directly over the motor cortex, by transcranial electrical stimulation, or by transcutaneous electromagnetic stimulation. A response is recorded in a peripheral nerve or muscle to assess the motor pathways during spinal surgery. Direct cerebral electrode placement for MEP monitoring is invasive, and it suffers from interference by most anesthetics. Transcranial electrical stimulation is unpleasant in awake individuals, although well tolerated by patients under anesthesia. Volatile anesthetics depress the MEP response at <1 MAC, whereas nitrous-narcotic techniques, ketamine, and etomidate have little effect. The existence of hypothermia, hypoxia, and hypotension adversely affect MEPs. If electromyographic responses are used to assess MEPs, muscle relaxant infusions must be kept at 1 to 2 twitches to detect the response accurately while avoiding overt movement. The advantage of electromagnetic stimulation lies in the noninvasive character of the monitor.

Electromyography

Electromyography (EMG) is used by some neurosurgeons to monitor fifth and seventh cranial nerve function during posterior fossa surgery. The facial nerve (seventh) is most commonly monitored at the orbicularis oris, orbicularis oculi, and frontalis muscles.

The trigeminal nerve (fifth) is monitored via the masseter muscle. Complete transection of a nerve results in dense discharges followed by electrical silence. The location of the nerve during neurosurgical dissection can be ascertained via direct stimulation even during partial paralysis (25% to 30%). EMGs are also used during dorsal rhizotomy for spastic cerebral palsy to decide whether to section a particular nerve based on the response of the nerve to stimulation.

Suggested Readings

Friedman WA, Grundy BL: Monitoring of sensory evoked potentials is highly reliable and helpful in the OR, *J Clin Monit* 3:38, 1987.

Kalkman CJ, Drummond JC, Riberink AA: Low concentrations of isoflurane abolish motor evoked responses to transcranial electrical stimulation during nitrous oxide/opioid anesthesia in humans, *Anesth Analg* 73:410, 1991.

Kofke W, Dong M, Bloom M, et al: Transcranial Doppler ultrasonography with induction of anesthesia for neurosurgery, *J Neurosurg Anesthesiol* 6(2):89, 1994.

Levy WJ: Intraoperative EEG patterns: implications for EEG monitoring, *Anesthesiology* 60:430, 1984.

Levy WJ, Shapiro HM, Maruchak G, et al: Automated EEG processing for intraoperative monitoring: a comparison of techniques, *Anesthesiology* 53:223, 1980.

Michenfelder JD: Intraoperative monitoring as sensory evoked potentials may be neither a proven nor an indicated technique, *J Clin Monit* 3:45, 1987.

Sperry RS, Johnson JO, Stanley TH, editors: *Anesthesia and the central nervous system,* The Netherlands, 1993, Kluwer Academic Publishers.

Sundt TM, Sharbrough FW, Piepgras DC, et al: Correlation of cerebral blood flow and electroencephalographic changes during carotid endarterectomy. With results of surgery and hemodynamics of cerebral ischemia, *Mayo Clin Proc* 56:533, 1981.

FLUID MANAGEMENT   *5*

Burkhard F. Spiekermann
Scott A. Thompson

Proper fluid and electrolyte management during neurosurgery requires knowledge of the patient's underlying pathophysiologic condition. The general principles of fluid management often do not take into account the effects of fluids on cerebral edema, cerebral perfusion, ischemic insults, and water and electrolyte homeostasis.

This chapter addresses the role of the blood-brain barrier in cerebral fluid balance, the influence of isotonic and hypertonic crystalloid and colloid solutions on cerebral edema, the use of mannitol for osmotic therapy, and the potential dangers associated with administration of glucose-containing solutions. Fluid management in selected clinical settings and the most common disturbances of water and sodium homeostasis in the neurosurgical patient are also briefly discussed.

BLOOD-BRAIN BARRIER

Early observations from intravascular dye studies demonstrated that, unlike other organs of the body, the brain is essentially "protected" from the extravasation of dye into its tissue. These and other findings led to the concept of the blood-brain barrier (BBB). However, it was not until modern electron microscopy became available that the capillary endothelium lining the inside of the cerebral capillary system was defined as the anatomic basis for the BBB.

The cerebral capillary endothelium differs from the capillary endothelium in the rest of the body: the cells are "glued" to one another by intercellular tight junctions that form a five-layered ring of adhesions around all cerebral blood vessels, preventing any passage of molecules between individual cells. Thus, in the healthy brain, the only way for molecules to cross the BBB is to pass through the endothelial cell itself. In contrast, capillaries outside the CNS have so-called gap junctions that provide a means for molecules to pass from the intravascular to the extravascular space.

Transcellular movement of molecules across the BBB depends on the molecular weight, ionic charge, lipid solubility, protein-binding capacity, concentration gradient, and availability of specific carrier molecules within the endothelium. In general, the BBB excludes the passive movement of molecules >8000 dalton. Lipophilic molecules cross the BBB by simple diffusion across the cells, whereas water-soluble ions characteristically do not cross the endothelium. Specific carrier proteins within the endothelial cells of the BBB are responsible for the transport of glucose and amino acids. This carrier-mediated transport differs from active transport in that it does not require energy and can go only in the direction of a concentration gradient. Other molecules that undergo carrier-mediated transport include other sugars, biogenic amines, specific neurotransmitters, and penicillin. Active transport mechanisms (which require cAMP [cyclic adenosine monophosphate] and are able to work against a concentration gradient) for glucose and certain amino acids have also been identified in the cerebral endothelium.

Mechanical separation of the capillary endothelial cells along their tight junctions (junctional uncoupling) causes a functional disruption of the BBB that allows the abnormal passage of molecules and water into the brain parenchyma. Many pathologic and physiologic conditions, and specific pharmacologic therapy may alter the permeability of the BBB.

A disrupted BBB is commonly found in patients with intracranial tumors. The capillaries supplying cerebral tumor tissue exhibit ultrastructural features more typical of the extracranial capillary system. They have intercellular fenestrations and gap junctions and allow for the passage of water and larger molecules.

Hypertension that exceeds cerebral autoregulation may cause junctional uncoupling: the cerebral capillaries are forcefully dilated, causing gaps in the intercellular tight junctions. Hyperthermia, prolonged hypercarbia, and head trauma have also been found to cause junctional uncoupling.

The BBB is highly resistant to hypoxic damage, but prolonged hypoxia may cause irreversible capillary endothelial cell death and BBB disruption. The effects of hypoxia are often seen only 6 to 12 hours after the initial hypoxic insult.

Reversible opening of tight junctions in the cerebral endothelium has been seen experimentally after the administration of hyperosmolar agents such as mannitol and urea. Shrinkage of the capillary endothelial cells secondary to the osmolar gradient is thought to cause a disruption of the tight junctions. This phenomenon may be partially responsible for the development of rebound intracranial hypertension observed with the administration of large doses of mannitol.

Care of the patient with a disrupted BBB, whatever the cause, is aimed at preventing cerebral edema. The same principles should be followed as for care of the patient with increased intracranial pressure (ICP). Dexamethasone may stabilize the BBB that is damaged as a result of intracranial tumors or pseudotumor cerebri. However, steroid therapy in patients who have sustained head trauma or cerebral ischemic events has not been shown to improve cerebral edema or patient outcome.

CRYSTALLOID, COLLOID, AND HYPERTONIC SOLUTIONS

There is long-standing debate in the literature concerning whether to use crystalloid or colloid solutions for volume replacement in the neurosurgical patient. The controversy revolves around the influence of various solutions on osmotic pressure and colloid oncotic pressure (COP) in the intravascular and extravascular compartments and their influence on the formation of cerebral edema.

Patient with Intact Blood-Brain Barrier

In the intact BBB, the tight junctions of the capillary endothelium prevent passive movement of electrolytes and larger molecules into the cerebral tissue. Water molecules can pass freely, and the net movement of water across the normal BBB is governed by the Starling's principle, which applies to fluid movement between any intravascular and extravascular compartments in the body: Net fluid movement depends on the difference between the hydrostatic pressure and the osmotic pressure of the intravascular and extravascular spaces.

Reduction of serum osmolarity by administration of free water (0.45% sodium chloride or D5W) will cause cerebral edema since water moves across the BBB along the altered osmotic pressure gradient. Even small (<5%) changes in serum osmolarity will increase cerebral edema, increase ICP, and decrease cerebral perfusion in patients with a normal or altered BBB. It is therefore imperative to avoid the administration of hypotonic solutions, and one of the goals of neurosurgical fluid management should be to prevent any decrease in serum osmolarity.

Historically it was thought that the administration of large amounts of isotonic crystalloid solutions would be detrimental to the neurosurgical patient by decreasing COP, thus favoring the flux of water across the BBB and causing cerebral edema. However, recent studies have shown that COP is actually a very weak force, relative to serum osmolarity, in driving water across the BBB. A 50% reduction in COP (from 20 to 10 mm Hg) causes less free water flow across the intact BBB than a 1 mmol/L decrease in serum osmolarity. Many investigations have shown that there is no evidence of increased brain edema when COP is reduced as long as serum osmolarity is carefully maintained at a normal value. Some studies have suggested the opposite—that a decrease in COP can cause cerebral edema even when serum osmolarity is normal. These studies, however, may have been flawed by the fact that lactated Ringer's was used as the hemodiluting solution. This solution is not strictly isotonic (osmolarity: 273), and the increase in cerebral edema seen in these studies, which was attributed to a decrease in COP, may have been caused by a decrease in serum osmolarity.

Patient with Disrupted Blood-Brain Barrier

Unlike the intact BBB, in the disrupted BBB, both colloid and crystalloid solutions extravasate into the cerebral tissue and may worsen cerebral edema. There is no agreement in the literature as to whether colloid or crystalloid is better for volume replacement in the setting of a disrupted BBB. Some studies suggest that colloid is less prone to cause cerebral edema, but most studies show no significant difference between the two classes of solutions. Unfortunately, all trials have focused on the outcome of volume resuscitation only during the first 24 hours after brain injury. The long-term effects have yet to be investigated. There is no proof that infusion of large volumes of isotonic crystalloid (with secondary reduction of COP) in a patient with a disrupted BBB will not augment further brain edema. Therefore it is probably wise to avoid substantial reductions in COP during volume replacement in the patient with acute cerebral injury.

If the primary goal is to achieve hemodynamic stability and rapid volume resuscitation is necessary, colloid solutions (and blood products, if indicated) may be more appropriate than crystalloid solutions. Colloid is (milliliter for milliliter) more effective in rapidly restoring intravascular volume than is crystalloid: 1 L of isotonic saline causes approximately a 200 ml increase in intravascular volume, 1 L of 5% albumin causes a 500 ml increase, and 1 L of hetastarch causes a 750 ml increase. Consequently, to achieve the same increase in intravascular volume, about three times as much crystalloid must be infused as colloid.

If the decision is made to infuse colloid, which colloid should be used? Albumin (5%) is safe and acceptable but expensive. Hetastarch (hydroxyethylstarch, MW 450 dalton) is a much less expensive alternative, but in large doses it may have adverse effects on normal coagulation by interfering with factor VIII function. Anecdotally, hetastarch has been linked to the development of postoperative cerebral hematomas, and its administration should be limited to no more than 20 ml/kg/day. Pentastarch, a low-molecular-weight hydroxyethylstarch (264 dalton) apparently has fewer effects than hetastarch on the coagulation cascade, but clinical data for the use of pentastarch for volume resuscitation are sparse. Dextran interferes with normal platelet function and is therefore not desirable in patients with intracranial pathology.

The use of hypertonic saline solutions (3% to 7.5% saline) has recently been studied in the context of fluid resuscitation in patients with brain injury. Theoretically, hypertonic saline, like mannitol, through its osmotic effect on the brain, should decrease brain edema and potentially decrease ICP when used for volume resuscitation. This assumption is supported by several laboratory studies and one clinical study that reported improved survival when hypertonic saline was compared to isotonic crystalloid solutions for initial fluid replacement in patients with severe head injury. A decrease in CSF production with the use of hypertonic saline also has been reported. However, the resultant hypernatremia may have a negative impact on myocardial, renal, and other physiologic functions, and further clinical studies need to be undertaken before hypertonic solutions can be recommended for clinical use.

At our institution we use isotonic crystalloid for fluid administration in almost all situations. If faced with the need for rapid-volume resuscitation secondary to hypovolemic shock, we also administer albumin or hetastarch. As mentioned, any decrease in serum osmolarity resulting from the use of hypotonic solutions should be strictly avoided.

How much fluid should be given? Historically a neurosurgical patient was kept "dry" to avoid the exacerbation of brain edema. However, keeping a patient dry may aggravate cerebral damage if this state interferes with hemodynamic stability and the maintenance of a normal cerebral perfusion pressure. An already compromised brain is very sensitive to secondary insults such as hypotension, hypoxia, and ischemia. Replacement of overnight fluid deficits is necessary in neurosurgical patients who have undergone angiographic dye studies with hyperosmolar agents or who have had mannitol therapy and are substantially volume depleted preoperatively. It would be unwise to avoid fluid replacement in such patients for fear of worsening cerebral edema. On the other hand, overhydration of the neurosurgical patient should be avoided (except with vasospasm, as discussed later).

MANNITOL THERAPY

Typically, the BBB maintains a 3 mOsm/L osmotic gradient between blood and brain parenchyma, and the brain parenchyma has a slightly higher osmolarity than the usual serum osmolarity of about 290 mOsm/L. However, with disruption of the BBB, fluids and osmotically active substances move freely into the brain and may cause cerebral edema.

If the BBB is sufficiently intact, intravenous administration of hyperosmolar agents reverses the osmotic gradient between the brain and blood and, following Starling's principle, water is drawn out of the brain parenchyma. In the early 1960s urea was used as the hypertonic medium to establish an osmolar gradient and to decrease increased ICP associated with brain edema effectively. However, it was subsequently shown that urea is able to cross the BBB and reverse the osmotic gradient, causing severe rebound intracranial hypertension a few hours after administration. This result and other side effects of urea led to its abandonment in favor of mannitol. Today, osmotherapy with mannitol is one of the mainstays of neuroanesthetic practice in the treatment of patients with increased ICP and cerebral edema.

The clinical effect of mannitol is related to the amount infused. A 20% solution of mannitol is usually administered in a dose range between 0.25 to 1 g/kg body weight over 40 to 60 minutes. A dose of 0.25 g/kg increases the serum osmolarity by 10 mOsm/L and can remove 100 to 150 ml of water from the brain. A dose of 1g/kg of mannitol causes a 40 mOsm/L rise in serum osmolarity.

The ability of mannitol to withdraw water from brain tissue is solely related to osmolar (not to diuretic) effects. However, if the loop diuretic furosemide is administered 10 to15 minutes after mannitol (at a dose of 0.5 mg/kg), the duration of action of mannitol can be prolonged. Furosemide produces a large volume of hypotonic urine, thereby maintaining a favorable osmotic gradient for an extended period.

The administration of mannitol may have beneficial effects on cerebral perfusion in addition to establishing an osmolar gradient. Mannitol reduces blood viscosity by decreasing red cell rigidity and by lowering the hematocrit secondary to hemodilution. This action tends to increase cerebral blood flow, and, if autoregulation is intact, may lead to reflex cerebral vasoconstriction with an overall decrease in cerebral blood volume and ICP.

Mannitol therapy, however, is associated with side effects and potential systemic and cerebral complications. Systemic complications of prolonged mannitol therapy include metabolic acidosis, electrolyte abnormalities (with associated cardiac arrhythmias), and transient or permanent renal damage. Mannitol is excreted renally, and hyperosmolar therapy should not be instituted in the anephric patient. Extreme caution is also required when mannitol is administered to the patient with limited cardiac reserve because the acute intravascular volume expansion may increase cardiac filling pressures to the point where congestive heart failure and pulmonary edema may develop. Mannitol crosses the placenta and can cause fetal cell dehydration. It should therefore be administered in reduced doses, if needed, in the pregnant patient.

Cerebral complications of mannitol therapy have also been described. Mannitol is a weak systemic and cerebral vasodilator and can initially decrease mean arterial pressure, increase cerebral blood volume and ICP, and therefore decrease cerebral perfusion pressure. The ICP rise usually occurs within the first 1 to 2 minutes and is only transient, but it can be significant. The administration of mannitol to patients with an already disrupted BBB worsens cerebral edema since mannitol and free water will accumulate in the brain parenchyma. Some recent studies also suggest that mannitol, like urea, is able to cross the BBB and may cause rebound intracranial hypertension in up to 12% of patients with an apparently normal BBB a few hours after intravenous administration of a single dose. However, at our institution, mannitol is used routinely at a dose range of 0.25 to 1 g/kg, unless specifically contraindicated.

GLUCOSE-CONTAINING SOLUTIONS

Glucose is the major substrate metabolized by the brain to meet its energy requirements during aerobic and anaerobic conditions. Many recent investigations have shown that an elevated serum glucose level present before an ischemic insult to the brain worsens neurologic outcome.

The mechanism for glucose-induced aggravation of neurologic injury is not clear. The favored hypothesis is that in the presence of ischemia glucose is metabolized anaerobically and lactic acid accumulates. Increased lactate is thought to decrease intracellular pH, compromise cellular function, and ultimately cause cell death. However, some recent studies have failed to correlate serum lactate levels with severity of neurologic outcome, and an alternative explanation proposes that hyperglycemia worsens ischemia by decreasing global cerebral blood flow. Other studies suggest that hyperglycemia decreases cerebral adenosine levels. Adenosine is an inhibitor of the release of excitatory amino acids that are thought to play a major role in ischemic cell death.

In spite of the controversies regarding the mechanism of hyperglycemia-induced neurologic damage, the overwhelming amount of data suggest that it is prudent to withhold glucose-containing solutions in neurosurgery unless it is specifically indicated (i.e., for treatment of hypoglycemia). It has been repeatedly shown that intraoperative hypoglycemia does not occur in operations of < 4 hours' duration in a nondiabetic adult patient.

Occasionally, although no exogenous glucose is administered, intraoperative hyperglycemia develops (i.e., in patients with diabetes mellitus or patients receiving corticosteroid therapy). There is no experimental evidence suggesting that treatment of hyperglycemia with insulin improves neurologic outcome during neurosurgery. However, hyperglycemia has many undesirable effects on the body's homeostatic mechanisms, and we recommend carefully treating elevated serum glucose levels (>200 to 250 mg/dl) with small doses of intravenous insulin. It is important to avoid hypoglycemia, and glucose levels should be measured regularly to adjust the therapeutic regimen.

FLUID MANAGEMENT IN SPECIFIC CLINICAL SETTINGS
Vasospasm

Vasospasm is one of the major factors contributing to postoperative morbidity and mortality after a subarachnoid hemorrhage. Treatment and prophylaxis of vasospasm involves the use of calcium channel blockers and (once the aneurysm has been clipped and there is no further risk of rupture) the so-called "triple H" therapy of hypertension, hypervolemia, and hemodilution. Hypertension is achieved through volume expansion and/or administration of vasopressors (phenylephrine or dopamine are commonly used agents). Hypervolemia is achieved by the administration of some combination of colloids, crystalloids, and blood products. Hypervolemia causes hemodilution, which in turn causes decreased blood viscosity, increased cerebral perfusion, and improved cerebral tissue oxygenation. Because it is difficult to maintain this hypervolemic state in a patient without cardiovascular compromise, some centers advocate the use of DDAVP (desmopressin) in combination with volume administration to counteract the excessive diuresis encountered in such a patient. Colloid may at times be superior to crystalloid solutions in maintaining hypervolemia. Pulmonary edema is a potential complication (7% to 17%) of triple H therapy, and we suggest invasive monitoring of the cardiovascular system (CVP or pulmonary artery catheter), especially in the patient with known cardiac disease.

Sitting Position

Placing a patient in the sitting position may substantially decrease cardiac preload, resulting in decreased cardiac output and hypotension with an associated decrease in cerebral blood flow. The decreased effective intravascular volume that results from the decreased preload also favors air entrainment through open venous channels and therefore increases the risk of venous air embolism. Furthermore, a reversal of the normal right atrial–to–pulmonary artery occlusion pressure (PAOP) gradient has been observed with the patient in the sitting position, which increases the risk of paradoxical air embolism in patients with a probe-patent foramen ovale. Intravenous fluid loading with a bolus of 500 ml of crystalloid or 250 ml of colloid given before the patient is placed in the sitting position (along with leg wrapping and slow institution of the final position) should reduce the incidence of cardiovascular instability and venous air embolism and prevent the reversal of the right atrial–PAOP gradient. However, there are no conclusive studies to support this assumption, and in our experience fluid loading does not predictably reduce hemodynamic instability when the patient moves from the supine to the sitting position.

ABNORMAL WATER AND SODIUM HOMEOSTASIS

Syndrome of Inappropriate Antidiuretic Hormone

Head injury and other intracranial pathologic conditions can lead to increased perioperative secretion of antidiuretic hormone (ADH). The diagnosis of syndrome of inappropriate antidiuretic hormone (SIADH) depends on the finding of increased urinary sodium (> 20 mEq/L) in the face of decreased serum sodium and a relative increase of free total body water. An acute decrease in serum sodium to <120 mEq/L can be associated with confusion, ataxia, seizures, hyporeflexia or hyperreflexia, coma, and irreversible brain damage. Initial management of SIADH includes fluid restriction. If serum hyponatremia is severe (<110 mEq/L), hypertonic saline solution (3% to 5%) should be administered, usually in combination with 10 to 20 mg of intravenous furosemide to induce a negative free water balance. Alternatively, sodium bicarbonate (a 6% solution of sodium) can be administered. A dose of 2 ml/kg administered over 1 to 2 minutes will increase the serum sodium concentration approximately 6 mEq/L. Once the patient's neurologic symptoms are stabilized, overly rapid correction to normal serum sodium should be avoided since this practice has been linked to the development of central pontine myelinolysis. A good rule of thumb is to limit the administration of hypertonic saline to no more than 100 ml/hr and to restore serum sodium levels at a rate of no more than 2 mEq/L/hr. Hypertonic saline should never be administered without careful cardiovascular monitoring since it can precipitate pulmonary edema and intracerebral hemorrhage.

Diabetes Insipidus

Diabetes Insipidus (DI) most commonly occurs in the setting of pituitary surgery, but it can be caused by other intracranial pathologic conditions, especially head trauma. The primary underlying defect in this syndrome is decreased or absent ADH secretion, resulting in polyuria and dehydration. Urine will have a low specific gravity and osmolarity, and serum will have a high osmolarity and sodium. Although cases of intraoperative DI have been reported, DI usually manifests itself postoperatively and should be suspected in any patient with polyuria. DI is generally self-limited, resolving spontaneously over a few days.

Once the diagnosis of DI has been established, the goal of fluid therapy is to maintain intravascular volume and a normal electrolyte profile. A simple regimen is the hourly administration of maintenance fluids plus three quarters of the previous hour's urine output. Alternatively, the patient's fluid deficit can be estimated by the following calculation:

$$\text{Fluid deficit (L)} = \text{Normal total body water} - \text{Actual body water}$$

$$\text{Actual body water} = \frac{[\text{Desired serum Na}^+]}{[\text{Actual serum Na}^+]} \times \text{Normal total body water}$$

$$\text{Normal total body water} = 60\% \text{ of body weight (kg)}$$

The choice of fluids depends on the patient's electrolyte status. Since the patient is losing hypoosmolar fluid (free water), half-normal or quarter-normal saline solutions are typically used. We do not advocate the use of D5W because of the danger of inducing hyperglycemia with administration of large volumes of this solution.

Pharmacologic therapy with ADH analogs is often used (in addition to fluid administration) if urine output is >300 mL/h for 2 hours. Vasopressin is available in a short-acting aqueous form that can be administered subcutaneously at 5 to10 IU every 4 hours, and in a long-acting oil-based form (pitressin tannate) that can be given subcutaneously or intramuscularly at 5 IU every 24 to 36 hours. A synthetic analog, DDAVP (desmopressin), is being used with increasing frequency, given either intranasally (10 to 20 μg) or intravenously (1 to 2 μg) every 8-24 hours.

Cerebral Salt-Wasting Syndrome

This little understood entity is seen most often in patients with subarachnoid hemorrhage. The syndrome is diagnosed by the triad of serum hyponatremia, dehydration, and high urine sodium (>50 mEq/L). It is thought that increased release of atrial natriuretic factor from the brain is the causative factor. Although the serum electrolyte profile of the two syndromes is similar, it is very important not to confuse this syndrome with SIADH. SIADH is a state of increased intravascular volume and dilutional hyponatremia and is treated with volume restriction. Cerebral salt-wasting syndrome is a state of decreased intravascular volume and hyponatremia and is treated by reestablishing normovolemia with the administration of sodium-containing isotonic solutions.

Suggested Readings

Claes Y, Van Hemelrijck J, Van Gerven M, et al: Influence of hydroxyethyl starch on coagulation in patients during the perioperative period, *Anesth Analg* 75:24, 1992.

Cottrell JE, Robustelli A, Post K, et al: Furosemide- and mannitol-induced changes in intracranial pressure and serum osmolality and electrolytes, *Anesthesiology* 47:28, 1977.

Drummond JC: Fluid management for neurosurgical patients, *ASA annual refresher course lecture* 511, 1993.

Drummond JC, Moore SS: The influence of dextrose administration on neurologic outcome after temporary spinal cord ischemia in the rabbit, *Anesthesiology* 70:64, 1989.

Joo F: The blood-brain barrier, *Nature* 321:197, 1986.

Kaieda R, Todd MM, Cook LN, et al: Acute effects of changing plasma osmolality and colloid oncotic pressure on the formation of brain edema after cryogenic injury, *Neurosurgery* 24:671, 1989.

Kaieda R, Todd MM, Warner DS: Prolonged reduction in colloid oncotic pressure does not increase brain edema following cryogenic injury in rabbits, *Anesthesiology* 71:554, 1989.

Kaufmann AM, Cardoso ER: Aggravation of vasogenic cerebral edema by multiple-dose mannitol, *J Neurosurg* 77: 584, 1992.

Kofke WA: Mannitol: potential for rebound intracranial hypertension? *J Neurosurg Anesth* 5:1, 1993.

Korosue K, Heros RC, Ogilvy CS, et al: Comparison of crystalloid and colloid for hemodilution in a model of focal cerebral ischemia, *J Neurosurg* 73:576, 1990.

Lanier WL, Stangland KJ, Scheithauer BW, et al: The effects of dextrose infusion and head position on neurologic outcome after complete cerebral ischemia in primates: examination of a model, *Anesthesiology* 66:39, 1987.

Nakakimura K, Fleischer JE, Drummond JC, et al: Glucose administration before cardiac arrest worsens neurologic outcome in cats, *Anesthesiology* 72:1005, 1990.

Origitano TC, Wascher TM, Reichman OH, et al: Sustained increased cerebral blood flow with prophylactic hypertensive hemodilution ("Triple-H" therapy) after subarachnoid hemorrhage, *Neurosurgery* 27:729, 1990.

Prough DS, Johnson C, Poole GV, et al: Effects on intracranial pressure of resuscitation from hemorrhagic shock with hypertonic saline versus lactated Ringer's solution, *Crit Care Med* 13:407, 1985.

Prough DS, Johnson C, Stump DA, et al: Effects of hypertonic saline versus lactated Ringer's solution on cerebral oxygen transport during resuscitation from hemorrhagic shock, *J Neurosurg* 64:627, 1986.

Pulsinelli WA, Waldman S, Rawlinson D, et al: Moderate hyperglycemia augments ischemic brain damage: a neuropathologic study in the rat, *Neurology* 32:1239, 1982.

Rudehill A, Gordon E, Ohman G, et al: Pharmacokinetics and effects of mannitol on hemodynamics, blood and cerebrospinal fluid electrolytes, and osmolality during intracranial surgery, *J Neurosurg Anesth* 5:4, 1993.

Scheller MS, Zorrow MH, Oh YS: A comparison of the cerebral and hemodynamic effects of mannitol and hypertonic saline in a rabbit model of acute cryogenic brain injury, *J Neurosurg Anesth* 3:291, 1991.

Sieber FE, Smith DS, Traystman RJ, et al: Glucose: a reevaluation of its intraoperative use, *Anesthesiology* 67:72, 1987.

Smerling A: Hypertonic saline in head trauma: a new recipe for drying and salting, *J Neurosurg Anesth* 4:1, 1992.

Trammer BI, Iacobacci RI, Kindt GW: Effects of crystalloid and colloid infusions on intracranial pressure and computerized electroencephalographic data in dogs with vasogenic brain edema, *Neurosurgery* 25:173, 1989.

Weinand ME, O'Boynick PL, Goetz KL: A study of serum antidiuretic hormone and atrial natriuretic peptide levels in a series of patients with intracranial disease and hyponatremia, *Neurosurgery* 25:781, 1989.

POSITIONING IN NEUROSURGERY

6

Richard J. Sperry

Proper patient positioning and the physiologic consequences of positioning are not given specific attention in most anesthesiology training programs. These issues are usually left for residents to deal with on their own. However, many preventable injuries occur when an anesthesiologist does not pay scrupulous attention to details during patient positioning. Also, the consequences of positioning need to be anticipated so that adequate preparations can be made.

This chapter discusses the proper ways to place a patient in the supine, prone, and sitting positions. The physiology of these positions and the associated common injuries and complications are also addressed. No suggestion is made that these are the only ways to safely position a patient. Rather, one or two safe and proven methods are presented.

SUPINE POSITION

Although the supine position is not unique to neurosurgery, many neurosurgical procedures are performed with the patient in this position. Therefore this common position can be used as a benchmark for comparing the effects of other positions.

The physiologic alterations seen with positioning the healthy awake patient may be different from those noted in a patient under anesthesia. The compensatory actions of the central nervous system and the cardiovascular system are depressed in direct proportion to the anesthetic concentration. The picture of depression varies, depending on the anesthetic techniques and the patient's disease, age, and medication regimen. Therefore it is vital that the patient be closely monitored during any major position change, especially if significant cardiovascular or pulmonary disease is present.

The major physiologic changes seen in the supine patient take place in the cardiovascular and respiratory systems.

Cardiovascular Effects

When the patient is in the supine position, venous return increases, producing increases in stroke volume and cardiac output. Sympathetic tone decreases, yielding a decrease in mean arterial blood pressure, heart rate, and peripheral vascular resistance. The systolic blood pressure remains at about the same level; however, the diastolic blood pressure is decreased, and the pulse pressure is therefore increased.

Respiratory Effects

A reduction of the functional residual capacity (FRC) occurs when the patient is in the supine position, and further reduction takes place when general anesthesia is induced. The supine anesthetized patient has an FRC decrement of approximately 1 L. This situation may have significant implications for some patients in regard to oxygen exchange in the lung.

Closing capacity is important as it relates to FRC. It is equivalent to the lung volume when distal airways begin to close, excluding distal lung units from ventilatory gas exchange. Units that remain closed during tidal ventilation become atelectatic and contribute to intrapulmonary shunt. Units that close early are poorly ventilated and contribute to ventilation-perfusion mismatch. Small airway closure normally occurs at a significantly lesser lung volume than FRC, and all lung units remain functionally patent. However, if FRC is reduced, as in the supine anesthetized patient, or if closing capacity is increased by age or disease, airways may begin to close, producing relative hypoxia.

Anesthesia administered with the patient in the supine position may also alter normal ventilation-perfusion relationships. In the upright position, gravitational influences provide a gradient of blood flow in the lung (least in the apex and greatest in the base). Because of an intrapleural pressure gradient from apex to base and as a result of the shape of the pulmonary compliance curve, ventilation is also greatest in the bases. Thus ventilation and perfusion are normally well matched.

In the supine position, gravity causes perfusion to be greatest in the dorsal aspect of the lung. The abdominal contents force the dorsal portion of the diaphragm in a more cephalad direction, placing it on an advantageous part of its length-tension curve. Thus a spontaneously breathing patient ventilates the dorsal lung best and ventilation-perfusion relationships remain intact.

However, during controlled ventilation the abdominal contents decrease the compliance of the dorsal lung. The ventral lung thus receives more ventilation but the same amount of perfusion. Thus ventilation and perfusion are not well matched, and hypoxemia may result.

Central Nervous System Effects

Since many neurosurgical patients undergo surgery in the supine position and nearly all hospitalized patients are kept in this position, it is important to discuss the effects of the supine position on cerebral blood volume (CBV) and intracranial pressure (ICP).

In any patient position used, adequate venous drainage must be ensured. Cerebral venous congestion will lead to an increase in both CBV and ICP if intracranial compliance is reduced. The patient's head must be maintained in an unobstructing posture, allowing the internal jugular veins to drain properly. Extremes of neck flexion and rotation must be avoided in patients with an intracranial mass. Elevation of the head 15 to 30 degrees promotes venous drainage.

Complications

All positions are associated with potential trauma or other complications. This section discusses the complications associated with the supine position. However, many of these complications also apply to other positions.

It is important to determine the points of weight bearing imposed by a given position. These points must be appropriately padded and protected. The weight of the supine patient is borne by the occiput, scapulae, elbows, sacrum, calves, and heels. These points should be padded and should rest on soft material that is not wrinkled. Wrinkled material can produce secondary skin and subcutaneous tissue pressure that may lead to an ischemic insult. Several case reports exist that describe tissue necrosis at these weight-bearing points following prolonged surgical procedures.

After the induction of general anesthesia and the onset of muscle relaxation, the musculoskeletal system is susceptible to abnormal stress. Joints are normally protected from hyperextension by muscle tone, pain sensation, and proprioceptive reflexes. Since all these protections are lost when the patient is under anesthesia, the joints may be placed in abnormal flexion or extension, and injury may result. This effect occurs in particular when a patient is turned, placed prone, or moved to the sitting position.

The cervical spine is of special concern during positioning because it is highly susceptible to injury, and such injury can have grave consequences. The head forms a pendulum on the end of the neck and can produce great torque and other disruptive forces. The head must be stabilized and held in the midline during positioning.

Stress and stretch can be placed on the elements of the thoracic and lumbar spine with the onset of muscle relaxation. If a flat operating table is used, the normal lumbar lordosis is lost and ligaments can be stretched. Backache is a common postoperative complication. This effect can be minimized by providing lumbar support or placing pillows under the legs.

The peripheral nerves are also vulnerable in an anesthetized patient and are common sites of injury. The brachial plexus and its branches are the nerves most often injured. The ulnar nerve passes along the medial side of the humerus and becomes very superficial at the medial epicondyle. Compression of the ulnar nerve at the elbow is likely if the elbow is not protected. The ulnar nerve is most vulnerable when the hand and the forearm are in pronation. Supination places the ulnar nerve in a more protected position.

The brachial plexus is also subject to stretch injury during extreme abduction of the arm. The radial and axillary nerves may be compressed by the screen poles or other attachments to the operating table. The median nerve is adjacent to major blood vessels at the elbow and can be injured during attempts at vascular cannulation. The brachial plexus and its branches can be protected by following these guidelines:

1. Pad the elbow.
2. Never abduct the arm more than 90 degrees.
3. Supinate the hand and the forearm.
4. Protect the arm from compression by the operating table attachments.

Function of the various upper extremity peripheral nerves can be tested rapidly, as shown in Fig. 6-1.

PRONE POSITION

Most procedures involving the thoracic and lumbar spine, many procedures on the cervical spine, and some intracranial procedures

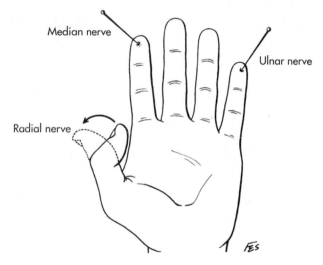

FIG 6-1.
Method to test function of major upper extremity nerves. Injury to musculocutaneous nerve causes loss of biceps function and inability to flex forearm. Injury to axillary nerve results in loss of deltoid function and inability to abduct arm. (From Martin JT: *Positioning in anesthesia and surgery,* ed 2, Philadelphia, 1987, WB Saunders.)

are performed with the patient in the prone position. Patients may be pronated either before or after the induction of anesthesia. Awake pronation can be useful in patients with a compromised spinal canal and a neurologic deficit that may be worsened with handling.

The patient may indicate that he is experiencing pain when a certain position is assumed. Also, a quick neurologic examination can be performed to document the absence or presence of progression of neurologic deficits. If progression of a deficit is found, the faulty positioning can be corrected.

Awake pronation requires adequate sedation and topical anesthesia to permit awake intubation. After adequate positioning has been achieved, general anesthesia is produced by the intravenous or inhalational method.

Pronation of the patient following the induction of anesthesia requires planning and the coordination of many members of the operating team. Injuries can occur to both the patient and the team members.

Optimal pronation of an anesthetized patient requires a level of anesthesia that blunts autonomic reflexes, but one that is not so deep as to risk hypotension. If narcotics are to be used as a part of the anesthetic, it is useful to administer a loading dose to the patient before pronation. A fluid bolus of about 500 ml can be used to stabilize the patient's hemodynamic condition. Neuromuscular blockade should also be achieved before pronation.

To pronate the patient, the bed is first moved parallel and directly adjacent to the operating table. Two assistants stand on the free side of the table to receive the patient, and two stand on the free side of the stretcher. One assistant manages the patient's feet. If the cervical spine is stable, the anesthesiologist manages the head and coordinates the turn. If the cervical spine is unstable, the neurosurgeon handles the head during pronation and coordinates the turn. The arms of the patient are placed and kept alongside the body. At the signal from the person managing the head, the patient is disconnected from the anesthesia machine and turned gradually onto the outstretched arms of the receiving assistants. The arms are held alongside the body and the head is kept in the sagittal plane during the turn.

After the turn is complete, the patient is reconnected to the anesthesia machine and the lung fields are auscultated for appropriate endotracheal tube position. The assistants then move their arms from under the patient, who remains supported by appropriate chest rolls. The chest rolls should support the lateral edge of the torso from clavicle to pelvis.

Next, the head is gently rotated toward the anesthesia machine and placed on the headrest. Special attention must be given to the downside eye and ear. No pressure should be placed on either of these two structures. Alternatively, the patient may be placed directly head down, leaving the cervical spine neutral.

The arms are secured either alongside or in front of the patient.

Cardiovascular Effects

The cardiovascular system usually adapts well to the prone position. Depending on the level of the legs in relation to the heart, venous pooling may reduce cardiac filling pressures and cardiac output. Improper positioning may obstruct the femoral veins or the inferior vena cava, causing a decrease in venous return and blood pressure. Wrapping the legs in elastic or pneumatic stockings helps prevent venous pooling. This method assists in maintaining cardiac filling pressures and thereby cardiac output and blood pressure.

Respiratory Effects

The respiratory system can be significantly compromised by incorrect prone positioning. A prone patient who is allowed to breathe spontaneously must raise the entire thoracic mass off the sternum to expand the pleural cavity. This effort can significantly increase the work of breathing. The work of breathing is increased further by the force exerted on the diaphragm by the abdominal contents, which are forced cephalad because of compression from the weight of the dorsal trunk.

If the patient is appropriately supported by chest rolls, the chest and abdomen will hang free. Ventilation is thus accomplished with normal pressures. The FRC decrement seen in the supine patient is not found in a properly positioned prone patient.

Central Nervous System Effects

The vertebral venous plexus forms an important anastomotic channel with the femoral veins and the inferior vena cava. When these venous channels are obstructed, blood will return from the lower extremity to the heart through the vertebral veins. Distention of the vertebral veins will lead to increased intraoperative bleeding and potentially decreased surgical visibility.

Proper positioning of a prone patient on chest rolls has many benefits. Ventilation is accomplished at lower airway pressures, decreasing the chance of barotrauma. As ventilation proceeds with a free abdomen and thorax, there is less motion of the back (exaggerated under the microscope) and cerebrospinal fluid flux in the wound is less. Proper support of the patient also decreases vertebral venous engorgement and bleeding.

Complications

The prone position has much potential for patient injury. The endotracheal tube may become displaced, and vascular access lines and monitors are more precarious. This equipment must be adequately secured before pronation and must be guarded during the turn.

Attention must be afforded various soft tissues such as breasts and genitalia. The breasts should be placed medially between the chest rolls. The delicate skin of the nipple and areola should not be stretched.

Both male and female genitalia should be placed in the midline. The genital tissues should have no stretch or pressure placed on them.

The eyes should be lubricated and taped shut to avoid drying and injury to the cornea. The padded head support must not place pressure on the eye, or ischemia may result. Multiple case reports have documented the potential for blindness following eye compression. This complication is of particular concern when a horseshoe headrest is used. The head supports must be spaced widely enough to keep pressure off both eyes. A pin-based head holder may be a better alternative for head fixation than a horseshoe headrest.

The down-side ear should lie flat, not folded on itself. Ischemic injury to the ear may result if this situation remains unnoticed. Plastic reconstruction of an external ear is difficult, and the results are often poor.

Additionally, pressure must not be placed in the preauricular area. The facial nerve is superficial in this area and can be injured easily.

During chest roll placement and arm positioning, care must be taken to protect the brachial plexus and its branches. The head of the humerus can be forced into the neurovascular bundle and may compress it if the arms and axillae are not relaxed. The ulnar nerve and the radial nerve are also susceptible to compression at the elbow and should be protected.

Undue neck rotation not only can cause postoperative neck pain but also may add to brachial plexus stretch.

Pathologic joints, found in the patient with rheumatoid arthritis, must not have force applied to them during positioning. All such patients should be considered to have pathologic cervical vertebrae.

SITTING POSITION

Perhaps no position has created more controversy and comment than the sitting position. Although some institutions use the sitting position only rarely, others perform procedures with the patient in this position almost daily.

The usual argument in favor of this position centers on better anatomic orientation for surgery, better visualization for the surgical assistant, and a drier surgical field (blood and cerebrospinal fluid drain away from the operative field). Some claim that these factors yield better operative results. The antecedents have basis in fact and consensus. The conclusion, however, has neither support nor refutation in the literature.

Arguments against the sitting position revolve around the added risk and the physiologic consequences produced by this position. The risks associated with the sitting position are not eliminated by using acceptable alternative positions for a given procedure. Hence the situation is not one of risk versus no risk but rather one of degree. The ultimate decision to use the sitting position should be one of judgment: Do the perceived benefits outweigh the possible risks for a given procedure in a given patient? Since the abilities and skills of both neurosurgeons and anesthesiologists vary, it is likely that the risk-benefit ratio will be unique in a given situation.

The patient's physiologic status and anatomy enter into the decision to use the sitting position. For patients who have poor cardiac reserve, an alternative may be preferred. The presence of a ventriculoatrial shunt is also a contraindication to the sitting position. Thus it would be unwise to make an all-encompassing statement about the use of the sitting position.

Although this discussion includes the technical aspects of the sitting position, the physiologic sequelae, and the injuries associated with the position, the major issues of venous air embolism and paradoxical air embolism along with special monitoring requirements are discussed in Chapter 11.

Following the application of the usual intraoperative monitors, general anesthesia is induced. Intraarterial monitoring, a urinary catheter, and a central catheter (if used) can be placed before or after the induction of anesthesia. Endotracheal intubation may be the safest approach if a reinforced nonkinkable tube is used.

The patient's legs are then wrapped to promote venous return and to prevent venous stasis. Compression boots may also be applied. The patient is then ready for gradual adjustment of the table to achieve the sitting position.

Although controversy exists concerning the best way to put a patient in the sitting position, a common method is described here.

First, a three-point skull clamp is placed on the patient while he is still in the supine position. With the blood pressure being continually monitored, the operating table is adjusted (Fig. 6-2). The table

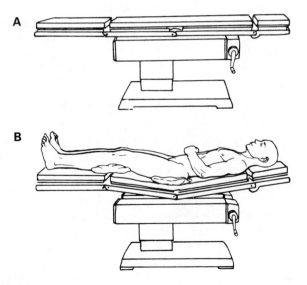

FIG 6-2.
A through D, Step-by-step procedure for establishing sitting position. **E,** Correct final sitting position. (From Martin JT: *Positioning in anesthesia and surgery,* Philadelphia, 1987, WB Saunders.)

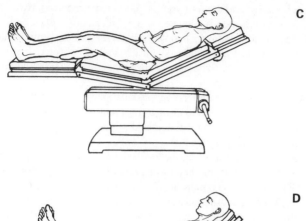

C

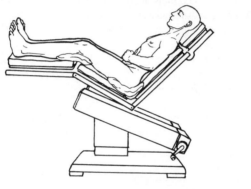

D

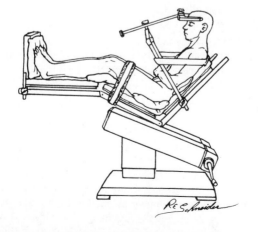

E

is flexed fully, and the foot section is lowered 45 degrees. Next, the back section is slowly elevated while the chassis is placed in the Trendelenburg position. Then the back is raised further until the desired sitting position is achieved. Finally, the foot section of the table is adjusted to the horizontal position. Optimally, the legs will rest at the level of the heart.

The headrest is removed and a skull clamp is attached to a U-shaped frame connected to the operating table. The U-frame and the skull clamp attachment are adjusted to produce the desired neck flexion and head position.

The U-frame can be attached to the back section of the operating table, which allows the head to be rapidly lowered by depressing the back section. Alternatively, if lateral access to the middle cranial fossa is required, the frame can be attached to the side of the thigh section. However, the latter placement may make it difficult to lower the head (if necessary).

Continuous monitoring of the blood pressure is essential while achieving the sitting position. Hemodynamic instability is usually not a problem if positioning is accomplished soon after the induction of anesthesia and if the level of anesthesia is not too deep. If hemodynamic instability is a problem, the level of anesthesia should be reduced and fluid should be administered. A fluid bolus of 500 ml of crystalloid or 250 ml of hetastarch or other isosmotic colloid is usually sufficient.

Once successful positioning is achieved, a precordial Doppler is applied and the patient is appropriately padded. Special care should be afforded such points as the heels, elbows, and portions of the legs or torso that may come in contact with the U-frame.

Pillows can be placed under the patient's knees to minimize sciatic stretch. The arms can be conveniently folded across the lap to give appropriate arm support, to allow access to venous and arterial lines, and to lift the shoulders to minimize brachial plexus stretch.

Cardiovascular Effects

The effects of the sitting position on the cardiovascular system can be profound. Intrathoracic blood volume may decrease by 500 ml or more, resulting in a decreased (right greater than left) atrial pressure. Cardiac output falls 12% to 20%, and systemic vascular resistance increases 50% to 80%, yielding decreased renal blood flow but a variable change in blood pressure. The heart rate is generally unchanged or slightly increased. Cerebral blood flow may be decreased by up to 15%.

These changes can produce a great strain on an individual with significant cardiovascular disease. Therefore the ability to tolerate these hemodynamic alterations must be considered in the preoperative decision to use the sitting position.

Anesthetics administered when the patient is in the sitting position may depress the myocardium, enhance venous pooling, and decrease systemic vascular resistance. If the blood pressure is not closely monitored, these anesthetic agents may produce rapid cardiovascular deterioration. Neuromuscular relaxation should be provided to prevent potentially dangerous movement, and the anesthetic should be titrated to optimal hemodynamic response. Hypotension should be treated promptly by giving vasopressors, adjusting the depth of anesthesia, and cautiously administering fluids.

Respiratory Effects

The respiratory system is not significantly stressed when the patient is in the sitting position. In fact, the FRC decrement that occurs in the supine position is not found in the sitting position. However, one author has reported a decrease in the diffusing capacity for oxygen. This decrease is thought to be secondary to an increased zone 1 of the lung that results from decreased pulmonary perfusion. The clinical significance of this finding is uncertain.

Complications

The sitting position is associated with some interesting potential complications. The problems of venous air embolism, paradoxical air embolism, and arrhythmias are discussed in Chapter 11.

The head-elevated position can be associated with decreased cerebral perfusion pressure. Therefore the arterial line transducer is placed at head level. The cerebral mean arterial pressure (MAP) differs from that measured at another (lower) reference point in a predictable manner:

Cerebral MAP = Measured MAP − Height difference (cm)/1.3

As cerebrospinal fluid drains from the cranial compartment, the brain tends to sag, placing traction on veins that bridge the brain and the venous sinuses. These bridging veins can tear, resulting in bleeding and a way for air to enter the venous circulation.

Air enters the cranial cavity as cerebrospinal fluid drains, creating pneumocephalus. This development is generally not an immediate threat to the patient. Rarely, delayed emergence from anesthesia is caused by pneumocephalus. The chief concern about pneumocephalus is the ability of nitrous oxide to expand the mass of air and create tension pneumocephalus.

Edema of the face and tongue have been reported following surgery in the sitting position. Presumably flexion and rotation of the head and neck can obstruct veins and impede lymphatic drainage.

Brachial plexus and sciatic nerve injury can result from improper positioning. The weight of the arms pulling down on the brachial plexus, combined with a fixed and rotated head, can stretch the neck and brachial plexus. To prevent this complication, extremes of head rotation should be avoided and the arms should be gently supported in the patient's lap. The sciatic nerve can be injured if the thighs and knees are not gently bent and supported.

Rare but potentially devastating injuries to the cervical spine and the spinal cord can occur when the patient is in the sitting position. Pathologic cervical vertebrae can be injured easily with neck flexion and rotation. Flexion and rotation of the neck can also stretch the spinal cord and compromise spinal blood flow, resulting in quadriplegia. It is customary to limit neck flexion so that two fingers can be placed between the chin and the sternum.

Suggested Readings

Bagshaw RJ, Smith DS, Young MS, et al: Anesthetic management of surgery in the vertebral canal, *Anesth Rev* 12:13, 1985.

Black S, Ockert DB, Oliver WC, et al: Outcome following posterior fossa craniectomy in patients in the sitting or horizontal positions, *Anesthesiology* 69:49, 1988.

Marshall WK, Bedford RF, Miller ED: Cardiovascular responses in the seated position—impact of four anesthetic techniques, *Anesth Analg* 62:648, 1983.

Martin JT: The head-elevated positions. In Martin JT, editor: *Positioning in anesthesia and surgery,* ed 2, Philadelphia, 1987, WB Saunders.

Martin JT: The prone position. In Martin JT, editor: *Positioning in anesthesia and surgery,* ed 2, Philadelphia, 1987, WB Saunders.

Matjasko J, Petrozza P, Cohen M, et al: Anesthesia and surgery in the seated position: analysis of 554 cases, *Neurosurgery* 17:645, 1985.

Standefer M, Bay JW, Trusso R: The sitting position in neurosurgery: a retrospective analysis of 488 cases, *Neurosurgery* 14:649, 1984.

ANESTHESIA FOR THE PATIENT WITH NEUROLOGIC DISEASE

7

George S. Leisure
Lawrence H. Phillips II

DUCHENNE'S MUSCULAR DYSTROPHY
   Anesthetic Considerations
AMYOTROPHIC LATERAL SCLEROSIS
   Anesthetic Considerations
FRIEDREICH'S ATAXIA
   Anesthetic Considerations
MULTIPLE SCLEROSIS
   Anesthetic Considerations
PARKINSON'S DISEASE
   Anesthetic Considerations
MYASTHENIA GRAVIS
   Anesthetic Considerations
SHY-DRAGER SYNDROME
   Anesthetic Considerations
STROKE
   Anesthetic Considerations

Providing anesthesia for the patient with neurologic disease presents a challenge to the clinician. Neurologic illnesses often have associated cardiopulmonary and neuromuscular pathologic features that are of special interest to the anesthesiologist. In addition, these patients may be taking medications that have important anesthetic interactions. We will discuss the following diseases because of these unique concerns: Duchenne's muscular dystrophy, amyotrophic lateral sclerosis, Friedreich's ataxia, multiple sclerosis, Parkinson's syndrome, myasthenia gravis, and the Shy-Drager syndrome. We will conclude with a discussion of the patient with a history of a previous stroke or cerebrovascular accident.

DUCHENNE'S MUSCULAR DYSTROPHY

Duchenne's muscular dystrophy (DMD) is the most common of all the muscular dystrophies. It occurs with an incidence of three per 10,000 live births and is inherited as an X-linked recessive disorder. The condition is usually clinically suspected when a child around the age of 3 years presents with proximal muscle weakness, pseudohypertrophy of the calf muscles, and an abnormal waddling gait. The predictable sequelae of this disease include a relentlessly progressive kyphoscoliosis leading to a restrictive pulmonary disease, progressive muscle weakness, dystrophic cardiomyopathy, pharyngeal dysfunction, pneumonia, and finally death by the third decade. Death is often the result of myocardial insufficiency. Although males are primarily affected by this disease, some female carriers may have mild symptoms.

Anesthetic Considerations

The primary anesthetic considerations for the patient with DMD include cardiopulmonary dysfunction and an abnormal response to depolarizing muscle relaxants. Dystrophic cardiomyopathy, which is characterized by a loss of myocardium with near-normal performance of the remaining sarcomeres, may occur in these patients. Histopathologic findings include myofibrillar loss with fibrous replacement. Intraoperative cardiac arrest and death from dystrophic cardiomyopathy have been reported. Teenagers with DMD undergoing general anesthesia, especially for spinal fusion, should be evaluated preoperatively for myocardial dysfunction. Clinical evidence of cardiac disease may be difficult to detect in the wheelchair-bound patient. However, Doppler and two-dimensional echocardiography may be helpful in determining the need for a thermodilution–flow-directed pulmonary artery catheter. Myocardial depressants such as halothane and thiopental should be used with caution. In addition, prolonged postoperative ventilatory support may be required in those with advanced stages of the disease. Diminution of respiratory function in DMD has been related to both thoracic scoliosis and respiratory muscle weakness, with muscle weakness being the major determinant of worsening respiratory function.

The administration of intravenous succinylcholine has led to massive hyperkalemia in patients with DMD, leading to cardiac arrest, rhabdomyolysis, hypermetabolism, and a syndrome similar to malignant hyperthermia. As a result, succinylcholine should not be used in these patients. The link between this hyperkalemic response and the syndrome of malignant hyperthermia is suggested in halothane-caffeine contracture testing. However, it remains unknown whether the structural protein abnormalities found in DMD are equivalent to those of malignant hyperthermia.

AMYOTROPHIC LATERAL SCLEROSIS

Charcot is credited with the original description of amyotrophic lateral sclerosis (ALS) around 1872. It is an uncommon disease with an annual incidence rate of 0.4 to 1.76 per 100,000 population, affecting males more frequently than females. Most patients are more than 55 years old when symptoms begin, and about 10% of cases are familial with an autosomal dominant inheritance pattern.

The principal pathologic finding is loss of nerve cells in the anterior horns of the spinal cord and motor nuclei of the lower brainstem and cortical motoneurons. These lost cells are then replaced by fibrous astrocytes. The subsequent degeneration of the corticospinal tract is most evident in the lower parts of the spinal cord but can be traced up through the brainstem to the posterior limb of the internal capsule and corona radiata.

The pathogenesis of this disease remains unclear. Some have postulated a relationship between an attack of paralytic poliomyelitis and the subsequent development of ALS. However, this occurrence is probably a chance event and does not represent the reactivation of the poliovirus or any other slow virus. Trauma, disordered immune function, and intoxication with heavy metals such as lead, mercury, and aluminum have all been linked to the development of ALS, but again the relationship is unclear. Unfortunately, there is no specific treatment for the disease nor therapy to halt its inexorable progression to death, with a median survival of 2 to 4 years after diagnosis.

The clinical manifestations of ALS include both upper and lower motor neuron symptoms. Typically the initial signs are asymmetric, with the patient complaining of weakness in one extremity. Tasks requiring fine motor control may become difficult. Fasciculations and atrophy of the muscles may be evident. The disease progresses to other extremities, and the triad of atrophic weakness, spasticity, and generalized hyperreflexia in the absence of sensory changes makes the diagnosis clear. The disease eventually progresses to involve the entire upper extremities. In later stages the atrophic weakness spreads to the neck, tongue, pharyngeal and laryngeal muscles, and finally to muscles in the trunk and lower extremities. As a result of the truncal and pharyngeal muscle weakness, respiratory insufficiency and aspiration are common complications. In approximately one third of patients the onset of symptoms is in a bulbar distribution. Disease progression and death typically occur more rapidly in such patients.

Anesthetic Considerations

General anesthetics possess numerous characteristics that may make their administration hazardous in the patient with ALS. First, general anesthetics depress the swallowing reflex in a dose-related manner, which may further predispose these patients to aspiration and airway obstruction, especially if bulbar involvement is profound. Second, many anesthetics depress ventilation, which may predispose to alveolar hypoventilation and make weaning and extubation difficult. In one study 86% of patients with ALS at presentation had evidence of respiratory muscle weakness according to pulmonary function studies, although only 19% were symptomatic. In addition, there is one case report of a patient with ALS whose initial symptoms were those of the obesity-hypoventilation syndrome. In general, if a patient has any amount of respiratory muscle weakness or bulbar dysfunction, endotracheal intubation and mechanical ventilation, even for brief periods, is extremely risky. Such patients, once intubated, are rarely weaned from the ventilator. There is no known cardiac involvement that is unique to ALS patients.

The potential for massive hyperkalemia and cardiac arrest in patients with lower motor neuron disease receiving succinylcholine is well known, and the drug should therefore be avoided. In addition, these patients may be sensitive to the effects of nondepolarizing muscle relaxants. These agents should be used judiciously if needed, titrating to clinical effect with a nerve stimulator.

The safe use of epidural anesthesia in patients with ALS has been reported. One of the primary advantages of the regional technique is that many of the potential hazards of general anesthesia can be avoided. However, if the sensory level rises above T6, ventilatory impairment may occur as a result of decreases in expiratory reserve volume and difficulty clearing secretions, which occur because of the inability to cough effectively. Although there are no data to suggest that regional anesthesia causes exacerbations of neurologic disease in patients with degenerative disease of the spinal cord, before proceeding, it may be wise to discuss in more detail the risks and benefits of regional versus general anesthesia with the patient and to document neurologic deficits.

FRIEDREICH'S ATAXIA

In 1861 Friedreich of Heidelberg described a type of familial progressive ataxia that he observed among nearby villagers, and by 1882 this new clinical entity bore his name. Freidreich's ataxia (FA) is a familial neuromuscular disorder characterized by degeneration of the posterior columns and the corticospinal and spinocerebellar tracts. The disease exhibits two inheritance patterns. The most common one is autosomal recessive, with an average age of onset at 11.75 years, and the other dominant, with an average age of onset at 20.4 years. The disease is steadily progressive, with a median age at death of 26.5 years for those with the recessive form and 39.5 years for those with the dominant form.

The initial presentation is ataxia of gait, which usually affects both lower extremities simultaneously. Early symptoms include difficulty with standing steady and running. Consistent with the pathologic findings in the disease, the ataxia is of mixed sensory and cerebellar types. In many cases walking is no longer possible within 5 years of the onset of symptoms. The hands become clumsy months or years after the gait disorder appears. Dysarthria, impaired deglutition, tremor, pes cavus, emotional lability, diabetes mellitus, and kyphoscoliosis are all features of the disease.

Cardiomyopathy is an important aspect of FA. Freidreich recognized an associated heart disease in his original description of the disorder. A form of cardiomyopathy that develops in 50% to 90% of patients represents the most common cause of death. In fact, long-term follow-up shows cardiac involvement in 100% of cases. Cardiomyopathy may be the presenting feature of the disease without ataxia or other neurologic symptoms, and the severity of the cardiomyopathy may not correlate with that of the neurologic condition. Cardiac symptoms include palpitations, chest pain, and progressive heart failure.

The most common echocardiographic finding in FA is that of concentric left ventricular thickening, which was found in 68% of patients in one study. The histologic findings are primarily diffuse myocardial fibrosis, cellular hypertrophy, and necrosis of cardiac muscle fibers. Hearts with left ventricular hypertrophy may exhibit diastolic function abnormalities.

Other cardiac defects have also been described in FA. A small proportion of patients have a hypertrophic obstructive cardiomyopathy with asymmetric septal hypertrophy and left ventricular outflow obstruction. Also rarely reported includes a group of patients with a nondilated, globally hypofunctional left ventricle, or so-called *dystrophic* heart. It is interesting to note that a cardiomyopathy seems specifically associated with FA and not with other spino-cerebellar–posterior column–corticospinal degenerative diseases.

Anesthetic Considerations

In the preoperative period attention should be focused primarily on the cardiovascular system. It is essential to realize that no correlation has been found between the duration or severity of the disease and the degree of left ventricular hypertrophy. Finley and Campbell suggest performing an echocardiogram as a minimum investigation before general or major regional anesthesia in those with FA. Furthermore, an electrocardiogram may be important because in a study of fatal cases of FA atrial arrhythmias were found in 50% of the patients before death. Furthermore, Alboliras et al. reported that the presence of atrial dysrhythmias in FA is a marker of left ventricular dysfunction and has negative prognostic implications. The use of invasive monitoring and the choice of specific anesthetic techniques must be based on the patient's full cardiac evaluation.

Kyphoscoliosis may be present in up to 80% of cases, progressing rapidly once the patient becomes wheelchair bound. The result is a progressive restrictive pulmonary disease pattern with a decrease in vital and total lung capacity. Consequently, respiratory failure in the perioperative period is a hazard. In the advanced form of the disease, when deglutition becomes impaired, aspiration may also become a concern.

Response to muscle relaxants in FA is not fully understood. There are reports describing hypersensitivity to nondepolarizing muscle relaxants and reports describing a normal response to these agents. It is best to administer them judiciously while monitoring response with a nerve stimulator. As with any disease that involves denervation, the possibility of massive hyperkalemia after succinylcholine administration exists.

Finally, diabetes mellitus may occur in up to 18% of patients, with as many as 40% exhibiting abnormal glucose tolerance test results. Both insulin-dependent and non-insulin-dependent types are reported and can be managed in the usual careful manner.

MULTIPLE SCLEROSIS

Multiple sclerosis (MS) is a demyelinating disease of the central nervous system (CNS) characterized clinically by episodes of a focal disorder of the optic nerves, brain, and spinal cord that remit and recur over a period of many years. The diagnosis is usually secured by the history of a relapsing and remitting course and evidence on examination of more than one discrete lesion in the CNS. The lesions, or plaques, that characterize the disease principally affect the white matter of the brain and spinal cord and do not extend beyond the root entry zone of the cranial and spinal nerves. The lesions show no special preference for a particular system of fibers but rather are randomly spread throughout the brainstem, spinal cord, and cerebellar peduncles. These plaques destroy the myelin but usually leave nerve cells intact.

Despite numerous theories, the etiology of MS remains unclear. One popular belief holds that there may be a relationship between MS and some environmental factor such as a virus encountered in childhood. After years of latency a secondary factor either causes or somehow contributes to the development of the disease. This secondary factor may relate to an autoimmune reaction. Although the precise cause is unclear, there certainly exists an epidemiologic association with geographic location. The risk of MS developing rises with increasing latitude. For example, the disease has a prevalence of fewer than 1 per 100,000 in equatorial areas, 6 to 14 per 100,000 in the southern United States and southern Europe, and 30 to 80 per 100,000 in the northern United States, northern Europe, and Canada. A familial tendency toward MS is also well established.

The clinical presentation of MS is variable. Some patients exhibit an acute onset and others a more insidious, slow onset. About two thirds of cases have onset between the ages of 20 and 40 years. Weakness or numbness of one or more extremities is the initial complaint in about one half of patients. About 25% of cases will present with an episode of retrobulbar or optic neuritis, characterized by partial or total loss of vision in one eye. Other presentations and symptoms include gait ataxia, brainstem symptoms such as diplopia, vertigo, vomiting, trigeminal neuralgia, disorders of micturition, and impotence. Progression of the disease is variable. Long-term follow-up studies show that 20% to 35% of patients with MS have a benign disorder with minimal disability, 3% to 12% have a malignant course with a rapid and severe disabilty, and the majority have a course somewhere between, exhibiting a relapsing course with progressive neurologic impairment after each relapse. Finally, a few factors have been identified that may affect progression of the disease. Surgery, anesthesia, fever, emotional or physical trauma, and pregnancy have all been associated with relapses.

Anesthetic Considerations

Providing anesthesia to the patient with MS presents a challenge to the clinician because there are numerous factors to be taken into consideration. The current neurologic condition of the patient should be well documented so that any postoperative changes can be interpreted in the light of that knowledge. Pulmonary function needs to be addressed because kyphoscoliosis may be present, causing restrictive pulmonary disease. Furthermore, acute respiratory failure and respiratory weakness from diaphragmatic paralysis have been reported in MS. Lability of the autonomic nervous system has also been reported in these patients. Consequently, to avoid severe hypotension, special attention is required in anesthetic drug selection and during patient movement. In advanced forms of the disease succinylcholine may need to be avoided because of the possibility of massive hyperkalemia.

There is no evidence that any of the drugs used to induce general anesthesia, either intravenous or inhaled, cause exacerbations of MS. However, a rise in temperature may be associated with a temporary clinical deterioration. The mechanism of this deterioration is uncertain. It has been shown that demyelinated axons are capable of conduction but function optimally at a certain temperature. An increase in temperature may inhibit optimal function. Consequently, it may be advisable to avoid agents with anticholinergic properties, such as glycopyrrolate, which may increase the possibility of a temperature rise. Furthermore, antipyretics should be administered when indicated and causes of infection should be treated promptly.

The issue of regional anesthesia remains controversial. Numerous reports exist of exacerbations of MS after spinal anesthesia. The mechanism of this reaction is unclear but may be related to the potential neurotoxic effect of a drug exposed to a spinal cord lacking the protective nerve sheath as a result of demyelination. It does not appear that diagnostic lumbar puncture induces relapses. Successful lumbar epidural anesthesia has been reported in patients with MS, but again there exists the possibility of exacerbation of symptoms. Epidural anesthesia is not contraindicated in those with MS, but a full discussion of risks and benefits should be made with the patient before proceeding. Along these same lines, the pregnant patient with MS may be at even higher risk of relapse in the puerperium. Again, labor epidural anesthesia may be approached, but only with caution.

PARKINSON'S DISEASE

This relatively common disease was first described by James Parkinson in 1817. It is a disease that usually begins between the ages of 40 and 70 years and is uncommon below 30 years of age. It is estimated that 1% of the population of the United States over 50 years old is affected, men somewhat more often than women. The pathogenesis of the disease involves a loss of pigmented cells in the substantia nigra and other pigmented nuclei such as the locus ceruleus and dorsal motor nucleus of the vagus. Dopaminergic nerve fibers in the basal ganglia degenerate, leading to a depletion of dopamine in the basal ganglia of the brain. Dopamine acts by inhibiting the rate of firing of neurons that control the extrapyramidal motor system. Consequently, depletion of dopamine leads to decreased inhibition of this system, resulting in many of the clinical signs that will be discussed. Although many predisposing factors have been suggested, including environmental agents, the etiology of PD remains obscure.

The clinical picture is characterized by expressionless facies, slowness and poverty of voluntary movement, festinating gait, resting tremor, stooped posture, soft and monotonous voice, and rigidity. Clearly some of the early symptoms may be difficult to recognize because they may be attributed to advancing age. Resting tremor is the most characteristic abnormality in PD, and it is the presenting symptom in 70% of cases. The tremor, often referred to as a "pill-rolling" tremor, is noted to be prominent in the resting extremity, disappearing briefly with intentional movement. Bradykinesia, or slowness in both the initiation and execution of movement, is a hallmark of the disease. Patients are also noted to have facial immobility characterized by infrequent blinking and little emotional response. As the disease progresses, micrographia develops, the voice becomes progressively less audible, walking is reduced to shuffling, and the patient frequently loses balance. Dementia is also commonly associated with PD, occurring in 10% to 20% of cases.

Anesthetic Considerations

The primary anesthetic concerns for patients with PD involve fully understanding the medications used and their side effects. Levodopa is a commonly used drug in this disease. It is administered in an effort to increase brain concentrations of dopamine because it is an immediate precursor of dopamine. The side effects of levodopa may involve the cardiovascular, gastrointestinal, and CNS. Dopamine that results from levodopa administration can augment cardiac rate and contractility, possibly predisposing to cardiac irritability. As a result, cardiac arrhythmias may occur more frequently under halothane anesthesia, although this has not proved to be clinically significant. Orthostatic hypotension may also occur in those being treated with levodopa for two reasons. First, dopamine will inhibit renin release and promote increases in renal blood flow, glomerular filtration rate, and sodium excretion. Second, dopamine will inhibit norepinephrine production in the sympathetic nervous system through a negative feedback loop. In addition, dopamine will replace norepinephrine at some sites, and, because of its weaker pressor action, fail to support the blood pressure adequately. Levodopa affects the gastrointestinal system by causing nausea and vomiting, probably through dopaminergic stimulation of the chemoreceptor trigger zone. This effect is especially prominent at the beginning of treatment. Consequently, if patients are symptomatic, the usual considerations apply to decreasing the risk of aspiration on induction. Long-term levodopa treament can also cause CNS dysfunction, such as dyskinesis. Agitation, confusion, and overt psychosis have been reported in the postoperative period with an increased incidence in those with PD. It is important to continue treatment with levodopa throughout the perioperative period to avoid skeletal muscle rigidity. Drugs with dopamine antagonizing properties such as phenothiazines and butyrophenones should also be avoided.

Bromocriptine, lisuride, and pergolide are all drugs that may be used in PD. The side-effect profile is similar to that of levodopa: nausea, vomiting, hallucinations, and hypotension are all possible. Amantadine is sometimes used, and side effects are rare. Anticholinergics are also used and are especially useful for reducing tremor but are less effective for treating bradykinesia and postural instability. The side effects of dry mouth, urinary retention, and confusion, especially in the elderly, can be troublesome.

The choice of muscle relaxants does not seem to be influenced by the presence of PD. However, succinylcholine should be used with caution because there has been one case report of succinylcholine-induced hyperkalemia in a patient with PD. The use of ketamine has been questioned in those being treated with levodopa because of the possibility of an exaggerated sympathetic response. However, its successful use has also been reported. Finally, one case report exists of an exacerbation of PD after alfentanil administration. It was suggested that alfentanil may have precipitated this reaction through a dopaminergic-blocking action in the nigrostriatal system.

MYASTHENIA GRAVIS

Myasthenia gravis is an autoimmune disease resulting from the production of antibodies against the acetylcholine receptors (AChR) of the motor end plate. The incidence of the disease is about one in every 20,000 adults. It may occur in any age group, but the incidence in those under 10 years is low, about 10% of all cases. The peak onset for women is between the ages of 20 to 30 years, whereas the peak onset for men is in the sixth to seventh decade. It remains unknown what triggers this autoimmune disease. However, a genetic predisposition exists, as well as an association with other autoimmune disorders such as systemic lupus erythematosus, thyrotoxicosis, polymyositis, and rheumatoid arthritis. The disease is frequently associated with morphologic abnormalities of the thymus gland such as thymoma and thymic hyperplasia. Hyperplasia occurs more often in younger patients, and thymomas are more common in those over 30 years old. In fact, 15% to 20% of patients with MG have thymomas, especially older men.

Antibodies to the AChR protein are present in the sera of approximately 85% of patients with MG. The majority of these antibodies are of the immunoglobulin G class and bind to the primary immunogenic region of the alpha subunit of the AChR. These antibodies reduce the number of active receptors by a functional block of the receptor, by increasing the rate of receptor degradation, or by a complement-mediated lysis of the postsynaptic membrane. The level of circulating receptor antibody does not correlate well with the clinical severity of disease. Furthermore, those patients with MG who fail to demonstrate AChR antibodies may possess different antibodies that bind to other yet-to-be-identified end plate determinants.

A clinical hallmark of this disease is that repeated or persistent activity of a muscle group leads to exhaustion of its contractile power, and rest at least partially restores the power. The onset of the disease is usually insidious, and progression is marked by periods of exacerbations and remissions. The muscles of the eyes, face, jaws, throat, and neck are affected first. As the disease progresses, the muscles of the trunk and limbs may become involved, proximal muscles being more affected than distal ones. Patients may complain of drooping eyelids and diplopia, and altered facial mobility and expression. Weakness of pharyngeal and laryngeal muscles results in dysarthria, dysphagia, and difficulty with clearing secretions. Weakness tends to increase as the day progresses, and temporary increases in weakness have been reported with vaccinations, menstruation, pregnancy, and extremes of temperature. Smooth and cardiac muscles are not involved. It should also be recognized that 15% to 20% of neonates born to mothers with MG will exhibit transient myasthenia. This situation is likely because of the passage of AChR antibodies across the placenta.

Anesthetic Considerations

Perioperative care of the patient with MG begins with adequate preoperative preparation. The severity of myasthenia and involvement of respiratory and bulbar muscles must be assessed. Pulmonary function studies should be performed to identify those with little respiratory reserve and to help predict the need for postoperative respiratory support. The medical control of the myasthenic patient will determine the need for preoperative preparation. That is, if the patient is responding well to the use of pyridostigmine, no further therapy may be needed. However, if the response is poor, preoperative plasmapheresis should be considered. For example, it has been suggested that patients with severe forms of the disease treated with prethymectomy plasma exchange required less mechanical ventilation and less time in the intensive care unit postoperatively.

Patients with MG may need postoperative mechanical ventilation for respiratory failure. After transsternal thymectomy 33% to 50% of patients may require prolonged postoperative ventilation. Four risk factors for the need for postoperative ventilation have been identified:

1. Duration of MG longer than 6 years
2. History of chronic respiratory disease other than respiratory dysfunction related to MG
3. Dose of pyridostigmine >750 mg/day
4. Preoperative vital capacity <2.9 L

Clearly the location of surgery may be important because only 7.4% of patients undergoing transcervical thymectomy required prolonged postoperative ventilation. In any case, return of adequate muscle strength and ability to protect the airway must be ensured by the usual clinical criteria before extubation is initiated.

The use of regional or local anesthesia is certainly prudent when possible. Theoretically, large doses of ester-type local anesthetics should be avoided in those myasthenic patients receiving anticholinesterase therapy because plasma cholinesterase activity is decreased and toxicity may be enhanced. Tetracaine may be used for spinal anesthesia because only small doses are needed. There is no evidence that the metabolism of amide-type local anesthetics is altered in MG.

Muscle relaxants must be used carefully in MG. Because of a decreased number of functional AChR in MG, patients exhibit a decreased response to depolarizing agents and a marked sensitivity to nondepolarizing relaxants. This abnormal response is seen even in patients who have localized ocular myasthenia and in those in remission. The median effective dose and the dose required for 95% response for succinylcholine in patients with MG is 2.0 and 2.6 times normal, respectively. Therefore a large dose may be needed for intubation. However, anticholinesterases used preoperatively can reduce plasma cholinesterase activity, causing a delayed hydrolysis of succinylcholine and potentiation of neuromuscular blockade.

Nondepolarizing drugs must be used with extreme caution in MG. The intermediate-acting drugs atracurium and vecuronium can be used, but it must be emphasized that, despite their rapid elimination, both exhibit prolonged effects in those with MG compared with controls. Response to muscle relaxants must be carefully titrated to clinical effect with the use of a nerve stimulator. Some clinicians choose to avoid muscle relaxants completely, and this approach may be an option. Finally, the clinician must be aware that certain drugs, especially the aminoglycoside antibiotics, potent inhaled agents, and magnesium, can potentiate the neuromuscular blocking actions of muscle relaxants.

SHY-DRAGER SYNDROME

In 1960 Shy and Drager described a group of patients with widespread neurologic disease associated with autonomic failure causing orthostatic hypotension. The Shy-Drager (SDS) syndrome presents between the fifth and seventh decades of life, is more common in men than women, and does not appear to be an inherited disorder. It is a slowly progressive illness that leads to death, often as a result of post-syncopal cerebral ischemia.

The principal pathologic finding is primary degeneration of the preganglionic lateral horn neurons of the thoracic spinal segments. Later there is a degeneration of the nerve cells in the vagal nuclei and the nuclei of the tractus solitarius, locus ceruleus, and sacral autonomic nuclei. The cause of this degeneration remains unknown.

These pathologic findings correlate with the clinical findings associated with loss of sympathetic and parasympathetic tone. The triad of orthostatic hypotension, anhidrosis, and impotence is common to most patients, as is urinary and fecal incontinence. The severity of the hypotension progresses and is associated with blurry vision, dizziness on standing, and fainting on walking. Not only do the patients with SDS exhibit a failure of compensatory vasoconstriction, but they also exhibit a minimal heart rate response to postural changes. Disordered thermoregulation, unequal pupils, stridor, and difficulty with speaking and swallowing are reported. Eventually, parkinsonian symptoms will develop in most of the patients.

Anesthetic Considerations

One of the primary concerns in the perioperative period is the autonomic failure associated with SDS. Preoperative preparation and meticulous intraoperative management are essential to prevent severe hypotension without causing massive volume overload. Management goals are aimed at decreasing venous pooling, increasing systemic vascular resistance, and increasing plasma volume.

Postural training by sleeping with a 25-degree head-up tilt and elastic stockings can be used to decrease venous pooling in the lower extremities. In addition, the application of 50 mm Hg positive pressure with a gravity suit has been used. However, this method is both uncomfortable and impractical. Preoperative use of sympathomimetic drugs to increase systemic vascular resistance has met with variable success. Amphetamines may actually exacerbate the symptoms of orthostatic hypotension by causing weight loss with a subsequent reduction in plasma volume. Monoamine oxidase inhibitors have been used, and they produce unpredictable responses. It is essential to realize that indirect-acting drugs such as atropine and ephedrine will provide little clinical response. Direct-acting drugs such as phenylephrine will work. However, these drugs need to be used cautiously because of the possible risk of an exaggerated hypertensive response reflecting denervation hypersensitivity. Finally, the mineralocorticoid, 9-alpha-fluorohydrocortisone has been used to help maintain plasma volume through its sodium-retaining properties. During long-term administration it may actually work by increasing the sensitivity of the resistance vessels to the low concentrations of circulating catecholamines. Clearly the possibility of steroid dependence and other side effects must be considered in these patients.

Intraoperative management is primarily concerned with avoidance of severe hypotension. Because of the possibility of abrupt blood pressure changes resulting from the absence of intact cardiovascular reflexes, placement of an intraarterial catheter should be considered. A central venous pressure monitor should also be considered to aid in volume assessment. Induction agents should be chosen that produce minimal cardiovascular changes. Volatile anesthetic agents can cause exaggerated hypotension because compensatory responses such as vasoconstriction and tachycardia may fail as a result of the absence of carotid sinus activity in these patients. Furthermore, placing the patient on positive pressure ventilation may profoundly depress cardiac output by inhibiting venous return. Maintenance of anesthesia may be complicated by the absence of signs of depth of anesthesia, hyperpyrexia because of poor sweating, and sluggish pupillary reflexes or unequal pupils. The latter finding should be recognized preoperatively to avoid making an erroneous diagnosis of a severe neurologic insult.

Vocal cord paralysis has also been reported in SDS, although it was not reported in Shy and Drager's original description. The vocal cord lesion is usually a bilateral abductor paralysis with resultant glottic obstruction and ventilatory failure. This sign may in fact be the presenting feature in some cases. The obstruction is not always total, and the patient may live uneventfully for some time after diagnosis. Of note, a patient with bilateral abductor vocal cord paralysis may have minimal stridor and normal phonation. Consequently, the diagnosis may not be considered in the preoperative evaluation. It may be prudent to arrange a vocal cord examination for any patient with SDS who is to undergo anesthesia and surgery.

STROKE

Strokes are caused by cerebral thrombosis, cerebral embolism, or intracranial hemorrhage. Cerebral thrombosis develops most often in those with extensive atherosclerosis. Other causes include profound hypotension, inflammatory diseases of the blood vessels, and hematologic conditions that predispose to poor microvascular blood flow, such as polycythemia and sickle cell anemia. Symptoms depend on the blood vessel affected, and the neurologic dysfunction may progress over minutes to hours. Sequelae can be minor and transient or severe and permanent.

Cerebral embolism is most often a result of embolization from the heart, especially in the face of bacterial endocarditis, prosthetic heart valves, and atrial fibrillation. Other sources of embolism occasionally include tumor cells, air, and fat. A paradoxical cerebral embolism is one in which an embolus passes from the right atrium into the left atrium through a patent foramen ovale, proceeding then directly to the brain. In contrast to cerebral thrombosis, the symptoms of embolism usually have an abrupt onset. The type of neurologic deficits depends on the vessel that becomes occluded.

Intracranial hemorrhage is most often the result of rupture of small aneurysms. These aneurysms result from a congenital weakness in the media of the cerebral arteries, predisposing them to rupture. Congenital cerebral aneurysms can be single or multiple. About 50% occur in the middle cerebral artery, and 30% are in the region where the anterior communicating artery joins the anterior cerebral arteries. Intracranial hemorrhage also may occur as a result of an arteriovenous malformation. Symptoms are related to the site and rapidity of bleeding and the development of increased ICP.

Anesthetic Considerations

Anesthesia for a patient who has recently had a cerebral vascular accident involves a thorough medical evaluation. In fact, those patients with cerebral embolus or thrombosis may require an extensive cardiac evaluation before surgery because significant cardiac pathologic features may be present. If a serious neurologic deficit with profound motor impairment exists, succinylcholine should not be used because of the possibility of a massive hyperkalemic response.

In the face of a recent cerebral vascular accident, it may be most prudent to delay elective surgery. Cerebral blood flow regulation undergoes changes after a stroke. Loss of carbon dioxide responsiveness and blood pressure autoregulation is common after the insult, and these changes may persist beyond a two-week period. In addition, blood-brain barrier abnormalities, as demonstrated by accumulation of computed tomography contrast agents, is still present 4 weeks after the injury. Histologic resolution of large infarcts may not be complete for several months. Consequently, it may be wise to delay elective surgery for 6 weeks to allow recovery of autoregulation, carbon dioxide responsiveness, and blood-brain barrier integrity.

Suggested Readings

Adams RD, Victor M: *Principles of neurology,* ed 5, New York,1993, McGraw-Hill.

Baraka A: Anaesthesia and myasthenia gravis, *Can J Anaesth* 39:476, 1992.

Birk K, Ford C, Smeltzer S et al: The clinical course of multiple sclerosis during pregnancy and the puerperium, *Arch Neurol* 47:738, 1990.

Campbell AM, Finley GA: Anesthesia for a patient with Friedreich's ataxia and cardiomyopathy, *Can J Anaesth* 36:89, 1989.

Drury PME, Weg N: Vocal cord paralysis in the Shy-Drager syndrome, *Anaesthesia* 46:466, 1991.

Gravlee GP: Succinylcholine-induced hyperkalemia in a patient with Parkinson's disease, *Anesth Analg* 59:444, 1980.

Hutchinson RC, Sugden JC: Anaesthesia for Shy-Drager syndrome, *Anaesthesia* 39:1229, 1984.

Leventhal SR, Orkin FK, Hirsh RA: Prediction of the need for postoperative mechanical ventilation in myasthenia gravis, *Anesthesiology* 53:26, 1980.

Mets B: Acute dystonia after alfentanil in untreated Parkinson's disease, *Anesth Analg* 72:557, 1991.

Rosenbaum KJ, Neigh JL, Strobel GE: Sensitivity to nondepolarizing muscle relaxants in amyotrophic lateral sclerosis, *Anesthesiology* 35:638, 1971.

Shapiro F, Sethna N, Colan S et al: Spinal fusion in Duchenne muscular dystrophy: a multidisciplinary approach, *Muscle & Nerve* 15:604, 1992.

Siemkowicz E: Multiple sclerosis and surgery, *Anaesthesia* 31:1211, 1976.

Warren TM, Datta S, Ostheimer GW: Lumbar epidural anesthesia in a patient with multiple sclerosis, *Anesth Analg* 61:1022, 1982.

ANESTHESIA FOR SPINAL CORD INJURY

8

Richard J. Sperry

Surgical procedures performed on the spine account for the majority of neurosurgical procedures in a typical anesthesiologist's practice. These procedures are usually associated with trauma or degenerative disease. Some procedures are performed on patients with spinal cord injury and significant neural deficits. These patients are at risk for developing autonomic hyperreflexia. A good understanding of the anesthetic challenges presented by surgery of the spine is an essential part of every anesthesiologist's knowledge base.

This chapter first focuses on the most common procedure, laminectomy. Next we discuss the management of the patient with spinal trauma. Then we address the management of patients with spinal deformities. Finally, we briefly discuss operations for management of pain.

LAMINECTOMY

Laminectomy may be performed for disc disease, bony spinal cord compression, neoplasm, abscess, or hematoma.

Disc disease most frequently occurs in the cervical and lumbar areas and generally causes symptoms of root compression, although a centrally herniated disc may cause cord or cauda equina compression.

Osteophytic projections may also compress the spinal cord or one of its major nerve roots. These bony projections are more common in older patients than in younger ones. Spinal stenosis is caused by these growths.

Although it is less common to find patients with spinal cord tumors, arteriovenous malformations, meningiomas, and neurofibromas, these conditions require a surgical laminectomy. Additionally, the spinal cord may be compressed by an extradural mass. The extradural mass may be produced by primary lymphoma, metastatic disease, epidural abscess, or hematoma. Epidural abscess may be caused by local disease (e.g., osteomyelitis) or spread of systemic infection (e.g., tuberculosis).

Preoperative Considerations

Many patients who undergo disc surgery are young and healthy and require only a basic preoperative evaluation. On the other hand, patients with cervical spondylosis and lumbar spinal stenosis are frequently elderly and require the special considerations of the geriatric patient. In general, these considerations include reduced reserve in the cardiac, pulmonary, and renal systems; altered drug responsiveness and metabolism; and frequently, the presence of underlying diseases and consequent polypharmacy. The coagulation status must be evaluated carefully in patients with malignant spinal cord compression and arteriovenous malformations. All patients should have an evaluation of baseline neurologic status.

Intraoperative Management

Regional anesthesia may be employed for operation in the lumbar area. However, general anesthesia is the most common anesthetic technique.

Cervical procedures may be performed with the patient in the supine position or even in the sitting position, depending on the preference of the surgical team. The patient may be transferred to the operating table before the induction of anesthesia. If, however, the patient is to be placed in the prone position, general anesthesia should be induced while the patient is supine on a stretcher, before being turned into the prone position on the operating room table. (See Chapter 6 for specific details on positioning.)

If the airway is perceived to be potentially difficult, the anesthesiologist may choose to employ one of the intubation techniques involving sedation and local anesthesia. These techniques are described later in this chapter in the discussion of cervical spine trauma.

Patients with rheumatoid arthritis frequently require cervical spine procedures. These patients may have multiple problems, including diminished cervical movement, potential for subluxation at the C1-C2 interface, inability to open the mouth widely, diminished mandibulohyoid distance caused by impaired mandibular growth, and a complex rotation of the larynx that can make direct visualization of the cords difficult. Fiberoptic bronchoscopy can be extremely useful in these patients.

Patients with metastatic disease who undergo laminectomy present a special problem because of their frequently debilitated state and the extensive blood loss associated with these procedures. Surgery is considered after the maximal radiation dose has been administered, if the spinal cord is compressed, or if it is required to prevent or treat fracture/dislocation. Preoperative evaluation in these situations may reveal pulmonary involvement from tumor, radiation, drugs, or infection; pancytopenia; tolerance to narcotics; pericardial or myocardial involvement by tumor; dehydration; and various degrees of neurologic dysfunction. Bleeding during the surgery may be severe and sudden. It is therefore essential to have accurate blood pressure monitoring and sufficient vascular access. Central venous or pulmonary artery catheters may be indicated in individual patients according to their cardiovascular status preoperatively. Coagulation should be assessed, and abnormalities should be corrected.

Although patients may be extubated while in a state of deep anesthesia or awake after lumbar laminectomy, they should be extubated awake after cervical laminectomy so no neck manipulation will be required to maintain the airway.

SPINAL CORD TRAUMA

Preoperative Evaluation

Patients with spinal cord trauma present a unique challenge for the anesthesiologist. It is important that these patients be thoroughly evaluated in the preoperative period. The neurologic, cardiovascular, and respiratory systems may be highly abnormal in these patients.

NEUROLOGIC SYSTEM

The findings of the neurologic examination are dependent on the level of the spinal cord involved by the trauma. A traumatic level between T2 and T12 causes paraplegia but leaves the upper extremities and the diaphragm intact. A level between C5 and T1 also causes a varying degree of upper extremity paralysis. The diaphragm is innervated by cervical roots 3 to 5; thus involvement at these levels causes various degrees of diaphragmatic dysfunction and ventilatory inadequacy in addition to the quadriparesis.

In patients with cervical spine trauma it is essential to avoid neck motion, which can produce further cord damage. Flexion at the neck is generally more deleterious than extension, but both should be avoided if possible.

In cases of spinal trauma the spinal cord is not usually severed; rather, it is injured by compression from bone, hematoma, edema, and ischemia. Currently, no pharmacologic treatment (steroid, mannitol, naloxone, thyroid-stimulating hormone) or physical measure (local hypothermia) has been clearly shown to be more beneficial than simply maintaining spinal cord perfusion. Spinal cord blood flow is controlled in a way similar to control of cerebral blood flow. As with head injury, severe hypercarbia should be avoided to prevent increases in intraspinal pressure that may result in ischemia.

The surgical treatment of spinal cord injuries is somewhat controversial. If there is clear-cut cord compression by bone or hematoma, most surgeons agree that decompression is necessary. Other surgeons take a more aggressive approach with early internal reduction and fixation, at least in part to accelerate rehabilitation.

CARDIOVASCULAR SYSTEM

A certain amount of cardioaccelerator and vasoconstrictor tone is lost as a result of cord injuries that involve the T1 to L1 levels. This loss may result in so-called spinal shock hours to weeks after the injury in patients with injury to levels above T6. Blood volume pools in the periphery, and the patient has unopposed parasympathetic tone, resulting in bradycardia and an inability to increase the chronotropic or inotropic state of the heart. The tendency to bradycardia is remarkable when such stimuli as suctioning or endotracheal intubation are used. This condition can be prevented with atropine, 0.6 to 1 mg IV.

Shock in this setting may have other causes, such as hemorrhage, pericardial tamponade, tension hemopneumothorax, or low blood pressure caused by a vascular injury (especially a tear of the aorta). The trauma team must be involved in this investigation. As a rule, the hypotension of spinal shock is associated with relative bradycardia, whereas that of hemorrhage is related to tachycardia. However, hemorrhage may coexist with spinal cord injury, resulting in blood loss without tachycardia.

Initially both forms of shock can be managed with fluids while preliminary evaluation proceeds. However, the patient with spinal shock will not handle large fluid challenges well because of an inability to increase heart rate and contractility. The Swan-Ganz (pulmonary artery) catheter may be used to avoid fluid overload. Spinal shock should be managed in part with doses of intravenous atropine and vasopressors to avoid the administration of large amounts of fluid. Some authors feel strongly that inotropes (e.g., dopamine), rather than pure vasopressors, should be used.

Hemorrhagic shock, by contrast, requires aggressive replacement of blood and crystalloid and surgical measures to stop the bleeding. Sorting these out in practice can be quite difficult, which is why the pulmonary artery catheter is useful. The patient with spinal shock is especially likely to have hypotension during anesthetic induction and maintenance and must be treated with special care. The rapid administration of a large dose of a cardiovascular depressant, such as thiopental, should be avoided.

The trauma patient may also have suffered a myocardial contusion that results in cardiac dysfunction and arrhythmia. Although electrocardiography and enzyme studies are unsatisfactorily nonspecific, two-dimensional echocardiography or a nuclear study may show areas of focal wall motion abnormalities otherwise inexplicable in a young, previously healthy patient. Treatment is directed toward the resulting abnormalities in heart rhythm and contractility.

RESPIRATORY SYSTEM

The degree of respiratory compromise depends on the level of spinal injury. However, even injury to levels below those involved in diaphragmatic innervation will affect respiratory function because the abdominal muscles are essential to produce a forceful cough. Even when secretions can be removed from large central airways by suction, a weak or nonexistent cough will predispose the patient to hypoxemia and recurrent atelectasis because of the accumulation of secretions in peripheral airways. Table 8-1 lists the innervation of the principal respiratory muscles. In addition to diaphragmatic and cough mechanism dysfunction, other pulmonary disorders may occur. Although underlying pulmonary disease is somewhat uncommon in this young population, some patients are smokers with baseline problems of cough, secretions, and bronchospasm, and others may have asthma or, less commonly, other underlying pulmonary disorders.

Patients with spinal cord injuries sometimes suffer pulmonary contusion, which is essentially a bruised area of lung that results in an area of very low V/Q distribution, leading to hypoxia. It also represents an area that is a good potential culture medium for pneumonia-producing bacteria. The chest wall above the contusion may be unstable, resulting in difficulty reexpanding the injured area of lung. This effect occurs when several adjacent ribs are broken in more than one place, causing a flail chest that does not expand with the remainder of the chest wall during inspiration. There is no specific treatment, but the patient should receive oxygen, positive airway pressure, and ventilation as required.

Other pulmonary problems include aspiration, neurogenic or cardiogenic pulmonary edema, inhalation injuries, fat embolism, and adult respiratory distress syndrome due to many causes, including sepsis. Neurogenic pulmonary edema can follow both spinal and intracranial trauma. This condition probably involves increased capillary permeability and increased pulmonary venous pressures.

Preoperative evaluation should include an appreciation of these superimposed problems as well as the current level of dysfunction caused by the spinal cord injury. Bronchospasm, if present, should

TABLE 8-1. Innervation of Muscles of Respiration

Muscle	Nerve
Sternocleidomastoid (CN XI, C2-3)	Accessory inspiratory
Trapezius (CN XI, C3-4)	Accessory inspiratory
Diaphragm (C3-5)	Accessory inspiratory
Scalenes (C4-8)	Inspiratory
Intercostals (T1-12)	Inspiratory and expiratory
Abdominal (T7-12, L1)	Expiratory

be treated with theophylline, beta-2 agonists, anticholinergics, and steroids. Secretions should be managed with adequate hydration, suction, and administration of a preoperative anticholinergic. If the spine is unstable, chest physical therapy may be contraindicated. Emergency surgery may need to be performed for patients in less than optimal pulmonary condition. In addition to devices for supplying intraoperative positive end-expiratory pressure, blood gases should be available. If lung compliance is severely diminished, a modern ventilator from the intensive care unit may be needed because many ventilators on anesthetic machines will not deliver adequate pressures for ventilation. Anesthesia can be provided intravenously in such a situation.

OTHER BODY SYSTEMS

In trauma patients other body systems may be involved with underlying disease or associated injuries. (Head trauma is discussed in detail in Chapter 18.) Injuries to the maxilla, skull base, and mandible in association with cervical spine trauma may produce great difficulties in airway management. For instance, the patient may have a basilar skull fracture that is a strong relative contraindication to nasal intubation and a mandibular injury that makes it impossible to open the mouth. Maxillary fractures may result in airway obstruction when the free-floating fragment falls backward when the patient is in the supine position and occludes the airway. Occasionally, these airways may need to be managed with cricothyroidotomy or tracheostomy. Cervical spine injuries may also be associated with injuries to the larynx and may present with various degrees of vocal dysfunction or airway obstruction.

Cardiac tamponade, tension pneumothorax, and rapid bleeding into the pleural spaces must be considered possible causes of hypotension. An aortic tear is an extremely serious injury that requires angiography for diagnosis and for guidance during surgical repair. An aortic tear is usually suspected when mediastinal widening is seen on the chest film.

Intraabdominal injuries may be immediately responsible for hemorrhage that can be detected by peritoneal lavage or computed tomographic (CT) scan. The CT scan will also detect retroperitoneal bleeding, which is frequently caused by pelvic fractures. Fractures, especially of the pelvis and femur, may account for a large amount of blood loss. Overall, injuries that are life-threatening because of hemorrhage, aortic rupture, or cardiac tamponade and those that are brain-threatening take precedence over less acute problems. In the chronically injured patient, calcium and renal function should be checked because the former may rise as a result of immobilization and the latter may be impaired by chronic and recurrent infections.

Intraoperative Considerations

ANESTHESIA INDUCTION AND MAINTENANCE

Airway Management.　The induction of anesthesia in patients with cervical spine injury requires special precautions. In some patients neck immobility is ensured by placement of a halo device, but other patients may require assistance by the surgeon to maintain neck immobility during intubation.

In general, intubation with careful topicalization and sedation is preferred. However, in children and uncooperative adults, a rapid-sequence intubation with the surgeon immobilizing the neck is preferable to having a thrashing patient who injures himself/herself further while resisting intubation. Intubation should be performed only by a skilled, experienced practitioner who has able assistance. The administration of an anticholinergic drug is highly recommended to reduce secretions and improve visualization.

Nasal intubation is contraindicated in the presence of significant coagulopathy and strongly contraindicated in the presence of basilar skull fracture. In some patients it is impossible to pass an adequately sized tube (at least no. 6 ID in women, no. 7 ID in men) through the nose.

Nasal, oral, and pharyngeal topicalization can be achieved with many different local anesthetic solutions. One that works well is 0.5% tetracaine (up to 1 mg/kg) prepared in a nebulizer. It is essential to use a vasoconstrictor in the nose to prevent bleeding and to facilitate passage of the endotracheal tube. If topical cocaine is used in the nose, this medication will serve as a vasoconstrictor. If, however, another local anesthetic is selected, a topical nasal decongestant should be used.

A local anesthetic can be introduced deeply into the nose with the plastic cannula of a 16- or 18-gauge intravenous line, or long cotton-tipped swabs (three or four) can be saturated with local anesthetic and placed until they touch the posterior wall of the nasopharynx. This can be comfortably accomplished with a slow twisting motion. Once the swabs are in place, further local anesthetic can be dripped in along the wooden sticks, which are slowly pulled out in stages to anesthetize the entire mucosa topically. When three cotton-tipped swabs can be introduced, a no. 7 ID endotracheal tube usually can be successfully passed into that nostril either directly or through a soft nasal airway guide.

If the cricothyroid membrane is accessible, laryngotracheal anesthesia can be supplied with the translaryngeal administration of local anesthetic through the cricothyroid membrane. If a cervical collar or other device is in place, it should not be removed without consultation with the responsible surgeons. Lidocaine (2 to 4 ml of 1% to 2%) is injected through the cricothyroid membrane with a 23-gauge needle after air is aspirated to ensure that the needle is within the lumen of the airway. Blind nasal intubation is accomplished by listening to the patient's breathing sounds through the tube until a position of maximal sound volume is achieved, which should represent a tip position just above the vocal cords. The tube can then be passed into the trachea during inspiration, when the vocal cords open. It is advisable to bend the tube to give it some anterior curvature before it is passed. This flexion can be done by placing the tube tip in the adaptor to form a circle of the tube or by placing a stylet in the tube in the shape desired and removing the stylet before tube placement.

Often the tube passes into the esophagus rather than into the trachea. If no cervical spine problem is involved, the neck can be manipulated with extension and rotation to help guide the tip into the trachea. Such manipulation cannot be done when there is any question of potential injury to the cervical cord. The fiberoptic bronchoscope is the preferred way to initiate nasal intubation in these situations. If fiberoptic bronchoscopy is planned, the transtracheal injection is not necessary since it does present a small risk (bleeding, mainly), and the lidocaine can be injected through the bronchoscope when the cords are visualized. Use of the fiberoptic scope is more difficult after bleeding and edema resulting from unsuccessful blind attempts. Successful use of the fiberoptic scope requires practice. Practice should be obtained before an attempt is made to use the fiberoptic scope in an emergency situation.

Blind nasal intubation may be facilitated by the use of an endotracheal tube in which tension on a loop near the proximal end pulls the endotracheal tube tip anteriorly (e.g., Endotrol, Mallinckrodt Critical Care). Gorback has described a technique of blind nasal intubation in which the cuff is inflated to bring the tip anteriorly and then deflated after the tip has been passed 2 cm into the larynx. Berry has described the use of a stylet in blind nasal intubation. In brief, the stylet is formed into a C-shape and passed into the tube, which has been introduced into the pharynx. The stylet is used to bring the tube tip anteriorly when the tube is slid off into the trachea.

Oral intubation can be accomplished with a fiberoptic scope, a light-wand stylet, direct laryngoscopy, or blind placement with the aid of a curved Macintosh laryngoscope blade. The mucosal surface of the tongue and pharynx can be topicalized with a local anesthetic solution as described for nasal intubation. However, this step does not blunt the discomfort of the laryngoscope blade pressure.

Glossopharyngeal blocks, as described by Woods and Lander, can be used to blunt this pressure response. Lidocaine (2 ml of 1% solution) with epinephrine injected through a 25-gauge needle at the point where the anterior tonsillar pillar approximates the base of the tongue on both sides. This block allows the laryngoscope to be comfortably placed in the usual way. When the cords are visualized, they can be topicalized with an "LTA" kit or with 4 to 5 ml of 1% lidocaine. Superior laryngeal nerve blocks topicalize the supraglottic area and are accomplished with 2 ml of 1% lidocaine given through a 25-gauge needle in the lateral portion of the thyrohyoid membrane. Thorough topicalization allows a reasonably comfortable intubation with minimal sedation.

Narcotics can be used to blunt discomfort; but the patient will be less responsive and less able to protect the airway. Fentanyl can be given in gradual (1 to 2 ml) increments and has the advantage of rapid and specific reversal with naloxone (which should be available). In addition to fentanyl, droperidol (1.25 to 5 mg IV) can be used to give additional sedation without producing further respiratory depression. Although some practitioners prefer to use a benzodiazepine, the action of these drugs is unpredictable (some patients are quickly oversedated), and the respiratory depression it produces is not reversible with naloxone. The action of benzodiazepines can be reversed with flumazenil. The inclusion of a narcotic is extremely helpful in blunting gag and cough responses. As noted previously, the use of an anticholinergic (glycopyrrolate, 0.4 to 0.5 mg IV) is essential to decrease the secretions that reduce visibility and increase airway irritability.

During direct oral laryngoscopy, the patient's head should be stabilized by the responsible surgical service. If the cords or the arytenoid (corniculate) cartilages cannot be visualized, a blind technique can be employed. A curved-blade laryngoscope is inserted to raise the epiglottis, and an endotracheal tube with a curved stylet is passed blindly through the cords. Because the clinician does not see the tube pass through the cords during blind techniques, it is advisable to confirm endotracheal intubation with a fiberoptic examination or analysis of end-tidal carbon dioxide because all the commonly used clinical signs (i.e., bilateral breath sounds and chest movement) may be unreliable.

The light-wand stylet can be used to facilitate blind oral intubation. Since the room must be darkened, the use of a pulse oximeter is strongly recommended because the patient's skin color is not observable. When the light is seen brightly in the midline, the tube is inserted another 2 cm and then slipped off the stylet into the trachea.

Retrograde intubation can be performed if other methods fail and there is no urgency to the situation. The cricothyroid membrane area is topicalized with 1 to 2 ml of 1% lidocaine injected with a 23-gauge needle. Either an epidural (17-gauge) or a central venous (16-gauge) needle is then inserted through the membrane, and the epidural or central venous catheter is inserted into the larynx to be coughed up through the cords by the patient. Nasal or oral intubation is then accomplished by sliding the endotracheal tube over the stretched-out catheter. The tube may be held up at the glottis, and this situation may be helped by rotating the tube or slackening the catheter.

If intubation cannot be performed, a cricothyroidotomy is indicated if air is needed urgently. This procedure is best performed by an experienced surgeon, but it may be done by the anesthesiologist if necessary. The cricothyroid membrane is incised, and a small endotracheal or tracheostomy tube is inserted. There is risk of laryngeal damage, but this life-saving procedure can be used when other measures fail or are impossible. Although some surgeons perform cricothyroidotomies electively, most choose to perform a formal tracheostomy if time permits. Even in the best of hands, it is extremely difficult to perform a tracheostomy quickly enough to deliver oxygen to the brain of a hypoxic patient.

Anesthesia Induction.   As previously noted, there may be compromise of the cardiovascular system caused by spinal shock, cardiac trauma, or hypovolemia. Thus anesthesia must be induced carefully. The use of atropine is strongly recommended before intubation. This drug is also helpful in an already intubated patient to reduce secretions, bronchospasm, and reflex bradycardia. If rapid-sequence intubation is chosen, it is reasonable to use ketamine (0.5

to 2 mg/kg) as an induction agent. Elevated intracranial pressure is a relative contraindication to the use of ketamine because cerebral blood flow is generally increased by this drug. Thiopental should be used with caution because of its potential to cause severe hypotension. Etomidate is also an excellent induction agent in these situations. Carefully chosen doses of midazolam or alfentanil are also options. The key to avoiding problems is to give the chosen drugs slowly and to observe for cardiovascular response carefully.

Anesthesia can be maintained with ketamine, narcotics, or propofol with nitrous oxide. A potent anesthetic agent such as isoflurane can be added if tolerated. Fluid and blood replacement should be exacting in order to avoid both overload and hypovolemia. The pulmonary artery catheter will reveal increasing pulmonary capillary wedge pressures that persist after a volume bolus when the left side of the heart is volume overloaded. At that point fluids are restricted and diuretics are given if judged necessary. Body temperature is carefully monitored since the patient may lose thermal regulation because of autonomic dysfunction. Warmed fluids, heated and humidified gases, a warming blanket, head covers, and an increase in the operating room temperature all help to manage body temperature.

Use of succinylcholine generally should be avoided since a hyperkalemic response may develop that cannot be prevented by pretreatment with nondepolarizing relaxants. Succinylcholine may be acceptable to use in the acutely injured patient (up to 24 hours after injury). However, we recommend that succinylcholine not be used in such a patient, even long after the injury has passed. Any of the nondepolarizing drugs is acceptable. Pancuronium offers the advantage of sympathetic stimulation.

Autonomic Hyperreflexia.   After the period of spinal shock has ended, the deafferented spinal cord may produce a group of deleterious reflexes known as autonomic hyperreflexia. When areas are stimulated below the level of the lesion, the affected cord segments respond with neural transmission, resulting in muscular (hyperreflexia, rigidity, spasm) and autonomic (hypertension) responses. Normal cord segments compensate for the hypertension with bradycardia and vasodilation. With cord injury above T7, this compensation may not be adequate to prevent hypertension severe enough to cause intracranial hemorrhage. The patient may be sweaty, nauseous, and agitated and may complain of headache. Cardiac arrhythmias and block may occur. Pain, bladder or bowel distention, or surgical stimulation all may trigger this reflex. The reflex can be blunted by general, spinal, or epidural anesthesia.

General anesthesia does not block the reflex if the level of anesthesia is too light, but care must be taken to avoid hypotension with deep anesthesia. Epidural anesthesia is difficult because it is impossible to know the effect of a test dose if the spinal cord injury level is high enough to cause autonomic hyperreflexia. Therefore extreme care should be taken to avoid using a high spinal level if the dura has been inadvertently punctured. Spinal anesthesia may be technically difficult, and the patient must be carefully watched for hypotension and bradycardia. Spinal headache will not be a problem in the already bedridden patient. Drugs for treating hypertension should be available for treatment of autonomic hyperreflexia (if it occurs).

Other Considerations.   After control of the airway has been established, ventilation should be controlled with large tidal volume breaths (10 to 15 ml/kg) to avoid hypercarbia and atelectasis. Care should be taken to avoid hypotension caused by decreased venous return when mechanical ventilation is begun.

Patients with chronic spinal cord injury should be moved carefully to avoid fractures of weakened bones. Areas of pressure should be checked for and relieved.

Postoperative Recovery and Intensive Care

The general principles of recovery and intensive care are outlined in Chapters 19 and 20. This section specifically addresses the problems of the patient with spinal cord injury.

RESPIRATORY STATUS

Problems of the respiratory system are key in the management of patients in recovery and intensive care. Because general anesthesia reduces postoperative vital capacity by about half, the patient with respiratory impairment secondary to a high spinal cord lesion may require postoperative ventilation. Patients with an acute injury affecting the cervical segments should be left intubated and ventilated. As noted previously, lesions below C5 should not affect the diaphragm, but they will significantly affect the expiratory muscles necessary for generating a forceful cough. Therefore these patients are susceptible to retention of secretions with resulting atelectasis and lobar collapse. After thoracic or upper abdominal surgery, vital capacity (and functional residual capacity) is reduced for days, and the patient with borderline preoperative lung function may require more prolonged mechanical ventilation.

In general, a patient with chronic injury who undergoes surgery for a single problem is less likely to have difficulty than an acutely injured patient operated on for multiple traumatic injuries. We often employ spinal anesthesia for orthopedic and urologic procedures in patients with chronic injury so that the patient's ability to ventilate himself/herself has been demonstrated throughout the case. In the multiply injured patient, there is little question about continuing postoperative intubation and ventilation.

In chronically injured patients with major procedures or in acutely injured patients with lower levels and minor procedures, the best way to proceed may be less clear. It is reasonable to bring such a patient to the recovery area while intubated and to wean the patient slowly from support while monitoring oxygenation and ventilation. Some sedation may be necessary to allow the patient to tolerate the tube and pain above the level of the injury. This approach may delay weaning and may even necessitate resumption of mechanical ventilation, but the process cannot be rushed.

As noted, the critical problems in these patients are loss of ventilatory capacity as a result of cervical injury and loss of forceful cough due to expiratory muscle weakness. Even lower cord lesions (T7 to T12, L1) affect the abdominal muscles and therefore the ability to cough. Loss of ventilatory capacity limits the patient's ability to expel carbon dioxide and to cough since coughing is less effective with low lung volumes. Secretions pool because suction does not remove them from the noncentral airway. If not contraindicated by an unstable injury, chest physical therapy (percussion, vibration, postural drainage, cough amplification) will bring secretions to the central airway, where they can be suctioned. Although bronchoscopic treatment of major atelectasis can usually be avoided in other populations, fiberoptic removal of plugs and secretions is very helpful in this group because these patients suffer from recurrent lung collapses, which cause severe V/Q abnormalities and hypoxemia.

CARDIOVASCULAR STATUS

Spinal shock and autonomic hyperreflexia have been discussed previously. Autonomic hyperreflexia may appear postoperatively as general or regional anesthesia is wearing off. During the spinal shock period, bradycardia is a recurrent problem. Asystole in response to stimuli, such as suctioning, may also occur because of an unopposed vagal reflex in patients who have lost all or most of the cardioaccelerator input (T1 to T6) of their sympathetic nervous system. The reflex can be blunted with the administration of atropine (0.4 to 1 mg IV), which blocks the vagus. Atropine is also useful because it reduces secretion volume (but not viscosity) and is a bronchodilator. Hypoxemia should be carefully avoided because it exacerbates the reflex. A small dose of intravenous narcotic or intravenous or intratracheal (1 to 1.5 mg/kg) lidocaine will make suctioning more comfortable for the patient. We have had patients who have required temporary pacemaker insertion to tolerate suctioning safely.

GENITOURINARY STATUS

An indwelling Foley catheter is generally left in place during the acute phase, but it is eventually replaced by intermittent catheterization. The patient consequently has recurrent urinary tract infections leading to renal dysfunction from tubulointerstitial nephritis and amyloidosis.

OTHER PROBLEMS

Other problems include deep venous thrombosis, which can be prevented with the use of elastic stockings, external pneumatic compression, and physical therapy; upper gastrointestinal bleeding, which can be minimized with antacids, H_2 blockers, or sucralfate; contractures; psychologic problems; and osteoporosis and pressure sores resulting from immobility.

CORRECTION OF SPINAL DEFORMITIES

Spinal deformities generally fall into the province of the orthopedic surgeon, but they are discussed briefly here.

Preoperative Evaluation
RESPIRATORY SYSTEM

Patients with spinal curvature severe enough to require surgery often have reduced lung volumes because of chest wall deformity. If neuromuscular disease is present, respiratory function also may be limited on this basis. Although there are grading systems for the degree of skeletal deformity, the anesthesiologist is primarily interested in the functional result, which can be examined through arterial blood gases and pulmonary function tests, including vital capacity and peak inspiratory and expiratory pressures.

If vital capacity is < 40% of the predicted level, postoperative ventilation is required. Although patients with higher vital capacities may not require postoperative ventilation, their condition must be judged on an individual basis. For instance, low peak inspiratory and expiratory pressures indicating respiratory muscle weakness may lead one to prophylactically ventilate the postoperative patient who had a borderline preoperative vital capacity. The arterial blood gas is useful for gauging the degree of resting hypercarbia that may be present and for evaluating the alveolar-arterial oxygen gradient.

Preoperative measures include teaching patients a deep breathing and cough regimen—which may include incentive spirometry, elimination of infection, treatment of bronchospasm, removal of secretions—and informing patients about what they can expect and how they can help themselves.

CARDIOVASCULAR SYSTEM

The low lung volumes of chest wall deformity may result in pulmonary hypertension and cor pulmonale. Hypoxemia may contribute to pulmonary hypertension and also may result in polycythemia. Patients with underlying muscular dystrophy may have an associated cardiomyopathy with the problems of cardiac muscle dysfunction, arrhythmias, and heart block. There is a high incidence of mitral valve prolapse in these patients. Because exercise tolerance is often not helpful in cardiac evaluation of these patients, echocardiography may be indicated to screen for myocardial and valvular abnormalities.

NEUROLOGIC SYSTEM

A screening examination should be performed by the anesthesiologist to document preoperatively any degree of gross neurologic impairments, such as baseline mental retardation, neuropathies, myopathy, and spinal cord dysfunction.

Anesthesia Induction and Maintenance

The two outstanding problems of anesthesia induction are blood loss and neurologic injury (about 1%). Preparation for induction should include consideration of avoiding succinylcholine in patients with neurologic deficits and the higher incidence of malignant hyperthermia in patients with muscular dystrophies. An arterial line and two intravenous catheters are placed. Many anesthetists also place a central venous pressure monitor to measure intravascular volume. The patient is carefully turned prone onto the chosen frame, with care taken to ensure that the abdomen lies free and that there are no pressure points.

HYPOTENSIVE ANESTHESIA

In order to minimize blood loss and provide better surgical conditions, some degree of controlled hypotension is often employed. If a wake-up test is planned, deep levels of anesthesia cannot be used for hypotension, and specific hypotensive agents are added to a nitrous-narcotic anesthetic. The patient may be pretreated with propranolol, captopril (3 mg kg PO), or clonidine (0.05 mg/kg PO).

Moderate hypotension (mean blood pressure 60 mm Hg) is the goal, and sodium nitroprusside (SNP) is the most commonly used drug in this setting. After pretreatment with one of the above drugs, which moderate the sympathetic and/or angiotensin response to hypotension, tolerable doses of SNP (0 to 8 μg/kg/min) usually result in the desired blood pressure. Small increments of labetalol (starting with 2.5 mg IV), a combined alpha- and beta-blocker, help if the SNP doses required are unacceptable.

OTHER MEASURES TO REDUCE BLOOD LOSS OR EXOGENOUS TRANSFUSIONS

Good positioning is the key to avoiding vena caval compression and excessive blood flow through epidural veins. Recently desmopressin (DDAVP) has been found to reduce blood loss in Harrington rod cases. This drug is a modified form of vasopressin that improves the function of what are presumably normal platelets in this setting.

The dose of DDAVP is 0.3 μg/kg and must be given over 20 to 30 minutes to avoid hypotension. Patients may donate their own blood preoperatively for intraoperative administration. Hematocrits in the mid-20s are tolerable if intravascular volume and cardiac function are normal. Lost blood may be recycled in a blood salvage device for transfusion. If blood loss is severe, blood should be given as indicated because the risk of death from hemorrhagic shock is still less acceptable than the extremely unlikely acquisition of AIDS or hepatitis.

MONITORING

There are two main techniques for monitoring spinal cord function during these operations: the wake-up test and somatosensory evoked potentials (SSEPs). The wake-up test awakens the patient and allows him/her to demonstrate movement of the lower extremities. Many still consider this test the gold standard of intraoperative spinal cord monitoring. The SSEP involves stimuli to sensory nerves in the lower extremities and recordings from the scalp. The results are found in the cerebral recording with the help of a computer, and they are evaluated for amplitude and latency. Details of evoked potential monitoring are given in Chapter 4.

In the wake-up test, the patient is informed preoperatively that it will occur, that he/she will be asked to move his/her legs, and that he/she will feel little or no pain. Preoperative sedation should be minimal, and the anesthetic is performed with nitrous oxide and a narcotic that is short-acting in moderate doses (fentanyl, sufentanil, alfentanil). The trachea may be sprayed with lidocaine to help the awakened patient tolerate the tube, which should be securely taped in place to avoid dislodgment during the wake-up. The surgeon should give about a 45-minute warning so that no further narcotic or relaxant is given before the test.

When the surgeon is ready for the test, the relaxant is reversed and the nitrous oxide is turned off. The patient is asked to move his/her feet and toes and is watched carefully to avoid injuring self. Once motion has been demonstrated, anesthesia can be reinduced with thiopental and continued with inhalation agents. The wake-up test is not a true monitor in the sense that it is not continuous, but it does provide assurance that damage has not been done up to the time of the test. The wake-up test should be used with caution, if at all, in patients with bronchospastic disease, emotional disorders, or mental retardation.

The main problem with SSEPs is that they may remain normal while motor function is lost. Motor potentials are being developed to deal with this problem. The SSEPs may also become abnormal (false-positive) when no damage has been done to the spinal cord. Since inhaled and intravenous agents may affect the tracing, the monitoring neurologist should be informed of their use. With conventional SSEP monitoring, deep inhalational anesthesia alters the tracing unacceptably, but a new spinal epidural recording technique may allow for use of deep inhalational anesthesia. The opposing opinions of Freedman and Grundy and Michenfelder (see Suggested Readings) regarding the use of the wake-up test and SSEPs in this setting is enlightening.

Postoperative Care

As noted earlier, patients with severe compromise of respiratory function should be ventilated postoperatively. Borderline patients can be brought to recovery or the intensive care unit with the tube in place and evaluated on an individual basis with the help of arterial blood gas determinations. Patients with muscular dystrophies may be extraordinarily sensitive to sedation and are best left intubated until their prolonged wake-up is accomplished. Blood loss needs to be monitored.

Postoperative lung expansive maneuvers are begun. These may simply involve chest physical therapy, cough, and deep breathing. Incentive spirometry may be used to help the patient take deep breaths to expand atelectatic areas and produce good coughs. In the uncooperative patient, mask continuous positive airway pressure (5 to 15 cm H_2O) will expand the lungs without the patient's help. It should not be used until the patient is wide awake in order to avoid aspiration. In patients with chest wall deformity or muscular weakness, intermittent positive pressure breathing may be helpful. This technique gives the patient a gas volume limited by the peak pressure generated.

OPERATIONS FOR MANAGEMENT OF PAIN

Operations for pain, which are not performed commonly, involve surgical interruption of pain pathways. They are usually performed in patients with terminal disease because the effect of cordotomy diminishes with time. Interruption of the anterolateral track in the high cervical or thoracic areas requires a laminectomy and general anesthesia. The previously noted principles of anesthesia for laminectomy apply. After operations of the high cervical spine, impairment of respiration and circulation may occur because of the nerve roots involved. Hypotension may be noted even after unilateral cordotomy. Cordotomy also can be performed with a percutaneous stereotactic technique that does not require general anesthesia.

Suggested Readings

Benumof JL: *Anesthesia for thoracic surgery,* Philadelphia, 1987, WB Saunders.

Berry FA: The use of a stylet in blind nasotracheal intubation, *Anesthesiology* 61:469, 1984.

Colice GL: Neurogenic pulmonary edema, *Clin Chest Med* 6:473, 1985.

Ebert TJ, Kotrly KJ, Masden KE et al: Fentanyl-diazepam anesthesia with or without N20 does not attenuate cardiopulmonary baroreflex-medicated vasoconstrictor responses to controlled hypovolemia in humans, *Anesth Analg* 67:548, 1988.

Fox DJ, Castro T, Rastrelli AJ: Comparison of intubation techniques on the awake patient: the Flexilum™ surgical light (lightwand) versus blind nasal approach, *Anesthesiology* 66:69, 1987.

Freedman WA, Grundy BL: Are the sensory evoked potentials useful in the operating room? Monitoring of sensory evoked potentials is highly reliable and helpful in the operating room, *J Clin Monit* 3:38, 1987.

Gorback M: Inflation of the endotracheal tube cuff as an aid to blind nasotracheal intubation, *Anesth Analg* 66:917, 1987.

Grande CM et al: Appropriate techniques for airway management of emergency patients with suspected spinal cord injury, *Anesth Analg* 67:714, 1988.

Gronert GA, Theye RA: Pathology of hyperkalemia induced by succinylcholine, *Anesthesiology* 43:89, 1975.

Kaffir ER: Respiratory and cardiovascular functions in scoliosis and the principles of anesthetic management, *Anesthesiology* 52:339, 1980.

Kallos T, Smith TC: The respiratory effects of Innovar given for premedication, *Br J Anaesth* 41:303, 1969.

Keenan MA, Stiles CM, Kaufman RL: Acquired laryngeal deviation associated with cervical spine disease in erosive polyarticular arthritis, *Anesthesiology* 58:441, 1983.

Kobrinsky NL: 1-desamino-8-0-arginine vasopressin (desmopressin) decreases operative blood loss in patients having Harrington rod surgery, *Ann Intern Med* 107:446, 1987.

Levy JH: *Anaphylactic reactions in anesthesia and intensive care,* Boston, 1986, Butterworth.

Mackenzie CF: Assessment of cardiac and respiratory function during surgery on patients with acute quadriplegia, *J Neurosurg* 62:843, 1985.

Mackenzie CF, Drucker TB: Cervical spinal cord injury. In Matjasko J, editor: *Clinical controversies in neuroanesthesia and neurosurgery,* New York, 1986, Grune & Stratton.

Michenfelder JD: Are the sensory evoked potentials useful in the operating room? Intraoperative monitoring of sensory evoked potentials may be neither a proven nor an indicated technique, *J Clin Monit* 3:45, 1987.

Pathak KS, Ammadio M, Kalamchi et al: Effects of halothane, enflurane, and isoflurane on somatosensory evoked potentials during nitrous oxide anesthesia, *Anesthesiology* 66:753, 1987.

Patil VU: *Fiberoptic endoscopy in anesthesia,* Chicago, 1983, Year Book.

Schonwald G, Fish KJ, Perkash I: Cardiovascular complications during anesthesia in chronic spinal cord injured patients, *Anesthesiology* 55:550, 1981.

Smith DS: Anesthetic management of patients with spinal cord injury, *ASA annual refresher course lecture,* no. 521, 1987.

Sutherland GR, Sibbald WS: Blunt traumatic myocardial injury, *Crit Care Clin* 1:663, 1985.

Tindal S: Anesthesia for spinal decompression in metastatic disease, *Anesth Analg* 66:894, 1987.

Woods AM, Lander CJ: Abolition of gagging and the hemodynamic response to awake laryngoscopy, *Anesthesiology* 67:220A, 1987.

SUPRATENTORIAL SURGERY

9

Steven T. Farnsworth
Joel O. Johnson

The majority of intracranial neurosurgical procedures are performed because of the presence of a mass lesion. Supratentorial procedures include those for tumor, hematoma, and trauma. Although the underlying pathologic features may be different for different lesions, the anesthetic considerations are similar.

PREOPERATIVE EVALUATION

The preoperative evaluation should begin much the same as for other anesthetic procedures, with a complete medical history that emphasizes heart and lung function. In neurosurgical procedures, as in other surgical procedures, most perioperative anesthetic morbidity and mortality are the result of cardiac or pulmonary dysfunction. Disease of either of these organ systems needs to be defined and then addressed in the preoperative patient preparation and the anesthetic plan.

Neurosurgical patients also need to be questioned specifically about central nervous system (CNS) diseases. Symptoms of increased intracranial pressure (ICP) should be discussed (headache, decreased level of consciousness, or visual disturbances). Cerebral hemorrhages or prior cerebrovascular accidents are noted, as are any residual neurologic deficits. A careful review of the results of previous intracranial surgery or diagnostic procedures and consideration of the possibility of residual pneumocephalus or other anesthetic interactions should be undertaken.

A review of the patient's medications is essential, with particular attention paid to those drugs that may have perioperative effects. Multiple medications and treatment regimens in neurosurgical patients can lead to decreased intravascular volume status. Mannitol and other diuretics used preoperatively to reduce cerebral edema can lead to hypovolemia and electrolyte imbalances, causing profound hypotension and cardiac arrhythmias on induction of anesthesia. Corticosteroids, also used to decrease cerebral edema, increase serum glucose levels by stimulating gluconeogenesis and cause direct adrenal suppression that may lead to hypotension and cardiovascular insufficiency with surgical stress. Antihypertensive medications may alter the patient's intravascular volume. Tricyclic antidepressants and levodopa have been incriminated for inducing intraoperative hypertension and cardiac arrhythmias. Benzodiazepines, phenothiazines, and butyrophenones can contribute to hypotension and cloud the sensorium perioperatively.

The preoperative physical examination is directed toward the airway, lungs, and cardiovascular and neurologic systems. In addition to the patient's underlying medical condition, the examiner needs to look especially for signs of hypovolemia. Neurosurgical patients are often somnolent and have inadequate oral intake, leading to another cause for hypovolemia. They may also have increased urinary water loss resulting from diabetes insipidus, x-ray dye, or diuretics. Mild to moderate hypovolemia is usually well tolerated and desirable in this patient population. However, significant hypovolemia should be corrected before induction of anesthesia.

A brief neurologic examination needs to be performed. The level of consciousness and any focal motor or sensory deficits should be documented. This neurologic examination can be briefly repeated in the operating suite just before the induction of anesthesia. This brief repeat examination may be the means of identifying a rapidly progressing lesion.

The patient should be questioned regarding symptoms and examined for signs of increased ICP. These signs include headache, nausea, vomiting, unilateral mydriasis, papilledema, and oculomotor or abducens nerve palsies. As ICP increases further, the patient's mental status deteriorates and is followed by respiratory and cardiac dysfunction. A Cheyne-Stokes breathing pattern or bradycardia with hypertension are ominous signs of brainstem compression.

Routine preoperative laboratory work includes a complete blood cell count and serum chemistry and coagulation studies. Other tests are ordered as indicated. Hyperventilation and diuresis will decrease the serum potassium level. Thus potassium supplementation should be considered early. A serum glucose level >200 mg/dl is unacceptable and requires monitored insulin therapy to lower the glucose level to within the normal range (for both osmotic and cerebral protective reasons). Serum osmolarity should be measured in patients being treated for increased ICP. Patients with head injury often have electrocardiographic (ECG) abnormalities, and a baseline ECG can be especially valuable because the diagnosis of intraoperative or postoperative myocardial ischemia will depend partly on ECG changes from this baseline.

Preoperative radiologic studies provide essential information about tumor or hemorrhage size and location, cerebral edema, and midline shift. Although anesthesiologists are generally not expert in interpretation of computed tomography (CT) or magnetic resonance imaging (MRI), they can obtain a good appreciation for the extent of surgery to be performed and associated potential problems. A midline shift of 0.5 cm noted on CT or MRI or encroachment of brain tissue on the basal cisterns indicates significantly elevated ICP.

Preoperative sedation is contraindicated in patients with a decreased mental status. If preoperative medication is appropriate and desired, benzodiazepines (diazepam, lorazepam, or midazolam) are recommended. Diazepam 5 to10 mg or lorazepam 1 to 2 mg can be given orally 1 to 2 hours before surgery. Both diazepam and lorazepam have half-lives long enough to potentially delay awakening in the patient postoperatively, however, and intravenous, intramuscular, or oral midazolam is a better choice. Narcotics are best avoided because they increase the risk of vomiting and hypoventilation, both of which will increase ICP. Perhaps the best alternative is to withhold all preoperative sedatives until the patient is in the operating suite and then administer an intravenous sedative while preparing the patient for surgery. In this way the anesthesiologist can readily address any adverse drug effects that may arise.

MONITORING

Routine monitoring for supratentorial procedures includes ECG, noninvasive blood pressure cuff, arterial line, esophageal stethoscope, fraction of inspired oxygen (FIO_2) monitor, pulse oximeter, temperature probe, peripheral nerve stimulator, and an indwelling urinary catheter. Ideally, ECG monitoring should include both leads II and V_5, and a modified V_5 should be placed for any patient with ischemic heart disease. The arterial line can be used not only for beat-to-beat blood pressure monitoring but also for obtaining blood for laboratory analysis. In addition, it can be valuable in helping to assess the patient's volume status. The external auditory meatus serves as a good landmark for the level of the circle of Willis and, to measure cerebral perfusion pressure accurately, the arterial line transducer should be placed at this height.

End-tidal CO_2 monitoring should also be considered essential. In addition to its usual function of helping to diagnose airway disconnection and obstruction, it is used to monitor hyperventilation (in conjunction with arterial blood gases). End-tidal nitrogen monitoring is not essential, but, if nitrous oxide (N_2O) and O_2 are the only inspired gases, a rise in end-tidal nitrogen suggests an air embolism or room air inadvertently entering the inspired gases somewhere in the anesthesia machine or circuit. For patients expected to have significant blood loss or patients with compromised cardiopulmonary status, central venous pressure (CVP) monitoring is used and pulmonary artery pressure monitoring should be considered. Acute fluid shifts caused by diuretics or mannitol also may mandate the use of CVP monitoring because of the unreliability of urine output in predicting hypovolemia.

ICP monitoring for supratentorial surgery is controversial. Although some advocate its routine use, others think that no outcome studies have proved its efficacy. If a patient does have an ICP monitor, the anesthesiologist can be more selective in the administration of aggressive diuresis and other decompressive therapy and subject only those patients with high ICPs to the potential side effects of this therapy. An ICP monitor also allows detection of what would otherwise have been occult increases in ICP during surgery. For example, changes in head positioning can obstruct venous drainage and lead to increases in ICP. Also, hemorrhage can lead to a rapid increase in ICP requiring immediate surgical decompression. The use of ICP monitors does carry risks, including damage to brain tissue, bleeding, and infection. These potential risks preclude its use in all patients undergoing craniotomy. However, in the subgroup of patients at risk for a large increase in ICP (tumor size >3 cm with midline shift or significant edema), there are potential advantages to ICP monitoring.

PHYSIOLOGIC MECHANISMS OF INTRACRANIAL PRESSURE

The cranium is a semirigid structure that houses the brain, blood, and cerebrospinal fluid (CSF). The brain accounts for 2% of total body weight (1400 g for a 70 kg person) and is composed of approximately 50% neurons and 50% glial cells. The normal cerebral blood volume (CBV) is 3% to 7% of intracranial volume, or 40 to 90 ml. The total volume of CSF is approximately 150 ml, divided roughly equally between the intracerebral and spinal compartments. The approximately 75 ml of intracerebral CSF is again split evenly between the ventricular system and the cerebral subarachnoid space.

CSF is formed at a rate of approximately 20 to 25 ml/hr in adults. Certain drugs and pathologic conditions can alter CSF production and absorption kinetics and thus alter CSF volume and ICP. Drugs that inhibit CSF production include acetazolamide, corticosteroids, furosemide, ouabain, spironolactone, and vasopressin. Hypothermia also decreases CSF production. Halothane decreases both CSF production and absorption. Enflurane increases CSF production and decreases absorption. Isoflurane does not affect CSF production significantly but does increase CSF absorption (by decreasing the resistance to reabsorption). Sevoflurane and desflurane appear to have CNS actions similar to those of isoflurane. However, at 1 MAC (minimum alveolar concentration), desflurane may increase ICP in patients with supratentorial mass lesion more than isoflurane does.

The ICP can remain normal in the presence of an intracranial mass because of compensatory mechanisms. The expansion of non-CSF tissue initially results in the displacement of venous blood and then in displacement of CSF from within the cranium into the distensible spinal subarachnoid space. Additional compensation may be provided by increased CSF reabsorption, which is a pressure-dependent process up to an ICP of 30 mm Hg. Once CSF volume buffering is exhausted, further spatial compensation must be achieved by a reduction in CBV or ICP will increase further. However, the homeostatic mechanisms for the maintenance of CBF are given priority over those of ICP.

An exhaustible buffer system generates an intracranial compliance curve like the one shown in Fig. 9-1. Two areas of the curve are marked. The area between points *1* and *2* indicates the period of CSF and CBV buffering. In this area the increase in intracranial mass is compensated by reduction of intracranial blood volume and displacement of CSF into the spinal subarachnoid space. Once this spatial buffering is exhausted (point *2*), the ICP increases markedly with small increases in intracranial mass. Many neurosurgical patients may have a normal ICP but sit at, or near, point *2* of the compliance curve. Although ICP is normal in these patients, a small increase in intracranial volume will increase ICP. A vicious cycle ensues as CBF is impaired and systemic mean arterial pressure is driven up, resulting in increased intracranial blood volume and possibly edema. Compensatory mechanisms fail and ICP rises, and vascular structures are compressed, inducing ischemia, shifting brain tissue, and producing brain death.

There are four possible supratentorial herniation sites as brain tissue is subjected to increasing pressure (Fig. 9-2). Subfalcine herniation occurs across the midline beneath the falx in the anterior portion of the brain, resulting in loss of movement and sensation in the lower extremities. Transtentorial herniation causes impairment

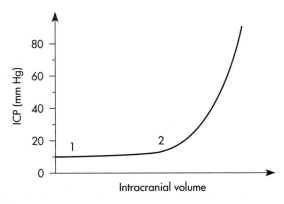

FIG 9-1.
Intracranial compliance curve.

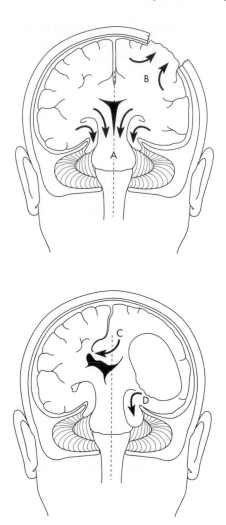

FIG 9-2.
Sites of supratentorial herniation. *A,* Transtentorial, causing pressure on brainstem; *B,* cranial, resulting in local tissue destruction; *C,* subfalcine, affecting sensory and motor areas subserving lower extremities; *D,* uncal, resulting in pressure on third cranial nerve. *Dotted line,* Midline.

of the level of consciousness, paralysis of eye movement, respiratory irregularity, and abnormal extemity posturing. Brain tissue is pushed through the tentorial incisura into the posterior fossa, leading to pressure on and damage to the brainstem. A subtype of transtentorial herniation, uncal herniation is the unilateral shift of the uncus, a temporal lobe structure, under the tentorium leading to anisocoria (early), ptosis, and lateral deviation of the eye. Finally, brain tissue may herniate through a traumatic or surgical opening in the cranial vault.

Therapy for increased ICP is multifaceted (Box 9-1). One simple but often overlooked principle is to ensure optimal venous drainage. Venous congestion of the brain increases blood volume and, subsequently, ICP. The optimal head position for venous drainage is midline with the head elevated 15 to 30 degrees.

Proper general medical care, such as seizure prophylaxis, treatment of hypoxia and hypertension or hypotension, is important in maintaining a normal CBV and ICP. There are times when mild hypotension of hypertension is desirable, but in patients with increased ICP normotension is the goal. If antihypertensive drugs are required to achieve normotension, care should be taken to avoid cerebral vasodilators, which will increase CBV and ICP while decreasing mean arterial (and cerebral perfusion) pressure. Such an alteration in intracranial dynamics could prove fatal. A good choice for antihypertensive therapy is a sympathetic blocker such as labetalol or esmolol.

Hyperosmolar therapy extracts water from and reduces the volume of brain tissue. The latency from administration of osmotic

---

BOX 9-1.
Preoperative and Intraoperative Control of Intracranial Hypertension in Patients Undergoing Supratentorial Surgery

Positioning (to improve venous drainage)
Fluid restriction
Diuretics (mannitol, furosemide, ethacrynic acid)
Corticosteroids (to reduce swelling)
Seizure prophylaxis
Blood pressure control
Anesthetic agents
Hyperventilation
Avoidance of bucking and light anesthesia

agents to ICP reduction is several minutes, and a maximal reduction occurs at 20 to 60 minutes. The patient must be able to tolerate this transient increase in intravascular volume from a cardiopulmonary standpoint. Elevating the serum osmolarity by 10 mOsm/L (to about 300 mOsm/L) reduces ICP in most patients, although an elevation of up to 30 mOsm/L may be necessary. This increase can be achieved with mannitol 0.25 mg/kg every 2 to 3 hours or 1 mg/kg less frequently. An acute elevation in serum osmolarity of 10 mOsm/L will extract about 100 to 150 ml of water. The upper limit for hyperosmolar therapy is 315 to 320 mOsm/L. A greater serum osmolarity is associated with a reduction in brain volume but is also related to renal and neurologic dysfunction.

The loop diuretics furosemide and ethacrynic acid have been used to control ICP. These agents act by brain dehydration, reduction of CSF formation, and reduction of cerebral edema. The onset of action for loop diuretics is slower than that of osmotic agents. However, they are equally effective in reducing ICP. Additionally, they can be useful in attenuating the increased intravascular volume load seen with osmotic agents.

Furosemide 0.7 mg/kg administered 15 minutes after mannitol will potentiate the effect of mannitol by producing a large volume of hypotonic urine and thereby maintaining a favorable osmotic gradient for a longer time.

Acute therapeutic hyperventilation (arterial carbon dioxide partial pressure [$Paco_2$] 20 to 25 mm Hg) has a rapid and generally successful influence on elevated ICP. An acute reduction in $Paco_2$ from 35 to 29 mm Hg lowers the ICP 25% to 30% in most patients. A failure to respond to hyperventilation is a grave prognostic sign. CBV changes 1% to 1.5% (0.04 ml/100 g) for each 1 mm Hg change in $Paco_2$ over a range of 20 to 80 mm Hg or, in an average 1400 g brain, roughly 0.56 ml per 1 mm Hg change in $Paco_2$. Thus hyperventilation from a $Paco_2$ of 40 to 20 mm Hg will decrease cerebral blood flow (CBF) by 50% and decrease CBV by 10 to 15 ml. This is a small but important volume when the patient is on the bend of the intracranial compliance curve.

The effect of prolonged hypocarbia on ICP is unclear. Hyperventilation influences CBV by its effects on the pH of CSF. The pH of CSF returns to normal with persistent hypocapnia (half-life 6 hours). After 24 to 48 hours of hyperventilation, there should be no active vasoconstriction. Sustained hyperventilation should not be terminated until the underlying mass or edema has decreased in size, or a rebound increase in ICP will occur.

Stimulation of the CNS can also have a detrimental effect on ICP. Unresponsive patients can have pain and other CNS stimulation. This stimulation increases the O_2 consumption of the brain, thereby increasing CBF and CBV. Deafferentation drugs (analgesics, anxiolytics) must be used during painful procedures on comatose patients. A very light anesthetic is not optimal for a patient with increased ICP.

Preventive therapy is also mandatory during respiratory care maneuvers (intubation, suctioning). These maneuvers not only stimulate the CNS but also elicit reflexes such as bucking, which may impede cerebral venous drainage. Lidocaine (1.5 mg/kg), short-acting narcotics, and hyperventilation before suctioning can blunt the increase in ICP associated with airway care. Barbiturates and mannitol may occasionally be required.

ANESTHETIC MANAGEMENT

The primary goal during induction of anesthesia in a patient undergoing a supratentorial procedure is maintenance of normal levels of ICP while maintaining adequate cerebral perfusion pressure. This goal is most practically accomplished by reducing the intracranial volume. Decreases in CSF volume account for compensation to chronic intracranial hypertension. A lumbar drain can be placed to decrease CSF volume. However, in the short-term setting (the operating room), intracranial blood volume is usually modulated by pharmacologic or ventilation therapies.

Induction

Although induction of anesthesia for patients undergoing craniotomy can be performed with various agents, the best single class appears to be the barbiturates. Thiopental administration provides a profound reduction in cerebral metabolic rate of oxygen consumption (CMR_{O_2}), CBF, and ICP. Propofol also decreases the CMR_{O_2}, CBF, and ICP. Narcotics also reduce CMR_{O_2} but to a lesser extent than CBF. In theory, this could lead to ischemia. However, this effect has not been shown to be clinically relevant. Narcotics provide excellent control of blood pressure and heart rate, which makes them useful anesthetic adjuncts. Etomidate does not cause an increase in ICP when used for induction. It appears to temporarily depress the pituitary-adrenal axis, but this change has not been shown to be of clinical significance. Ketamine causes an indirect increase in heart rate, blood pressure, and ICP and produces a seizure pattern on the electrocephalogram. For these reasons, ketamine is a poor anesthetic agent for neuroanesthesia. The effect of anesthetic agents and other drugs on ICP and CBF is shown in Fig. 9-3.

A gentle, smooth induction of anesthesia is more important than the exact drug combination used. The patient should be preoxygenated and self-hyperventilated. Administration of thiopental (3 to 4 mg/kg), propofol (2 mg/kg), or etomidate (0.3 mg/kg) intravenously should be followed with mask ventilation to ensure air-

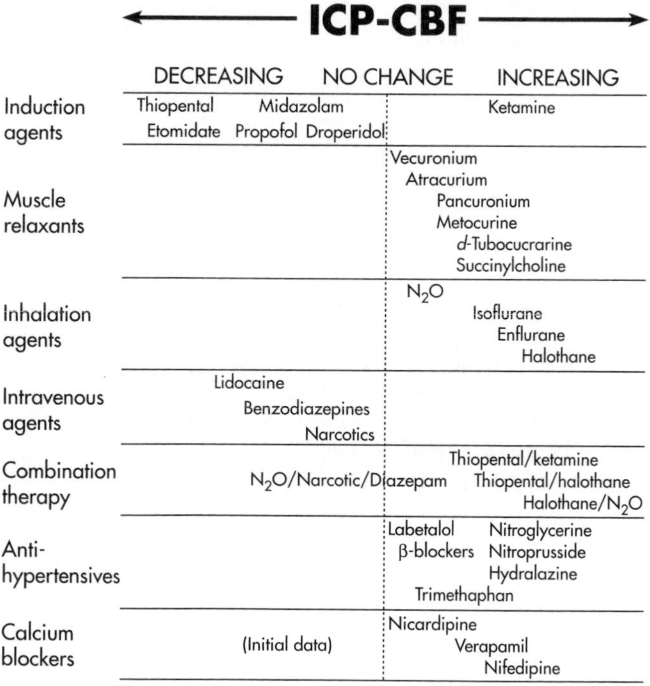

←——— ICP-CBF ———→

	DECREASING	NO CHANGE	INCREASING
Induction agents	Thiopental Etomidate	Midazolam Propofol Droperidol	Ketamine
Muscle relaxants			Vecuronium Atracurium Pancuronium Metocurine d-Tubocucrarine Succinylcholine
Inhalation agents		N$_2$O	Isoflurane Enflurane Halothane
Intravenous agents	Lidocaine Benzodiazepines Narcotics		
Combination therapy		N$_2$O/Narcotic/Diazepam	Thiopental/ketamine Thiopental/halothane Halothane/N$_2$O
Anti-hypertensives		Labetalol β-blockers Trimethaphan	Nitroglycerine Nitroprusside Hydralazine
Calcium blockers	(Initial data)	Nicardipine	Verapamil Nifedipine

FIG 9-3.
Effects of various drugs and drug combinations on ICP and CBF.

way patency and hyperventilation. Next, neuromuscular blockade is induced with vecuronium (0.1 to 0.15 mg/kg) or rocuronium (0.6 to 0.8 mg/kg) intravenously and continued mask hyperventilation with O_2 and N_2O (or O_2 and low-concentration isoflurane [if N_2O is contraindicated]). Intravenous lidocaine (1.5 mg/kg) and a small (one-half induction dose) amount of the intravenous induction agent should be given just before endotracheal intubation.

The dose of these induction agents needs to be adjusted for patients with cardiovascular instability. A combination of narcotics (fentanyl 5 μg/kg, or sufentanil 0.5 to 1 μg/kg) and a small dose of etomidate (6 to 10 mg) allows for ICP control and remarkable cardiovascular stability. Adequacy of ventilation must be closely assessed during a narcotic induction to avoid hypoventilation and subsequent increased CBF from hypercarbia. As always, the key to the appropriate use of anesthetic agents is close patient monitoring with titration of drug to effect.

A rapid-sequence induction can be performed with the same combination of drugs used in a routine induction. However, cricoid pressure is applied, mask ventilation is not delivered, and rocuronium 0.6 to 0.9 mg/kg or vecuronium 0.2 to 0.3 mg/kg is used to facilitate rapid endotracheal intubation. In a patient with a full stomach and a difficult airway, awake intubation should be performed. Heavy topical anesthesia and minimal intravenous sedation, with subsequent fiberoptic or oral endotracheal intubation with a lighted stylet, is extremely effective in these patients.

If narcotics are to be used as a part of the anesthetic, these agents should be administered slowly during induction. Fentanyl or sufentanil can make induction and endotracheal intubation very smooth. However, care must be taken when using narcotics. Neurosurgical patients may have a rapid clouding of sensorium with any sedative agent. Hence their protective airway reflexes may be blunted quickly. Narcotics induce hypoventilation, which can be dangerous in these patients. The combination of thiopental or propofol and narcotics (particularly sufentanil) can produce a dramatic decrease in blood pressure. Hence the dose of thiopental or propofol must be reduced for induction of anesthesia when a significant narcotic load has been given.

Esmolol or labetalol may also be given before intubation. These drugs blunt the hypertensive response to intubation. As with narcotics, the dose of thiopental must be adjusted if these drugs are administered or hypotension will result. The short half-life of esmolol is particularly advantageous in blunting the hypertensive response to intubation and stereotactic head-frame pin placement and not exacerbating postintubation hypotension during the relatively stimulus-free period of skin preparation.

Maintenance

Maintenance of anesthesia can be accomplished in a number of ways. These techniques generally fall into three categories: inhalational anesthetic agents, intravenous techniques, and "balanced" techniques. The most important feature in administering a given anesthetic is not which technique is used but, rather, how appropriately that technique is applied. This point cannot be overemphasized.

Many authorities think that a narcotic-based anesthetic technique with N_2O or low-dose isoflurane (<1%) in O_2 is optimal, but recently this technique has been associated with an increased incidence of postoperative nausea and vomiting when compared with inhalational or propofol-based anesthetics. If a narcotic-based anesthetic is chosen, either fentanyl, alfentanil, or sufentanil may be used. The place of remifentanil has not yet been well defined. Sufentanil may affect ICP and cerebral perfusion pressure unfavorably. However, we have extensive experience with sufentanil for intracranial procedures at our institution and have not found this concern to be of clinical significance.

Fentanyl 5 µg/kg, combined with <1% isoflurane in O_2 is an acceptable technique for anesthetic maintenance. Alternatively, sufentanil, 0.5 to 1 µg/kg load, followed by either incremental boluses (not to exceed 0.5 µg/kg/hr) or an intravenous infusion of 0.25 to 0.5 µg/kg/hr in combination with <1% isoflurane in O_2 may be used. The narcotic and the isoflurane dose are adjusted to yield the desired blood pressure. Sufentanil infusions must be discontinued approximately 1 hour before the end of surgery, or the patient may not awaken promptly and will require unacceptably high levels of hypercarbia to breathe spontaneously. Hypertension or tachycardia near the end of surgery is best treated with either labetalol or esmolol and not narcotics because this method will enable rapid awakening and neurologic examination at the end of the procedure.

A volatile agent, preferably isoflurane, with little or no narcotic supplementation, can also be used for maintenance of anesthesia. Hyperventilation in combination with <1% isoflurane generally results in stable intracranial dynamics. Because of the length of many intracranial procedures, it is best to treat hypertension and tachycardia at the end of the surgery with labetalol or esmolol rather than with increased levels of isoflurane. This approach allows more rapid awakening and assessment.

N_2O may be used in an anesthetic regimen if it is deemed desirable. However, if the patient is suspected of having a pneumocephalus (recent intracranial surgery or trauma) or air embolism, N_2O is contraindicated. Pneumocephalus under the influence of N_2O becomes a tension pneumocephalus and acts like a rapidly expanding mass lesion. In addition, a large venous air embolus can cause more rapid cardiovascular collapse in the presence of N_2O. However, worsened clinical outcomes after neurosurgery have not been shown. The use of N_2O also allows less narcotic and isoflurane to be used throughout surgery and helps smooth and quicken emergence.

Total intravenous anesthetic techniques have been described with propofol and fentanyl. After induction, a propofol infusion beginning at 200 μg/kg/min and reduced at the discretion of the anesthesiologist, along with a maintenance fentanyl infusion of 2 μg/kg/hr results in a stable anesthetic course and reasonably rapid emergence. The incidence of postoperative nausea and vomiting is acceptably low. In addition, there is no significant cost difference among well-conducted maintenance anesthetic techniques.

Each of these anesthetic techniques produces an acceptable anesthetic state. However, the art of anesthesia dictates that the anesthesiologist learn to properly evaluate the patient and not overmedicate or undermedicate, which can be difficult for the novice and, even occasionally, the seasoned anesthesiologist. If a patient does not awaken promptly at the end of surgery, an excess of either volatile agent or intravenous drug is part of the differential diagnosis. The anesthesiologist must rationally evaluate this possibility. Other common causes of delayed awakening in neurosurgery are brain tissue damage (surgical, hemorrhage, ischemia), electrolyte abnormalities, and hypothermia after a long procedure.

Hyperventilation is an important adjunct to any neuroanesthetic technique. Hypocapnia decreases ICP before the dura is opened, counteracts the vasodilation produced by the volatile anesthetic agents, and relaxes the brain during surgery. Optimal hyperventilation during surgery would yield Pa_{CO_2} of 25 to 30 mm Hg. If increased ICP remains a problem, it may be beneficial to reduce the Pa_{CO_2} to 20 to 25 mm Hg. The Pa_{CO_2} should be correlated, with the end-tidal CO_2 being monitored. Normally the Pa_{CO_2} will be 4 to 8 mm Hg higher than the end-tidal CO_2. Further reduction of Pa_{CO_2} results in no significant change in ICP (linearity exists between 20 and 80 mm Hg), and extreme hypocapnia may adversely affect cellular metabolism, cause a leftward shift of the oxyhemoglobin dissociation curve, or lead to maximal vasoconstriction.

Muscle relaxation prevents patient movement at critical times. It may also decrease ICP by relaxing the chest wall, which decreases intrathoracic pressure and encourages venous drainage. The agent used for muscle relaxation should be chosen on the basis of the length of the procedure and the impact of the drug on hemodynamics and ICP. For most supratentorial procedures pipecuronium and doxacurium are good choices because of their minimal hemodynamic effects and increased duration of action.

A peripheral nerve stimulator is used to monitor neuromuscular blockade in all patients. Lesions that involve the motor cortex or any of its outflow tracts can cause muscle dysfunction on the contralateral side. When such a lesion is resected, the patient may be positioned supine with the lesion away from the anesthesia machine to allow more room for the surgical team and equipment. In this way the affected muscle groups, usually of the patient's arm, are closest to the anesthesiologist and most convenient for neuromuscular monitoring. However, because of end-plate receptor proliferation, muscles that are functionally paretic are resistant to muscle relaxants. When a nerve stimulator is used on such a muscle, a much higher dose of relaxant is needed to produce the signs of neuromuscular blockade. The difference in sensitivity between normal and affected groups can lead to overdosing if one of the affected group's train-of-four is monitored.

The potential for overdose is partly advantageous because a deep level of relaxation is more likely to be maintained when a resistant muscle group is monitored. However, there is the problem of inability to reverse profound neuromuscular blockade in the normal muscles, which can be minimized by monitoring an unaffected muscle whenever possible. When such monitoring is not practical, good judgment regarding the dose of relaxant and constant vigilance for patient movement must be used. At the end of surgery neuromuscular blockade is tested on an unaffected muscle before the administration of reversal agents and extubation.

A balanced salt solution is the fluid of choice for neurosurgical procedures. The volume of fluid administered should be minimized during the induction of anesthesia and then kept as low as hemodynamic stability and urine output will allow. When volume resuscitation is needed and the hematocrit does not dictate the use of blood, 500 to 1000 ml of a colloid solution can be effective.

Emergence

Emergence from anesthesia after supratentorial surgery should be smooth and gentle. The decision to attempt a prompt awakening and extubation should include consideration of the patient's preoperative mental status, the location of the surgery, the extent of brain edema, and the quantity of intraoperative medication administered. A patient who was comatose preoperatively or who has undergone significant surgical manipulation for removal of a large centrally located tumor is not a candidate for early extubation. Such a patient should remain intubated and be allowed to awaken slowly in the intensive care unit after a period of monitoring and continued controlled ventilation. There are two clinical situations in which a previously comatose patient may be expected to wake up immediately after neurosurgery: (1) operative drainage of an acute subdural or epidural hematoma and (2) shunting of acute hydrocephalus relieves the condition immediately.

The majority of patients who undergo supratentorial surgery can be extubated in the operating suite on the termination of surgery. Labetalol or esmolol and intravenous lidocaine (1.5 mg/kg) can be used to treat the hypertension, tachycardia, and sympathetic stimulation associated with the period just before extubation.

The postoperative period may be associated with acute hypertension because of the need to have the patient awaken promptly for rapid assessment of neurologic function. Hypertension is a frequent occurrence and may result in postoperative intracerebral hemorrhage, possibly because of increased catecholamine levels. Appropriate treatment with alpha- and beta-sympatholytic agents or titration of a vasodilator (if ICP is monitored or is not significant) are approaches used in the postoperative period.

Suggested Readings

Bedford RF, Morris L, Jane JA: Intracranial hypertension during surgery for supratentorial tumor: correlation with preoperative computed tomography scans. *Anesth Analg* 61:430, 1982.

Felding M, Jakobsen CJ, Cold GE, et al: The effect of metoprolol upon blood pressure, cerebral blood flow and oxygen consumption in patients subjected to craniotomy for cerebral tumours, *Acta Anaesthesiol Scand* 38:271, 1994.

From RP, Warner DS, Todd MM, et al: Anesthesia for craniotomy: a double-blind comparison of alfentanil, fentanyl, and sufentanil, *Anesthesiology* 73:896, 1990.

Grosslight K, Colohan A, Bedford RF: Isoflurane anesthesia—risk factors for increases in ICP, *Anesthesiology* 63:533, 1985.

Jung R, Shah N, Reinsel R, et al: Cerebrospinal fluid pressure in patients with brain tumors: impact of fentanyl vs. alfentanil during nitrous oxide–oxygen anesthesia, *Anesth Analg* 71:419, 1990.

Madsen JB, Cold GE, Hansen ES, Bardrum B: The effect of isoflurane on cerebral blood flow and metabolism in humans during craniotomy for small supratentorial cerebral tumors, *Anesthesiology* 66:332, 1987.

Muzzi DA, Black S, Losasso TJ, et al: Labetalol and esmolol in the control of hypertension after intracranial surgery, *Anesth Analg* 70:68, 1990.

Muzzi DA, Losasso T, Dietz N, et al: The effect of desflurane and isoflurane on cerebrospinal fluid pressure in humans with supratentorial mass lesions. *Anesthesiology* 76:720, 1992.

Reasoner DK, Todd MM, Scamman FL, Warner DS: The incidence of pneumocephalus after supratentorial craniotomy, *Anesthesiology* 80:1008, 1994.

Todd MM, Warner DS, Sokoll MD, et al: A prospective, comparative trial of three anesthetics for elective supratentorial craniotomy, *Anesthesiology* 78:1005, 1993.

ANESTHESIA FOR EPILEPSY SURGERY AND STEREOTACTIC PROCEDURES

10

Joel O. Johnson

Anesthesia for epilepsy surgery and anesthetic care during stereotactic procedures share similar considerations. Many of these procedures are performed with the patient under mild sedation or under "awake" conditions requiring the cooperation of the patient during production of localized brain lesions or functional testing. Knowledge of the patient's disease and the interactions between therapeutic medications and anesthetic drugs are prerequisites to successful anesthesia.

EPILEPSY SURGERY

The incidence of epilepsy in the United States is 0.5%, amounting to more than 1 million patients. Approximately 10% of these have medically intractable seizure activity resulting in progressive neurologic impairment. These patients may benefit from surgical therapy, which should be carried out in a medical center with a well-organized program consisting of an epileptologist (neurologist), an experienced electroencephalographer and neurosurgeon, and the support team (including an anesthesiologist) necessary to perform prolonged electroencephalographic (EEG) studies and resultant neurosurgical procedures.

Preoperative Evaluation

The majority of the preoperative studies are done by a qualified sleep laboratory. Extensive EEG studies evaluate the seizure focus, attempting to localize it to a small discrete area, usually in the temporal lobe. If scalp recording is unable to identify a unilateral focus, 24-hour monitoring is instituted. Surgical implantation of subdural and possibly subcortical electrodes is sometimes needed. With the patient under general anesthesia, these are placed through a twist drill craniostomy and left in place for 2 weeks. Risks of surgery include hemorrhage, occlusion of blood vessels, and infection.

Two weeks after intracranial electrodes are placed, the patient may have a "thiopental test" consisting of an intravenous injection of 25 mg of thiopental every 30 seconds until the corneal reflex is gone. Although that dose of barbiturate normally produces β activity on the EEG, an absence of that response indicates focal cerebral dysfunction. Anesthetic care during this test consists of appropriate monitoring and airway management with a jaw thrust.

Preoperative computed tomography (CT) and magnetic resonance imaging (MRI) are initially used to rule out other causes of seizure (anatomic abnormalities or tumor) and to assist in stereotactic approaches to temporal lobe surgery. MRI is superior to CT in the identification of structural abnormalities implicated as seizure foci. Positron emission tomography (PET) has future potential for functional localization of epileptic foci.

Angiography is performed a number of days before surgery to delineate the blood supply of the area to be resected. A "Wada test," which is done to evaluate hemispheric dominance, involves the intracarotid infusion of sodium amobarbital while the patient is talking and holding both arms in the air. As the rapidly acting barbiturate exerts its effect, the contralateral arm falls. If the patient's speech simultaneously stops, the injected hemisphere is probably dominant. The test is repeated on both sides because of the possibility of mixed dominance of speech. In cases where the identified epileptogenic focus is located on the speech-dominant hemisphere, awake craniotomy during temporal lobectomy is carefully considered.

Surgical Issues

Procedures for seizure surgery involve excision of an epileptogenic focus or interruption of a seizure pathway. Awake craniotomy for surgical resection is requested when the proposed surgical excision places functionally important areas at risk for damage. These generally consist of Wernicke's area for speech and the motor strip. Excision of the anterior 5 to 6 cm of the temporal lobe on either side or 8 to 9 cm on the nondominant side can be done without risk to the speech areas. Careful functional testing during surgical resection may still result in temporary neurologic deficits because of edema around the surgical site. Surgical prognosis in carefully selected patients is good. One third will be mostly seizure free, one third will have diminished seizure frequency, and one third will be unchanged. The risk of death from surgery is <1%, and morbidity (including infection, aphasia, memory deficits, cranial nerve palsy, visual field deficits, and hemiparesis) is approximately 2%.

ANESTHETIC CONSIDERATIONS

A preoperative medical and physical examination allows for the identification of anesthetic-related issues. Patients on long-term anticonvulsant therapy should be evaluated for liver function because of the possibility of hepatocellular dysfunction. Bone marrow depression may be present, requiring a complete blood cell count (Table 10-1). Examination of the airway is important in the presence of gingival hyperplasia and poor dentition.

Anesthetic agents are proconvulsant or anticonvulsant; at times the classification of a drug depends on dose or physiologic conditions (Table 10-2). Anesthetic management involves the appreciation of the conditions under which seizure activity is more or less likely. This issue is particularly important during electrocorticography (ECoG) when the interpretation of the tracing is critical in iden-

TABLE 10-1. Pharmacologic Properties of Antiepileptic Medications Used for Simple and Complex Seizures

Drug	Adult Dose Range (mg)	Toxic Effects
Phenytoin	300-400	Neuropathy, blood dyscrasia, rash, lupus, Dupuytren's contracture
Phenobarbital	60-200	Rash
Carbamazepine	600-1200	Rash, blood dyscrasia, hepatitis, fluid retention
Primadone	750-1500	Rash
Clonazepam	1.5-20	Hair loss, nephritis, glaucoma
Methsuximide	500-1000	Rash, blood dyscrasia, nephritis
Valproic acid	1000-3000	Hair loss, hepatitis

TABLE 10-2. Electroencephalographic Effects of Anesthetics Used During Neurosurgery

	Effect on Electrocorticography	Convulsant Effects
Volatile anesthetics		
Isoflurane	Depresses	Anticonvulsant
Halothane	Depresses	Anticonvulsant
Enflurane	Activates	Proconvulsant
Desflurane	Depresses	?Similar to isoflurane
Sevoflurane	Depresses; activates in epileptic children	?Similar to isoflurane
Nitrous oxide	None	None
Barbiturates		
Thiopental	Depresses	Anticonvulsant
Methohexital	Activates	Proconvulsant
Amobarbital	Activates	Anticonvulsant
Etomidate	Activates	None
Benzodiazepines	Depresses	Anticonvulsant
Ketamine	Activates	Anticonvulsant, seizures in epileptics
Propofol	Depresses	Proconvulsant and anticonvulsant
Opioids		
Alfentanil	Activates	None
Fentanyl	Activates (high doses)	Proconvulsant?
Muscle relaxants	None	Laudanosine (atracurium), proconvulsant
Antihistamines	Activates	Proconvulsant

tifying the seizure focus. Medications that alter the cortical EEG should be avoided, if possible.

Potent inhalational anesthetics, which tend to be anticonvulsant, have a depressing effect on the EEG at higher concentrations. A notable exception is enflurane, which activates the electrocorticogram and at a concentration of >2.5% has been associated with seizure activity. Hyperventilation and sensory stimulation accentuate this effect. In contrast, nitrous oxide (N_2O) is not proconvulsant or anticonvulsant and is useful as a supplement to a balanced technique.

Intravenous sedative hypnotics exhibit a wide range of effects on patients with seizure activity. Barbiturates are traditionally anticonvulsant but may be avoided as bolus doses for treatment of seizure because of the rapid drug redistribution and subsequent reappearance of seizure activity. Methohexital in low doses (as small as 25 mg) activates the intraoperative cortical EEG and is at times used to "unmask" a seizure focus. Benzodiazepines are uniformly anticonvulsant through activation of the inhibitory gamma aminobutyric acid (GABA) channel and enhancement of chloride conductance. In the event of an intraoperative seizure, midazolam may be administered and ECoG continued in 10 to 15 minutes. Etomidate and ketamine activate epileptogenic foci and are ineffective as anticonvulsants. Propofol is reported to cause seizure activity but also is an anticonvulsant. In addition, it may interfere with ECoG by obscuring a seizure focus. The mechanism behind these contradictory effects of propofol is not known.

Opioids generate mu-opioid receptor-specific seizure activity in animals and possibly limbic system seizures in humans. Alfentanil in particular is used to enhance epileptiform discharges during ECoG. Activation of the EEG and epileptiform patterns are seen with high-dose opioid therapy.

Local anesthetics have an anticonvulsant effect at low blood levels but may cause seizure activity if a sudden large dose is administered. This effect is due to the marked inhibition of inhibitory neurons leading to excitatory predominance. Antihistamines activate seizure foci at levels below that causing sedation.

Positioning. Positioning is dependent on the surgical procedure and whether the patient is to be awake or under general anesthesia. The surgical setup for a right temporal lobectomy is shown in Fig. 10-1. Note the extensive use of padding. Most awake temporal lobectomies for epilepsy surgery involve the left hemisphere, necessitating a right lateral decubitus position. The patient's face should always be directed toward the anesthesiologist for awake procedures to facilitate communication and a reassuring environment.

Nonmovement of the head is desirable during awake procedures and the head holder varies with surgeon preference. Most prefer a three-pin Mayfield device, although surgery without head restraint is possible. The use of sufficient long-acting local anesthetic with epinephrine is mandatory for pin placement. Draping of the surgical field is done in a manner to allow a direct line of vision from the patient to the anesthesiologist. Appropriate padding consists of pillows between the legs, a small axillary roll, and padding of the cheek to prevent facial nerve palsy.

Monitoring. Standard intraoperative monitoring is supplemented by intraarterial pressure monitoring in all patients undergoing craniotomy. Careful control of intraoperative blood pressure during in-

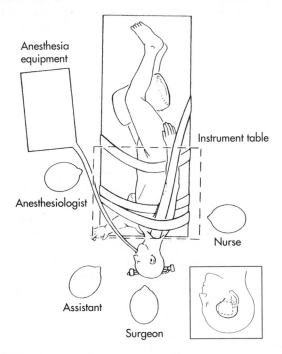

FIG 10-1.
Surgical approaches to lesions of cerebral convexity. For lesions of calvaria and intracerebral masses of posterior portion of frontal lobes and parietal and occipital lobes, free bone flap, centered over route used to reach lesion, is removed from cerebral convexity. Lateral decubitus patient position is used, with sagittal plane of patient's head parallel to floor. *Inset:* For large lesions in anterior aspect of temporal lobe or for temporal lobe seizure surgery, craniotomy is extended to include temporal bone superior to zygoma and anterior to external auditory meatus. (From O'Rourke DK, Oldfield EH: Supratentorial masses: surgical considerations. In Cottrell JE, Smith DS, editors: *Anesthesia and neurosurgery,* ed 3, St Louis, 1994, Mosby, p 298.)

tracranial surgery minimizes the risks of ischemia from retractor pressure, excessive surgical bleeding, and intraoperative brain swelling or edema. A surface lead EEG is generally not used. Further monitoring involves close and continuous interaction with the awake patient. An additional innovation is the use of an inexpensive microphone with an amplifier to enhance communication between the patient and the operating room team.

Perioperative anesthetic care for seizure surgery under general anesthesia begins with induction (barbiturate, etomidate, or propofol), muscle relaxation, and intubation. Long-term anticonvulsant therapy causes an increased dosage requirement for muscle relaxants. If intraoperative ECoG is to be used, a N_2O–narcotic technique is effective and potent inhalational agents should be avoided if possible. Hyperventilation may potentiate seizure activity and other methods (fluid restriction, mannitol, or furosemide with a urinary catheter) are used to improve operating conditions. Enflurane, methohexital, and alfentanil may be judiciously used to activate a seizure focus, although the appearance of "new" foci has been reported with methohexital.

For surgery in which ECoG is not planned, an anticonvulsant technique using potent inhalational agents is preferred. Supplemental opioids are given to decrease the total dose of inhalational agent and to facilitate a rapid awakening. Emergence in both cases should be planned to avoid hypertension and coughing. Postoperative care involves seizure precautions and planned treatment for seizures because blood levels of antiepileptic drugs may vary widely after general anesthesia. Carbemazepine and phenytoin levels increase dramatically in the postoperative period, resulting in toxic side effects.

Awake craniotomy requires a responsive patient who can safely and comfortably endure a prolonged neurosurgical procedure. Analgesia and sedation is achieved with medications and verbal reassurance. Neuroleptanesthesia consisting of fentanyl (0.5 to 0.75 μg/kg) and droperidol (0.15 mg/kg) has been used successfully for many years. We use intravenous propofol and alfentanil to successfully achieve patient cooperation, accurate electrocorticographic analysis, stable surgical conditions, and adequate ventilatory responses during monitored anesthesia care.

All patients are interviewed during the preoperative anesthetic evaluation and informed of the details of the anesthetic procedure. The exact nature of the intraoperative setup, the planned anesthetic regimen, and the use of arterial and urinary catheters are explained at length. All questions and concerns are discussed thoroughly to ensure patient cooperation and consent. The patient is instructed to take medications on schedule.

Preoperative sedation is not used. The patient is asked to lie on the operating table in a modified lateral decubitus position. Electrocardiogram leads, a noninvasive blood pressure cuff, a pulse oximeter, nasal cannulas, and pillows between the knees, at the abdomen, and under the left shoulder are arranged to ensure surgical exposure. The patient is asked to position the head comfortably on a foam doughnut, and oxygen is administered by nasal cannulas. An infusion of propofol (8 mg/ml) mixed with alfentanil (50 μg/ml) and lidocaine (2 to 4 mg/ml) is begun at 100 to 200 μg/kg/min, reading the propofol dosage (alfentanil is simultaneously administered at a ratio of 1:160 [i.e., when propofol is 80 μg/kg/min, alfentanil is 0.5 μg/kg/min]). This dose is occasionally supplemented with bolus doses through the infusion pump to achieve sedation. A radial arterial catheter is placed with local anesthesia, and a urinary catheter is introduced into the bladder because of the possible need to administer a diuretic during the surgical procedure. A soft nasal trumpet is inserted after preparation of the nares with a vasoconstrictor and viscous lidocaine. End-tidal CO_2 monitoring is instituted. The patient has little or no response to these maneuvers yet ventilates and oxygenates well. The infusion is typically decreased to 50 to 80 μg/kg/min propofol while the patient is unstimulated. Anesthesia setup time varies from 10 to 15 minutes. A three-pin head holder may be placed under local anesthesia; prepping and draping is done to ensure access to the patient's face by the anesthesiologist. The scalp is infiltrated with local anesthetic while the patient is sedated. Craniotomy and dural stimulation sometimes require additional bolus dosing of intravenous anesthetics.

Twenty minutes before the need for ECoG and brain stimulation the infusion is stopped. The patient awakens and functional testing is carried out during simultaneous brain stimulation. ECoG for the identification of spiking activity and occasionally placement of deeper electrodes is necessary to locate the seizure focus. Stimulation of the speech areas while a patient is talking causes an immediate cessation of speech in midsentence; the patient resumes talking (again from midsentence) when the stimulation is stopped. After the identification of the seizure focus and functional areas, the anterior temporal lobe is resected. During that time the infusion is increased and the patient is allowed to become more sedated.

Possible complications of awake craniotomy include restlessness and agitation. Good rapport with the patient in the preoperative period and, at times, a change in the level of sedation will resolve this complication. Intraoperative nausea and vomiting is rare with the use of propofol. Seizure control is sometimes necessary; methohexital (1 mg/kg) or a benzodiazepine (midazolam) is effective. At the completion of the surgery all patients are taken to the recovery room awake and responsive.

STEREOTACTIC PROCEDURES

Clinical use of stereotactic surgical techniques began in the late 1940s with the production of lesions in brain structures for treatment of psychiatric and movement disorders. The position of these structures in the brain was determined by the location of intracerebral landmarks and consultation with a published atlas. The use of the computer to combine CT and MRI into three-dimensional representations in space has led to its extensive use in directing stereotactic surgery.

Most stereotactic procedures are done with the patient awake. After appropriate local anesthesia for placement of the stereotactic head frame and burr hole, the rest of the operation is relatively painless. Advantages of this technique include the ability to perform functional assessment before the intracranial procedure, avoidance of postoperative hypertension associated with emergence, and immediate neurologic evaluation after surgery. Stereotactic surgery is used for treatment of movement disorders, cancer and chronic pain, psychosurgery, epilepsy, and biopsy of intracranial masses.

Preoperative Evaluation

A large proportion of patients who undergo stereotactic surgery have Parkinson's disease. Treatment with levodopa leads to drug resistance in some patients after 3 to 5 years. These patients are candidates for stereotactically guided thalamotomy or pallidotomy, which reduces tremor in about 90% and bradykinesia in >50%. Levodopa treatment may increase the risk of perioperative arrhythmias through sensitization of the cardiovascular system. In addition, butyrophenones and phenothiazines should be avoided because of their dopamine-blocking properties.

Pain-alleviating procedures are done in patients with chronic pain by interrupting the spinothalamic tract (mesencephalotomy), by thalamotomy, and by cingulotomy. These patients should be elevated for narcotic addiction. Psychosurgery on patients with obsessive-compulsive neurosis, anxiety, or depression involves cingulotomy. Preoperative evaluation includes documentation of psychotropic medications and consideration of anesthetic interactions.

Brain biopsies are associated with a mass lesion in a closed space. Estimate of intracranial pressure by clinical findings of headaches or visual disturbances is necessary, particularly for general anesthetic cases. Pretreatment with steroids and anticonvulsants should be considered.

Monitors

Routine monitors are used, including an electrocardiogram (ECG), noninvasive blood pressure, oxygen saturation, and precordial stethoscope. An arterial catheter for blood pressure monitoring is generally not required. If the patient is in a sitting position, precordial Doppler monitoring for venous air embolism is prudent. Placement of an ECG-guided right atrial catheter for evacuation of entrained air during venous air embolism is optional. If an air embolism is detected, N_2O is discontinued, 100% O_2 must be instituted, and other therapeutic measures (e.g., jugular venous compression, lowering the surgical field) should be considered.

Stereotactic Apparatus

The equipment used in stereotactic surgery poses the biggest problem for the anesthesiologist. There are many stereotactic devices, but the most common in use is the arc type (Fig. 10-2, *B* and *D,* and Fig. 10-3). The Brown-Roberts-Wells frame consists of a ring attached to the skull by four pins (Fig. 10-2, *D,* and Fig. 10-3). An interlocking arc is placed on the ring, and a computer is used to calculate the appropriate settings. This device lends itself to MRI- and CT-guided stereotactic localization.

The ring platform and arc may obscure the patient's airway. This matter is of concern for awake and general anesthesia procedures because access to the airway to assist ventilation or for tracheal intubation is restricted. If the patient is to undergo general anesthesia, tracheal intubation may be accomplished through fiberoptic or awake techniques. Before intubation is attempted, the wrench used to remove the platform must be available in the event of an emergency situation. Platforms have been developed with a hinged handle that may be moved to assist in airway access.

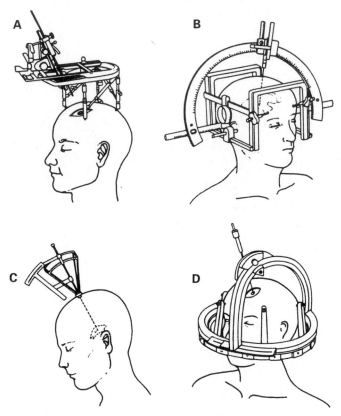

FIG 10-2.
Four types of stereotactic devices. **A,** Rectilinear. **B,** Arc type. **C,** Aiming device. **D,** System with interlocking arcs. (From Gildenberg PL, Katz J: Stereotactic surgery. In Frost EAM, editor: *Clinical anesthesia in neurosurgery*, Boston, 1991, Butterworth Heinemann, p 392.)

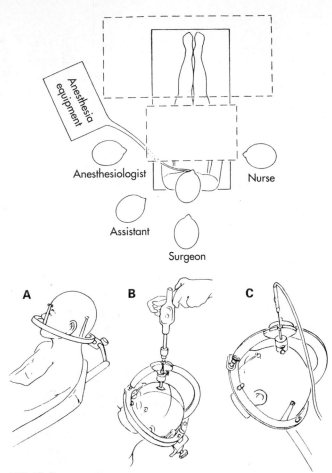

FIG 10-3.
A, Coordinates of target for CT- and MRI-guided stereotactic surgery are obtained by use of a head frame fixed to patient's skull by base ring. CT or MRI is performed with localizing frame (not shown) in place on base ring. **B,** For surgery, localizing frame is replaced with surgical frame. For stereotactic biopsy, small opening is drilled in skull (**B**) and biopsy needle is guided to target (**C**). (From O'Rourke DK, Oldfield EH: Supratentorial masses: surgical considerations. In Cottrell JE, Smith DS, editors: *Anesthesia and neurosurgery,* ed 3, St Louis, 1994, Mosby, p 298.)

Intraoperative Care

The stereotactic device is positioned, prepping and draping are performed, and a skin incision is made after infiltration of local anesthetic. A burr hole through the cranium and incision of the dura allow a probe to be placed along the predetermined trajectory. If a functional lesion is to be made, electrical stimulation at the tip of the probe reproduces the probable lesion and ensures appropriate placement. For instance, stimulation of the ventroposterolateral thalamus decreases tremor and rigidity in patients with Parkinson's disease. Lesions are generally produced with radiofrequency current, which causes ionic oscillations in the surrounding tissue and heat production. The usual lesioning temperature is 80°C for 1 to 2 minutes.

Suggested Readings

Archer DP, McKenna JM, Morin L, Ravussin P: Conscious sedation analgesia during craniotomy for intractable epilepsy, a review of 354 consecutive cases, *Can J Anaesth* 35:358, 1988.

Gignac E, Manninen PH, Gelb AW: Comparison of fentanyl, sufentanil, and alfentanil during awake craniotomy for epilepsy, *Can J Anaesth* 40:421, 1993.

Kelly PJ, Earnest F, Kall BA, et al: Surgical options for patients with deep-seated brain tumors: computer assisted stereotactic biopsy, *Mayo Clin Proc* 60:223, 1985.

Manninen PH, Contreras J: Anesthetic considerations for craniotomy in awake patients, *Int Anesthesiol Clin* 24:157, 1986.

Olivier A: Surgery of epilepsy: methods, *Acta Neurol Scand Suppl* 117:103, 1988.

Templehoff R, Modica PA, Berarno KL, et al: Fentanyl-induced electrocorticographic seizures in patients with complex partial epilepsy, *J Neurosurg* 77:201, 1992.

POSTERIOR FOSSA SURGERY

11

Richard J. Sperry

PREOPERATIVE EVALUATION
MONITORING
ANESTHETIC MANAGEMENT
SPECIAL PROBLEMS
 BRAINSTEM STIMULATION
 AIR EMBOLISM
 MONITORING FOR AIR EMBOLISM
USE OF NITROUS OXIDE
POSITIVE END-EXPIRATORY PRESSURE
CENTRAL VENOUS CANNULATION
THERAPY FOR AIR EMBOLISM
PARADOXICAL AIR EMBOLISM

Surgery in the posterior fossa can be a dramatic and dynamic experience. Constant vigilance on the part of the entire operating team and continuing "real-time" communication with the neurosurgeon are essential for an optimal result.

The contents of the posterior fossa explain the drama of surgery on this area of the brain. The posterior fossa, or infratentorial compartment, is home to the brainstem. The major motor and sensory pathways, the primary cardiovascular and respiratory centers, the reticular activating system, and the nuclei of the lower cranial nerves are all concentrated in the brainstem. All these vital structures are contained in a tight space with little room to accommodate edema, tumor, or blood.

This chapter first presents the preoperative patient management and monitoring decisions for patients having posterior fossa surgery. Intraoperative and postoperative patient management are then discussed. Finally, an outline of intraoperative problems, including air embolism, is presented.

PREOPERATIVE EVALUATION

The fundamentals of the preanesthetic visit for any surgical procedure have been abundantly discussed in the anesthesiology literature and should be followed for neurosurgery.

There are a few additional considerations in the patient with a posterior fossa mass lesion. First, these patients may have an unappreciated involvement of the brainstem. Hence sedative premedication before arrival in the operating room should be minimal, if administered at all, and prescribed judiciously. Involvement of the cardiovascular and respiratory centers may first become apparent with the administration of sedative medication, which is particularly true with respiratory depressants such as narcotics. Respiratory depression includes hypercarbia and thereby increases the mass effect of the patient's lesion.

Sedative agents or respiratory depressants are best avoided before the time when the patient receives constant attention from the anesthesiologist. This general principle can be appropriately modified in the cases of posterior fossa exploration for aneurysm or cranial nerve decompression. In these cases some preoperative analgesia and sedation may be desirable. However, prudence may dictate the administration of these drugs in the operating room holding area.

Position during surgery is the second consideration that must be addressed in patients with posterior fossa lesions. For various reasons the neurosurgeon may request that the patient be placed in the sitting position. This position places extra demands on the cardiovascular system. The patient's cardiovascular reserve must be evaluated adequately during the preoperative visit to determine whether the sitting position will be tolerated. Any objections should be raised with the neurosurgeon before surgery.

Some authors suggest that uncontrolled hypertension, advanced age, and American Society of Anesthesiologists physical status 3 or 4, all of which increase the risk of orthostatic hypotension, are relative contraindications to the sitting position. Significant hypovolemia would be considered an absolute contraindication.

The potential for venous and paradoxical air embolism is another major consideration for patients who are placed in the sitting position. Venous air entrainment is a common event during surgery in the sitting position. The incidence of detectable air embolism is reported at between 20% and 40% of all sitting cases. However, clinically significant air embolism is rare if appropriate monitoring is used and if prompt measures are undertaken to halt the entrainment of air, hence the need for preoperative decisions regarding monitors and therapy for air embolism. Also, as a part of obtaining informed consent, patients must be informed of the risks associated with air embolism.

The possibility of air crossing to the left side of the circulation from the right, creating a paradoxical air embolus, is real. The potential consequences of arterial air are so grave that everything possible must be done to prevent this complication. Known anatomic cardiac shunts or the presence of a ventriculoatrial cerebrospinal fluid (CSF) shunt, which would increase the total amount of air entering the right side of the heart, are absolute contraindications to the sitting position.

Technical aspects of the sitting position are discussed in the chapter on positioning. Further discussion of air embolism is presented later in this chapter in the section on special problems.

MONITORING

As for all patients receiving any anesthetic, neurosurgical patients should be given routine monitors: temperature probe, neuromuscular blockade, precordial or esophageal stethoscope, noninvasive blood pressure cuff, and continuous electrocardiographic (ECG) trace. For patients with ischemic heart disease it may be beneficial to simultaneously monitor ECG leads II and V. Pulse oximetry and respiratory gas monitoring are also standards of care.

In addition to the usual monitors, most neurosurgical procedures require an indwelling urinary catheter because of the length of many procedures and the occasional need to administer diuretics for brain relaxation.

An invasive blood pressure catheter is also highly desirable, if not mandatory, for all major intracranial procedures. Beat-to-beat blood pressure information is essential if the sitting position or techniques such as induced hypotension are used. An arterial catheter also allows rapid determination of arterial blood gas tensions and electrolyte levels.

Other monitors, such as the pulmonary artery catheter, may be required for certain patients if their conditions warrant. Also, if the sitting position is used, additional monitors should be used. Foremost among these monitors is precordial Doppler ultrasonography.

The section on venous air embolism later in this chapter contains a full discussion of monitoring modalities useful for detecting this complication.

As in all situations when monitoring is used, the anesthesiologist must guard against major patient management decisions as a reflex to isolated information. Monitors must never serve as a substitute for close patient observation and contact.

The decision to use a given monitor, especially an invasive one, must be made in light of the potential for morbidity associated with the monitoring system. Guidelines for the use of technology must never inhibit deliberate rational thought.

ANESTHETIC MANAGEMENT

Patients with posterior fossa lesions have the potential for development of obstruction of CSF outflow at the level of the aqueduct of Sylvius or fourth ventricle. This obstructive hydrocephalus results from compression by the lesion. Thus intracranial hypertension may even result from small, strategically placed lesions. Hence these patients must always be considered to be at risk for development of increased intracranial pressure and must be treated appropriately.

The anesthetic management for posterior fossa procedures is essentially the same as for supratentorial surgery. (See Chapter 9 for a detailed discussion of anesthetic management techniques.)

Intravenous fluid administration during posterior fossa surgery should be limited to deficit and maintenance quantities of a balanced salt solution. Major volume resuscitation may be accomplished with blood, colloid, or crystalloid (see Chapter 5 for a complete discussion of fluid therapy during neurosurgery).

Emergence from anesthesia should, like induction, be as smooth and gentle as possible. Coughing against an endotracheal tube may precipitate intracranial bleeding. However, vomiting and pulmonary aspiration of gastric contents are real dangers in a patient who is not sufficiently alert to protect the airway. An adequate blood level of narcotic generally produces an awake patient who does not cough or strain to any significant degree. Alternatively, lidocaine, 1.5 mg/kg given intravenously, decreases the amount of coughing and straining.

The decision to extubate a patient at the end of the procedure is not always an easy one. Generally, if a patient is alert preoperatively and the surgery is superficial and performed without much traction on the brainstem, extubation is assumed to be safe. However, deep-seated lesions or protracted surgery with frequent traction on the brainstem may place the patient in danger of apnea or a decreased sensorium with diminished airway reflexes. The patient should remain intubated and ventilated until he/she is out of danger.

SPECIAL PROBLEMS

Brainstem Stimulation

Historically, patients with posterior fossa lesions were allowed to ventilate spontaneously during surgery. This was thought to allow for monitoring of the pontine respiratory centers for surgical encroachment. However, changes in blood pressure and the presence of arrhythmias are equally sensitive indicators of brainstem manipulation. Therefore spontaneous ventilation during posterior fossa surgery can no longer be recommended.

Brainstem and cranial nerve stimulation can have dramatic effects. Profound hypertension results from stimulation of the fifth cranial nerve, the periventricular gray area, the reticular formation, or the nucleus of the tractus solitarius. Significant bradycardia and escape rhythms result from stimulation of the vagus nerve. Hypotension can be a result of pontine or medullary compression. Ventricular and supraventricular arrhythmias can occur from stimulation of many brainstem structures.

Close attention to cardiovascular parameters during critical periods of surgery is essential to the patient's well-being. Not only will life-threatening disorders be diagnosed, but also the surgeon may be informed of potential brainstem encroachment.

Air Embolism

Veins situated higher than the level of the right atrium have an intravascular pressure less than central venous pressure. The higher the vein is above the right atrium, the lower the intravascular pressure. At some elevation veins will have a negative intravascular pressure. When a patient is tilted head up 65 degrees, the pressure in the jugular bulb becomes subatmospheric. At this degree or greater of head-up tilt, the veins of the head and neck also have a subatmospheric pressure. If these veins are open to the atmosphere, they entrain air, causing a venous air embolus.

Once air enters the venous system, it can flow with the venous blood to the heart and subsequently to the pulmonary circulation. Venous air can occur as small or large bubbles. A capsule of platelets, lipid, and protein forms around the gas bubble. Additionally, gas exchange between the blood and the air bubble readily occurs.

Venous air can be entrained in either a slow or rapid fashion. Air entrained slowly, usually as a stream of small bubbles, is carried through the heart to lodge in the pulmonary capillary, which results in a functional decrease in the pulmonary capillary bed. Pulmonary artery and, subsequently, central venous pressures increase. If the pulmonary artery pressure increases enough, right ventricular failure may result and cardiac output will fall. However, a decrease in cardiac output is generally not seen until a large volume of air has been entrained, if it is entrained slowly.

Alveolar dead space increases with slow air embolization because of the decreased perfusion of the capillary bed. With constant ventilation the arterial carbon dioxide pressure (PCO_2) increases and the arterial oxygen pressure (PO_2) decreases.

Rapid air embolism, frequently occurring as a series of large bubbles, often produces a swirling vortex of air in the superior vena cava, right atrium, or right ventricle. The increase in pulmonary artery pressure is initially less than with slow air embolism. However, a rapid air embolus can severely impede flow through the right heart, and cardiac output and blood pressure subsequently decrease.

Air embolism is most likely to occur during dissection of neck muscles, turning of the craniotomy flap, and dissection of a vascular tumor bed. Particular vigilance is required at these times.

A large air embolus can be a fatal event. In the first half of the 1960s, 93 cases of venous air embolism were reported in the literature. In the 40 untreated cases there was a 93% mortality rate. In those patients treated with various combinations of pressor drugs, left lateral positioning, and open cardiac massage, the mortality rate was less but still a significant 58%.

In 1969 a report came from the Mayo Clinic of 2500 operations performed with the patient in the sitting position with no deaths attributable to venous air embolism. Thus venous air embolism was initially regarded as a rare but devastating complication. However, our understanding of the true incidence of air embolism during procedures performed with the patient in the sitting position changed dramatically because sensitive monitors for venous air were used.

In 1965 end-tidal carbon dioxide monitoring was introduced by Bethune and Brethren, followed in 1968 by the introduction of precordial Doppler ultrasonography by Maroon. With these sensitive monitors we soon learned that the incidence of detectable venous air embolism during procedures in the sitting position is 20% to 40%. The vast majority of these cases of air embolism are not clinically significant.

Monitoring for Air Embolism

Several methods are currently available to monitor for air embolism.

Precordial Doppler Ultrasonography

The precordial Doppler monitor is the most sensitive of the practical monitors and should be used during all procedures in which air embolism is likely to occur. This monitor generates an ultrasonic signal that is reflected by moving erythrocytes and cardiac structures. The reflected signal is received and processed to produce a characteristic rhythmic sound. When air, an excellent reflector, enters the Doppler detection field, a roaring noise is heard.

Doppler ultrasonography can detect a bolus of air as small as 0.25 ml and is an excellent early warning system for air entrainment. However, with this method there is no reliable way to quantitate the volume of air entrained.

The precordial Doppler monitor is effective as an early detector only if it is placed to "listen" over the right side of the heart. The Doppler probe should be placed to the right of the sternum in the third to sixth intercostal space. Placement of the probe should be done after the patient is positioned because the heart will move caudad when the patient is placed in the sitting position. Select the 2 Hz setting on the Doppler monitor and check the position of the probe by injecting a rapid bolus of 10 ml of agitated saline solution through a central line (or if necessary a peripheral intravenous line). This rapid bolus produces a noticeable change in the Doppler sound if the probe is placed correctly. Hold the probe firmly in place by tight taping or some other mechanism.

Precordial Doppler ultrasonography is an excellent early warning device. The vast majority of the air detected with the monitor is clinically unimportant. Detection of some air during a sitting procedure is to be expected and should not be cause for alarm. However, a continuous stream of air or frequent intermittent air should prompt a search for the source and elimination of further entrainment.

End-Tidal Carbon Dioxide Monitoring

End-tidal carbon dioxide monitoring is another sensitive indicator of venous air embolism. When air is trapped in the pulmonary capillary bed, alveolar dead space is created. If enough dead space is present, the diffusion gradient for carbon dioxide is increased. This causes an increased arterial PCO_2 value but a decreased alveolar PCO_2 value. Because the end-tidal PCO_2 reflects alveolar PCO_2, the end-tidal PCO_2 decreases with an air embolus.

End-tidal carbon dioxide monitoring is less sensitive than precordial Doppler monitoring. The end-tidal PCO_2 begins to fall significantly when 0.25 to 0.5 ml/kg of air has been entrained into the pulmonary system.

The major advantages of end-tidal carbon dioxide monitoring are that it is easy to use and noninvasive and it correlates closely with clinically significant air embolism. A disadvantage is that factors other than air embolism can affect an end-tidal carbon dioxide value. The most important of these is hypotension, which also increases the dead space in the lung.

End-Tidal Nitrogen Monitoring

End-tidal nitrogen determination is another monitoring technique for air embolism. When a patient is connected to a breathing circuit and no air is used in the inhalation gas mixture, the nitrogen in the lungs is quickly eliminated. Normal end-tidal nitrogen is, however, not identically zero because the body tissues continue to excrete dissolved nitrogen. When an air embolus occurs, nitrogen, a component of air, is excreted through the lungs, causing end-tidal nitrogen to rise. End-tidal nitrogen increases before end-tidal carbon dioxide decreases. However, end-tidal nitrogen returns to normal before resolution of the air embolus. One chief advantage of end-tidal nitrogen as a monitor for air embolism is the capacity to quantitate the amount of embolized air.

Pulmonary Artery Catheterization

The pulmonary artery catheter has been advocated as a technique to monitor for air embolism. It is true that pulmonary artery pressure usually does increase with air embolism. However, the sensitivity of the pulmonary artery catheter is probably no greater than that of the end-tidal carbon dioxide monitor. Because of the risk associated with the use of pulmonary artery catheters and because they provide little additional information, I cannot recommend the pulmonary artery catheter as a monitor for air embolism.

Echocardiography

Echocardiography has been used in various forms to monitor for air embolism. An echocardiogram can be obtained from the precordial or subxiphoid area or by a transesophageal probe. Although echocardiography may be slightly more sensitive as a monitor for intracardiac air than Doppler ultrasonography, it may interfere with the normal operation of the precordial Doppler monitor. Also, echocardiography currently requires constant visual attention to detect intracardiac air. A case of vocal cord paralysis from the transesophageal probe has been reported.

One major advantage of echocardiography is that it is the only monitor available to detect air that crosses into the left side of the heart. Despite this advantage I believe that echocardiography is currently a research tool and should not be considered standard for the monitoring of air embolism.

USE OF NITROUS OXIDE

The use of nitrous oxide (N_2O) as an anesthetic supplement during procedures in which air embolus is likely to occur has been controversial. N_2O is 34 times more soluble in blood than is nitrogen. It diffuses more rapidly into an air embolus than nitrogen diffuses out. Hence N_2O in the blood will increase the size of an air embolus, and the quantity of air causing morbidity or mortality will thus be decreased. The median lethal dose of air is 5.1 ml/kg in dogs and 0.5 ml/kg in rabbits. However, in rabbits breathing 75% N_2O the median lethal dose is decreased to 0.16 ml/kg.

For a controversy to exist there must be opposing views. The arguments for the use of N_2O are that (1) less volatile agent will be used and so patients may have less cardiovascular depression and may awaken more quickly and (2) because N_2O will increase the size of an air embolus, a smaller quantity of air will need to be entrained before identification and initiation of appropriate measures.

POSITIVE END-EXPIRATORY PRESSURE

Positive end-expiratory pressure (PEEP) has been suggested as a method to decrease the incidence of air embolism. The increase in intrathoracic pressure generated by PEEP would be transmitted to the cerebral veins and thereby decrease the entrainment of air. However, in animal models 10 cm H_2O PEEP is not always effective in accomplishing this goal.

There have been a few objections to the use of PEEP. It may decrease the mean arterial pressure and therefore cerebral perfusion pressure. Perkins and Bedford found that 10 cm H_2O of PEEP can reverse the normal left-to-right interatrial pressure gradient. This shift in the pressure gradient was postulated to increase the incidence of paradoxical air embolism. Subsequent work in pigs with a surgically created atrial septal defect demonstrated that a left-to-right pressure gradient may not always protect against paradoxical air embolism. This situation is so because a right-to-left pressure gradient develops at some point during the cardiac cycle, even when the mean pressure gradient is the opposite.

CENTRAL VENOUS CANNULATION

The last issue relating to venous air embolism is the issue of central venous catheters. There is no question that air can be aspirated from a properly placed central venous catheter during episodes of air embolism in both humans and experimental animals. The aspiration of air has been conclusively shown to decrease the mortality from a lethal injection of air in animals and has been suggested as a contribution to resuscitation from air embolism in humans. Recently developed multiorificed catheters may even improve previous results.

However, the need for a central catheter during procedures in the sitting position is not compelling. With correctly functioning Doppler and end-tidal carbon dioxide equipment, air embolism can usually be diagnosed and halted before the entrainment of a significant amount of air. With this early warning system in place, it is rare to aspirate more than a few bubbles of air. The therapeutic benefit of central catheters has been significantly negated by these new monitors.

With a diminishing benefit, the risks of central venous cannulation become a significant factor. Eisenhauer et al. reported a 13.7% complication rate in 554 attempts at internal jugular vein cannulation. Although most of these complications were minor, there was a 4% rate of major complications (arterial puncture, pneumothorax, venous air embolism).

In light of a shrinking benefit-to-risk ratio for central venous catheters during episodes of air embolism, the clinician should not view them as an absolute necessity and cry malpractice when they are not used. However, I believe that some benefit can accrue from the use of a central venous catheter, and therefore a reasonable effort should be made to place one before a sitting craniotomy is performed.

A small number of patients entrain a large quantity of air so quickly that other monitors do not serve as early warning devices, but merely confirm that something "bad" has occurred. Experimental evidence suggests that these patients will respond to air aspiration through a properly placed central catheter. Although the number of patients in this group is small, the risk is real and must not be ignored.

Another benefit of central catheters is that small amounts of air can be removed, thus decreasing the amount of air available for paradoxical embolization. Again, the number of patients who will benefit from this maneuver is small, but because it is impossible to predict who will or will not shunt air to the left side all patients must be considered as potential beneficiaries.

As a result of these arguments, a reasonable effort should be made to place a central venous catheter properly in all patients about to undergo a sitting craniotomy. The term *reasonable effort* needs some clarification. If accessible arm or neck veins can be identified, then I agree with Michenfelder than a 10 to 15 minute attempt constitutes a reasonable effort. Anesthesiologists must know their skills well enough to determine the point at which patient risk is increasing more than patient benefit and then quit if the attempt has been unsuccessful.

The issue of cannulation site (arm versus neck) has proponents on both sides. Although it is true that there is less risk associated with central venous cannulation through an antecubital vein, it is also true that antecubital catheters are frequently of a smaller diameter than catheters designed for the neck. In the case of massive air embolism, a larger catheter placed in a jugular vein may be more beneficial, although its placement may increase the risk associated with central venous cannulation. I prefer to use an antecubital vein but do not hesitate to move to a jugular vein if an antecubital vein is not available.

The last consideration for the placement of central catheters is where to locate the aspirating tip of the catheter. Early in the history of central vein cannulation for air embolism it was assumed that the catheter tip should be localized in the middle right atrium. This early recommendation was based on intuition. In 1981 Bunegin et al. evaluated the catheter aspiration of air in an in vivo model of the human right atrium. They determined that it is critical to place the aspirating tip of the catheter in the upper quarter of the right atrium. Although their study is important, it is an in vivo study and extrapolation to humans must be done with caution.

The tip of a central venous catheter can be placed in the high right atrium with ECG guidance. Once access to the central circulation is obtained, fill the catheter with sodium bicarbonate (1 mEq/ml) or normal saline solution. Then electrically couple either lead II or lead V of the ECG machine to the fluid inside the catheter. The tip of the catheter thus becomes an exploring electrode. Move the catheter until the P wave becomes biphasic, indicating correct placement. Confirm the position of the catheter by injecting a rapid bolus of 5 to 10 ml of saline solution through the catheter to elicit the typical Doppler sound.

THERAPY FOR AIR EMBOLISM

Finally, what should the anesthesiologist do when faced with a significant air embolism? First, the surgeon should be notified and N_2O discontinued if it is being used. The surgeon should inspect the surgical field for an open vein. If an open vein is not found, a Valsalva maneuver or bilateral compression of the jugular vein for 5 to 10 seconds will increase the cerebral venous pressure and induce bleeding. Compression of the jugular veins will also halt air embolism. If air entrainment continues, the anesthesiologist should ask for an assistant. A second pair of hands will allow simultaneous jugular vein compression and central catheter aspiration.

If the blood pressure falls, additional therapy should be instituted. Ephedrine, 10 to 20 mg given intravenously, and a bolus of fluid usually improve the blood pressure and propel the air into the pulmonary circulation. If this does not restore the blood pressure, the patient should be placed in the left lateral decubitus position with a 15-degree head-down tilt. This position may release an existing air lock and allow the cardiac output to increase.

PARADOXICAL AIR EMBOLISM

Paradoxical air embolism, air entering the left circulation, has occasionally occurred. Air may cross to the left side of the heart either through an intracardiac lesion or through other venous-arterial connections. From 20% to 30% of patients have a probe-patent foramen ovale that may become a gateway for paradoxical air. However, animal studies have demonstrated that air can cross from right to left with no demonstrable intracardiac lesion. Hence all patients with venous air embolism are at risk for paradoxical air embolism.

The two primary circulatory beds at risk are the coronary and cerebral vascular beds. As little as 0.6 ml of air injected into the carotid artery of a cat decreases electroencephalographic amplitude and causes cerebral edema and increased intracranial pressure. Just 0.2 ml of air injected into a dog's coronary circulation results in myocardial damage.

The intraoperative diagnosis of paradoxical air embolism is very difficult. Echocardiography allows for visualization of left-side air but is not always practical. ECG changes may reflect coronary air. However, air is only one of many possible causes for ECG changes. Occasionally air bubbles in the cerebral circulation may be seen by the surgeon.

The therapeutic options available to the anesthesiologist during paradoxical air embolism are very limited. The blood pressure and cardiac output should be supported if necessary. Effort should also be made to retrieve any venous air or to halt air entrainment that may be a source of continuing paradoxical air embolism.

Paradoxical air embolism became a major concern in the late 1970s. Although its actual incidence is not known, seven cases of clinically significant paradoxical air embolism were reported through 1981.

Suggested Readings

Artru AA, Colley PS: Bunegin-Albin CVP catheter improves resuscitation from lethal venous air embolism, *Anesth Rev* 12:32, 1985.

Artru AA, Colley PS: Placement of multiorificed CVP catheters via antecubital veins using intravascular electrocardiography, *Anesthesiology* 69:132, 1988.

Artru AA, Colley PS: The site of origin of the intravascular electrocardiogram recorded from multiorificed intravascular catheters, *Anesthesiology* 69:44, 1988.

Bedford RF: Perioperative venous air embolism, *Semin Anesthesia* 6:163, 1987.

Black S, Muzzi DA, Nishimura RA et al: Preoperative and intraoperative echocardiography to detect right-to-left shunt in patients undergoing neurosurgical procedures in the sitting position, *Anesthesiology* 72:436, 1990.

Bunegin L, Albin MS, Helsel PE et al: Positioning the right atrial catheter: a model for reappraisal, *Anesthesiology* 55:343, 1981.

Colley PS, Artru AA: ECG-guided placement of Sorenson CVP catheters via arm veins, *Anesth Analg* 63:953, 1984.

Cucchiara RF, Nugent M, Seward J et al: Air embolism in upright neurosurgical patients: detection and localization by two-dimensional transesophageal echocardiography, *Anesthesiology* 60:353, 1984.

Gottdiener JS, Papademetriou V, Notargiacomo A et al: Incidence and cardiac effects of systemic venous air embolism, *Arch Intern Med* 148:795, 1988.

Gronert GA, Messick JM, Cucchiara RF et al: Paradoxical air embolism from a patent foramen ovale, *Anesthesiology* 50:548, 1979.

Losasso TJ, Black S, Muzzi DA et al: Detection and hemodynamic consequences of venous air embolism: does nitrous oxide make a difference? *Anesthesiology* 77:148, 1992.

Losasso TJ, Muzzi DA, Dietz NM et al: Fifty percent nitrous oxide does not increase the risk of venous air embolism in neurosurgical patients operated upon in the sitting position, *Anesthesiology* 77:21, 1992.

Marshall WK, Bedford RF: Use of a pulmonary artery catheter for detection and treatment of venous air embolism: a prospective study in man, *Anesthesiology* 52:131, 1980.

Marshall WK, Bedford RF, Miller ED: Cardiovascular responses in the seated position—impact of four anesthetic techniques, *Anesth Analg* 62:648, 1983.

Michenfelder JD: Central venous catheters in the management of air embolism: whether as well as where, *Anesthesiology* 55:339, 1981.

Pearl RG, Larson CP: Hemodynamic effects of positive end-expiratory pressure during continuous venous air embolism in the dog, *Anesthesiology* 64:724, 1986.

Perkins NAK, Bedford RF: Hemodynamic consequences of PEEP in seated neurological patients: implications for paradoxical air embolism, *Anesth Analg* 63:429, 1984.

Perkins-Pearson NAK, Marshall WK, Bedford RF: Atrial pressures in the seated position: implication for paradoxical air embolism, *Anesthesiology* 57:493, 1982.

Toung TJK, Miyabe M, McShane AJ et al: Effect of PEEP and jugular venous compression on canine cerebral blood flow and oxygen consumption in the head elevated position, *Anesthesiology* 68:53, 1988.

Zasslow MA, Pearl RG, Larson CP et al: PEEP does not affect left atrial-right atrial pressure difference in neurosurgical patients, *Anesthesiology* 68:760, 1988.

PITUITARY SURGERY *12*

Burkhard F. Spiekermann
J. Michael Jaeger

The pituitary gland synthesizes and stores many hormones that are directly involved in regulating the body's homeostasis. Any pathologic disorder of the pituitary gland can have profound effects on the entire body. When medical therapy is insufficient to treat pituitary disease, surgery may be indicated.

In this chapter we review the normal anatomy and physiologic features of the pituitary gland and the most common pathophysiologic disorders that may require surgery. We discuss the special perioperative anesthetic concerns in patients with functioning pituitary tumors, the intraoperative management of patients undergoing transsphenoidal pituitary surgery, and the postoperative complications after surgery of the pituitary gland.

ANATOMY OF PITUITARY GLAND

The pituitary gland rests at the base of the skull within the sella turcica of the sphenoid bone (Fig. 12-1). The anterior pituitary (adenohypophysis) makes up the largest part (75%) of the gland and receives a rich vascular supply from the hypothalamus. The posterior pituitary (neurohypophysis) is connected to the hypothalamus by the pituitary stalk. The pituitary normally weighs between 500 and 600 mg and is largest in multiparous women.

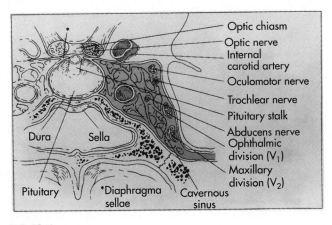

FIG 12-1.
Coronal section through sella turcica showing pituitary gland and its relationship to surrounding structures. (From Rengachary SS, Wilkins RH, editors: *Principles of neurosurgery,* London, 1994, Mosby-Year Book Europe, Ltd.)

Superiorly, the gland is separated from the optic chiasm by the diaphragm sella (composed of dura mater). The lateral walls of the sella separate the pituitary from the cavernous sinus and its contents: the internal carotid artery and third (oculomotor nerve), fourth (trochlear nerve), fifth (first division of the trigeminal nerve) and sixth (abducens nerve) cranial nerves.

Because of the close anatomic relationship of the pituitary gland to these important neurovascular structures, significant arterial and venous bleeding and cranial nerve injuries are potential complications of surgery in this area.

NORMAL PHYSIOLOGY OF PITUITARY GLAND

The activity of the pituitary gland is primarily controlled by the hypothalamus. Releasing and inhibiting factors from the hypothalamus influence the synthesis and release of pituitary hormones while positive and negative feedback loops tightly regulate serum hormone levels. The anatomic anterior and posterior lobes function physiologically as discrete entities.

Anterior Pituitary (Adenohypophysis)

Five different cell types within the anterior pituitary are responsible for the production of specific hormones. On the basis of their secretory products, modern immunochemistry allows for identification of these five cell types, which will be briefly described.

SOMATOTROPES

These cells secrete growth hormone (GH), which has anabolic effects on every organ system in the body, resulting in an increased rate of protein synthesis, mobilization of free fatty acids, and increased glycogen storage, whereas the rate of glucose uptake and utilization is decreased. The secretion of GH from the pituitary is under dual control by the hypothalamus through GH-releasing factors (somatomedin) and GH-inhibiting factors (somatostatin). Dopamine may also influence GH secretion by regulating somatostatin secretion. Hypersecretion of GH before puberty may lead to gigantism, whereas postpubertal hypersecretion results in acromegaly.

GH is also released as a result of physiologic stress such as surgery or anesthesia and from dopaminergic drugs. Corticosteroids suppress GH release.

LACTOTROPES

These prolactin (PRL)–secreting cells are responsible for the growth and development of breast tissue in preparation for lactation. They are controlled primarily by PRL-releasing factors from the hypothalamus and are normally under tonic inhibition by hypothalamic dopamine. Dopamine receptor antagonists, such as metoclopramide, alpha-methyldopa, and the phenothiazines, may increase serum PRL levels and cause galactorrhea.

CORTICOTROPES

Adrenocorticotropic hormone (ACTH) secreted by these anterior pituitary cells stimulates the zona fasciculata and zona reticularis of the adrenal cortex to produce and secrete corticosteroids. Absence of ACTH causes atrophy of the adrenal cortex (with symptoms of Addison's disease), whereas ACTH-producing tumors cause Cushing's disease. The serum level of ACTH is controlled by corticotropin-releasing hormone (CRH) secreted by the hypothalamus and arginine vasopressin from the paraventricular nucleus. High serum cortisol levels inhibit the release of CRH. Normally the release of ACTH is diurnal, but this diurnal release is frequently lost with pituitary disease.

GONADOTROPES

Gonadotropic cells produce luteinizing hormone (LH) and follicle-stimulating hormone (FSH). Both hormones, which are normally under hypothalamic control, play a major role in stimulating growth and maturation of the reproductive organs. They also regulate the menstrual cycle.

THYROTROPES

Thyrotropes secrete thyroid-stimulating hormone (TSH), which accelerates the formation of thyroid hormone by the thyroid gland. TSH is released from the anterior pituitary in response to thyrotropin-releasing factor (TRF) from the hypothalamus. TRF is released when circulating levels of thyroid hormone are low.

Posterior Pituitary (Neurohypophysis)

Unlike the anterior pituitary, the posterior pituitary does not produce hormones. It stores and releases two hormones, antidiuretic hormone (ADH) and oxytocin, which are synthesized within neuroendocrine hypothalamic nuclei and transported by an axonal connection along the pituitary stalk to the posterior pituitary gland.

ANTIDIURETIC HORMONE (ADH OR VASOPRESSIN)

ADH is produced in the supraoptic nuclei of the hypothalamus and is instrumental in regulating water and electrolyte homeostasis of the body. It acts on the distal tubule of the kidneys to increase the permeability of the epithelium to water (through a process mediated by cyclic adenosine monophosphate), thus increasing the reabsorption of free water and producing a concentrated urine.

Osmoreceptors located in the hypothalamus regulate the release of ADH from the pituitary. A decrease in total body water or an increase in serum osmolarity to >280 mOsm/L will stimulate ADH release. The most potent stimulus for ADH secretion is hemorrhagic shock. Other circumstances such as hypotension, angiotensin release, head injury, intracranial hypertension, and surgical stress can also cause the release of ADH. Inadequate or absent ADH secretion results in diabetes insipidus, whereas excessive ADH secretion causes the syndrome of inappropriate antidiuretic hormone (SIADH).

OXYTOCIN

Oxytocin is produced within the paraventricular nuclei of the hypothalamus. Its release is independently regulated from ADH secretion. Oxytocin augments uterine contractions and is one of the hormones responsible for lactation.

PATHOLOGIC DISORDERS OF PITUITARY GLAND
Pituitary Neoplasms

Pituitary neoplasms comprise approximately 15% of all intracranial tumors. At autopsy, pituitary tumors are found incidentally in as many as 10% of asymptomatic patients. Most pituitary tumors are histologically benign and originate in the anterior pituitary. Metastatic disease to the pituitary gland is very uncommon.

Hardy classified pituitary tumors on the basis of their size and the extent to which the sella is involved:

Grade 1—Microadenoma smaller than 10 mm, sella normal in size.

Grade 2—Sella enlarged but without extrasellar expansion.

Grade 3—Involvement of sphenoid sinus or suprasellar area, localized erosion of sellar floor.

Grade 4—Diffuse erosion of sellar floor, "phantom sella," involvement of sphenoid sinus or suprasellar space.

Pituitary tumors are most commonly classified according to whether they are functioning (e.g., endocrine active) or nonfunctioning (endocrine inactive) and named on the basis of their secretory products. About 70% of pituitary adenomas produce one or two hormones that become measurably elevated in the blood and result in clinically recognizable syndromes. An exception might be the ACTH-secreting and the gonadotropic adenomas, which can remain clinically silent. The remainder are mostly null cell adenomas (endocrine inactive) or a variant with little histologic, immunocytochemical, or ultrastructural clues as to their cell line of origin.

Symptoms from pituitary tumors can be due to physiologic effects of abnormal hormone secretion or physical effects of tumor mass. Progressive mass effect from large macroadenomas can produce hypothalamic symptoms, intracranial hypertension, epilepsy (very rare), and even motor or sensory loss, depending on the direction of expansion.

Functioning Pituitary Tumors and Their Medical Management

Immunoperoxidase staining of individual hormones or identification of specific messenger ribonucleic acid species allows for greater resolution of the functional classification of pituitary adenomas (Table 12-1). Many tumors previously classified as "nonsecretory" or null cell on the basis of clinical findings are now recognized as secretory tumors synthesizing subunits of glycoproteins, particularly gonadotropins. This knowledge has led to the development of new pharmacologic therapies to control or ameliorate symptoms and to arrest growth of many types of pituitary adenomas.

TABLE 12-1. Incidence of Pituitary Tumor Classified by Function

Hormone Secreted	Tumors (approx. %)
PRL	30
PRL + GH	10-12
GH	20
Null cell	20
ACTH	12-15
FSH/LH	1-2
TSH	1

PROLACTINOMAS

PRL-secreting adenomas comprise 30% of all secreting neoplasms of the pituitary and are the most common functioning pituitary lesion. The presenting symptoms depend on the sex and age of the patient. Women usually have galactorrhea (in up to 80% of patients), amenorrhea, menstrual disturbances, decreased libido, and sometimes infertility. Men most frequently complain of impotence, decreased libido, and infertility. Galactorrhea occurs in up to 30% of men with a prolactinoma. Headaches, visual disturbances, and signs of elevated intracranial pressure (ICP) are more common in males because males usually present with larger tumors at the time of diagnosis. Hyperprolactenemia during adolescence may interfere with puberty and may result in stunted growth.

Initial therapy for prolactinomas is often medical. Dopamine (D_2 receptor) agonist drugs such as bromocriptine (Parlodel) have been successful in suppressing PRL secretion in both normal individuals and patients with PRL-secreting adenomas. The incidence of side effects with bromocriptine, notably nausea, dizziness, headache, or orthostatic hypotension, can be as high as 50%. Prolactinomas unresponsive to bromocriptine therapy or those causing a mass effect may require surgical intervention.

GROWTH HORMONE–PRODUCING TUMORS

An excess production of GH is responsible for a disorder called acromegaly. GH affects the growth of all tissues and organ systems in the body, including heart, lungs, liver, and kidneys. Most affected are the bones and soft tissues of the hand, feet, and face. The cosecretion of excess PRL with GH, which can occur in up to 30% of cases, and somatomedin C (insulin-like growth factor I) helps to explain the diverse physiologic, biochemical, and clinical manifestations of acromegaly. Excess GH can lead to an increased incidence of coronary artery disease, hypertension, cardiomyopathy, and glucose intolerance. Patients may complain of heat intolerance, pronounced sweating, and signs of carpal tunnel syndrome. Acromegaly affects patients of both sexes, most commonly between the ages of 20 to 60 years. If the disease is left untreated, the mortality rate is 50% before age 50 years. The most common cause of death is cardiac arrhythmias.

Although surgery remains the primary therapy, patients are usually started on a long-acting somatostatin analog, octreotide (Sandostatin), to suppress growth of the tumor and GH secretion. In addition, octreotide reduces secretion of serotonin and numerous gastroenteropancreatic peptides producing dysfunction in glucose metabolism, progressive decline in serum thyroxine levels, reduction in splanchnic blood flow, and cholestasis. There are no reported interactions of octreotide with anesthetic drugs. Bromocriptine may be used as an adjunct medication. Acromegalic patients may also require drug treatment for associated cardiac failure, arrhythmias, hypertension, and diabetes.

ACTH-Producing Tumors

Abnormally increased production of ACTH by the pituitary gland with resultant bilateral adrenal hyperplasia is the cause of Cushing's disease. Cushing's syndrome refers to a group of disease states that have in common increased serum corticosteroid levels. Examples include adrenal adenoma or carcinoma, ectopic ACTH production (oat cell lung cancer), or iatrogenic administration of corticosteroids.

The clinical features of Cushing's disease and Cushing's syndrome include truncal obesity, moon facies, abdominal striae, acne, supraclavicular fat pads ("buffalo hump"), hirsutism, and easy bruising. Hypertension, diabetes mellitus, and subclinical proximal muscle weakness and osteoporosis may be present.

The standard treatment is surgical excision, but some patients may receive adjunctive treatment with drugs that either inhibit CRH-ACTH secretion (cyproheptadine, sodium valproate, bromocriptine, and octreotide), inhibit adrenal cortisol synthesis and secretion (aminoglutethimide, metyrapone, and ketoconazole), or adrenolytic agents (mitotane). Ketoconazole has proved to be most efficacious at achieving complete adrenal suppression. Therefore recipients require supplemental exogenous steroids. In addition, cushingoid patients are frequently treated with antihypertensive agents.

Glycoprotein (Thyroid-Stimulating Hormone, Follicle-Stimulating Hormone, Luteinizing Hormone)– Secreting tumors

The medical management of these tumors has not been fruitful. Early surgical resection offers the best chance of a cure. Delayed clinical presentation, however, can result in gross suprasellar tumor extension and involvement of the cavernous sinus with consequently poorer surgical results. Radiation therapy may be used to treat residual tumor.

Nonfunctioning Pituitary Tumors

The most common nonfunctioning tumors are null cell adenomas, craniopharyngiomas, and meningiomas. As already mentioned, metastatic tumors to the pituitary are rare. Craniopharyngiomas are often seen in children. Nonsecreting tumors usually present later than secreting tumors and therefore are often larger at diagnosis. Consequently, symptoms of panhypopituitarism and of increased ICP (i.e., bifrontal or bitemporal headache) are more frequent on presentation. Pressure from the tumor on neighboring structures may cause visual disturbances (classically a bitemporal hemianopsia) and symptoms related to the third, fourth, fifth, and sixth cranial nerves.

Panhypopituitarism

The complex manifestations of panhypopituitarism can be caused by tumors that destroy either normal pituitary or hypothalamic tissue or that exert pressure on vascular structures, interrupting the blood supply to these organs. Symptoms of panhypopituitarism may occur up to 2 years after radiation therapy to the pituitary gland for large tumors. Patients with panhypopituitarism show signs of anterior pituitary gland deficiency and are susceptible to hemodynamic instability and hypoglycemia during stressful periods, including surgery. Diabetes insipidus may not be present in these patients, in spite of ADH deficiency, because adrenocortical hormones are also necessary for the excretion of water. Only after steroid replacement therapy is initiated does massive diuresis begin. If panhypopituitarism develops acutely, hypothyroidism usually does not occur until later because of the long serum half-life of thyroxine.

Pituitary Apoplexy

Pituitary apoplexy (i.e., pituitary stroke) can be caused by hemorrhagic infarction and necrosis of a pituitary tumor (where large tumors compress and outgrow their blood supply or smaller adenomas bleed spontaneously). It can also be a consequence of head trauma and, although rare, may occur as a result of bromocriptine therapy.

Pituitary apoplexy can be acute or chronic. In the acute setting pituitary apoplexy may have the signs and symptoms of a subarachnoid hemorrhage. Hypotension, blindness, ophthalmoplegia, and manifestations of panhypopituitarism are other initial acute complications. Aggressive intervention is necessary, including steroid replacement and urgent surgery to decompress the surrounding structures.

SURGICAL APPROACH TO PITUITARY TUMORS

The timing of surgical removal of pituitary adenomas depends on the aggressiveness of the endocrinologist and the neurosurgeon. In general, surgical intervention is indicated for (1) pituitary apoplexy, (2) pituitary macroadenomas, (3) active acromegaly, (4) poorly responding or suprasellar prolactinomas, (5) active ACTH-secreting pituitary tumors, especially in adults, and (6) failure of prior therapy to control symptoms or growth of the adenoma.

Approximately 95% of pituitary adenomas can be treated surgically by the transsphenoidal approach, with the remainder requiring a frontal craniotomy. The choice is based on the anatomy of the lesion, the size of the sella, its mineralization, and the size and pneumatization of the sinuses. A craniotomy is generally performed if there is (1) minimal or disproportionately little enlargement of the sella relative to a large suprasellar mass, (2) extrasellar extension into the middle fossa with the extrasellar greater than the intrasellar volume, (3) presence of unrelated complicating pathologic features (e.g., a parasellar aneurysm), or (4) an unusually fibrous tumor.

The standard transsphenoidal approach allows direct visualization of the pituitary gland and pathologic features, is well tolerated by even the frail and elderly, and completely conceals all incisions. As a consequence of the removal of the bony confines of the sella turcica, any recurrence of disease tends to follow the path of least resistance into the sphenoid sinus rather than extending into intracranial regions.

In the transsphenoidal approach an incision is made in the nasal septum, and a submucosal plane of dissection is carried out posteriorly and inferiorly along the nasal septum. A second sublabial incision is made to create a large inferior submucosal tunnel along the floor of the nose. The two tunnels are joined posteriorly, the cartilaginous nasal septum is disarticulated from the maxillary ridge, and the entire nasal septum is dislocated to the side. The face of the sphenoid sinus is exposed and the bony septum removed. A speculum is inserted and aligned with the sella turcica under flouroscopic guidance (Fig. 12-2). The floor of the sella is exposed and carefully removed, usually laterally from one cavernous sinus to the other and superiorly near the junction of the floor of the anterior fossa and the sella. This method allows for excellent exposure of the anterior pituitary gland. Occasionally the more superior aspects of the gland are brought down into view by injecting air or nitrous oxide into the

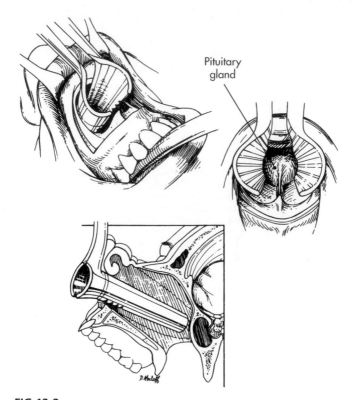

Pituitary
gland

FIG 12-2.
Schematic representation of sella turcica and pituitary gland as seen
during transsphenoidal surgery. Speculum is placed once bony septum of sphenoid sinus is removed. (Courtesy E.R. Laws, Jr., M.D.)

subarachnoid space or draining cerebrospinal fluid (CSF) through a
previously placed lumbar drain.

After excavation of the pituitary adenoma, closure of the wound
is achieved by packing the sella with muscle or fat, or in some instances, Gelfoam. This step prevents postoperative CSF rhinorrhea
and assists in achieving hemostasis of the sella. Next, the sellar floor
is reconstructed with remnants of the bony or cartilaginous nasal

---

BOX 12-1.
Complications of
Transsphenoidal
Hypophysectomy

Hemorrhage
Visual loss
Persistent CSF leak
Panhypopituitarism
Stroke/vascular injury
Meningitis/intracranial
    abscess
Oculomotor palsy
Facial numbness/pain
Diabetes insipidus
Nasal deformity

---

septum. The nasal septum is also reconstructed and the primary mucosal incisions closed. The nostrils are then packed with petroleum jelly or bacitracin-impregnated gauze rolls.

Complications of this surgery (Box 12-1) are uncommon but include hemorrhage, damage to the hypothalamus or other intracranial structures (e.g., internal carotid arteries, cavernous sinus, optic nerves, or other cranial nerves within the cavernous sinus), and CSF rhinorrhea with or without meningitis. Temporary or permanent anterior pituitary dysfunction and, occasionally, diabetes insipidus can be expected postoperatively. Stroke or aneurysm formation resulting from thrombosis, vasospasm, or surgical trauma to the internal carotid artery during the dissection occurs in <1% of cases.

PREOPERATIVE ASSESSMENT AND RELATED INTRAOPERATIVE CONCERNS

In addition to the routine assessment done on all neurosurgical patients, specific inquiries regarding symptoms and their progression or amelioration by pharmacologic intervention and any acute changes in their condition should be made. Details of the endocrine evaluation, current laboratory results of hormone replacement therapy and serum Ca^{2+}, Na^+, K^+, and glucose, and any report of visual field assessment should be noted. Reports of computed tomograms, magnetic resonance imaging, or cerebral angiograms are valuable and should be reviewed with the neurosurgeons before surgery. This information will help to determine the surgical approach and patient positioning and will suggest particular monitoring or intravascular access requirements. As always, a physical examination with particular attention paid to neurologic function is essential to enable comparison with postoperative findings in the operating room or postanesthesia care unit.

Headaches are generally associated with macroadenomas or craniopharyngiomas with extensive suprasellar extension. When accompanied by papilledema, nausea, and vomiting, headaches are highly suggestive of third ventricle obstruction and increased ICP. Note that cranial bone pain may be found in acromegaly. In either case ICP precautions should be taken during the perioperative anesthetic management (i.e., no preoperative sedation, the head and neck should be kept midline and maintained elevated at least 10 degrees), the patient should be hyperventilated on induction, and the use of diuretics to lower ICP should be considered.

Complaints of facial pain, facial numbness, or diplopia usually connote lateral extension of tumor into the cavernous sinus. Besides the concern for sparing any further damage to the cranial nerves involved, the possibility of catastrophic hemorrhage from the cavernous sinus or the internal carotid artery must be anticipated and adequate venous access obtained. Of special note, GH-secreting tumors can be associated with massive dilatation of all intracranial arteries and the possibility of a giant cavernous aneurysm must be ruled out. Venous air embolism is also a potential threat when dissection around the cavernous sinus is anticipated in the patient who is positioned with the operative field elevated above the right atrium of the heart. Precautions include the use of precordial Doppler monitoring, end-tidal nitrogen, and carbon dioxide monitoring, and placement of a multiorifice central venous catheter at the junction of the superior vena cava and right atrium. Nitrous oxide should be avoided.

The airway of the acromegalic patient must be carefully evaluated because the disease is associated with multiple alterations in the pharyngeal osseous and soft tissues (Box 12-2). Macroglossia; hypertrophy of the lips, epiglottis, and vocal cords; redundancy of pharyngeal and laryngeal mucosa; lengthening of the hypopharynx; and prognathism produce narrowing of the the airway and difficulty with mask ventilation and direct laryngoscopy. Any history of hoarseness, stridor, dyspnea, or obstructive sleep apnea should be

---

BOX 12-2.
Anesthetic Concerns in Acromegalic Patient

Airway
   Prognathism
   Macroglossia
   Hypertrophy of lips and epiglottis
   Thickened and stiff vocal cords
   Recurrent laryngeal nerve palsy
   Elongated hypopharynx
   Redundant and polypoid pharyngeal mucosa
   Subglottic narrowing
Cardiac failure, arrhythmias, coronary artery disease
Hypertension
Diabetes mellitus
Proximal muscle weakness, peripheral sensory loss
Carpal tunnel syndrome with poor collateral blood flow

---

sought. Occasionally recurrent laryngeal nerve paralysis occurs as a result of excessive thyroid cartilage growth. The difficult acromegalic airway should be managed awake either with direct laryngoscopy or fiberoptic bronchoscopy after appropriate topical anesthesia is established. The requirement for a smaller than usual endotracheal tube should be anticipated.

The anesthetic management of the patient with Cushing's disease is notable only for the physiologic effects engendered by excess cortisol secretion. Poorly controlled hypertension, hypokalemia, hyperglycemia, skeletal muscle weakness, and obesity will require the usual precautions with respect to blood pressure, serum electrolyte and glucose monitoring, and the monitoring of neuromuscular blockade.

ANESTHETIC MANAGEMENT
Choice of Anesthetic

The induction and maintenance of anesthesia is not limited to any one technique in pituitary surgery except, as already noted previously, in the case of the patient who requires ICP precautions. The only requirement is that the patient not move during the microdissection and that the patient be sufficiently lucid at the conclusion of surgery to allow a prompt, reliable neurologic exam. These conditions can be met with any combination of intravenous or inhalational agents now available.

Positioning

A frontal craniotomy usually requires the patient to be supine with the head supported either on a Mayfield horseshoe headrest or fixed in Mayfield tongs at a slight elevation. The transsphenoidal approach requires the patient to be in a semirecumbent position with the head elevated and turned slightly to the right while supported on a Mayfield horseshoe headrest. This position allows the surgeon to stand at the patient's right side and directly view the pituitary gland with the operating microscope while simultaneously permitting the head to be centered within the C-arm of a fluoroscopic image intensifier (Fig. 12-3). This setup requires that the endotracheal tube be carefully taped to the lower jaw or sutured to the teeth on the left side of the mouth. In addition, we recommend the placement of an orogastric tube for evacuation of blood and other contents of the stomach before extubation. Good eye protection with commercially available disposable goggles is also highly recommended.

Monitoring

In general, routine noninvasive monitors are acceptable for transsphenoidal surgery. An arterial line for continuous monitoring of blood pressure and frequent blood gases is placed in accordance with the usual indications (e.g., significant history of coronary artery disease, cardiac arrhythmias, severe pulmonary disease, or if intracranial vascular structures are involved in the dissection and massive bleeding is likely). In a frontal craniotomy approach we routinely place an arterial catheter. Particular care must be taken when such monitors are placed in the acromegalic patient. These patients have a high incidence of carpal tunnel syndrome and have a higher chance of arterial thrombosis and poorer collateral blood flow with radial artery cannulation.

As previously noted, precordial Doppler ultrasound, and end-tidal nitrogen and carbon dioxide monitoring is valuable in situations where considerable dissection around the cavernous sinus or an extreme head-up position is required. Similar monitoring might be considered at any time in patients with a history of cardiac septal defects where even subclinical air embolism could be catastrophic.

Although rarely used in our institution, visual evoked potentials could be used to monitor the integrity of the visual system during

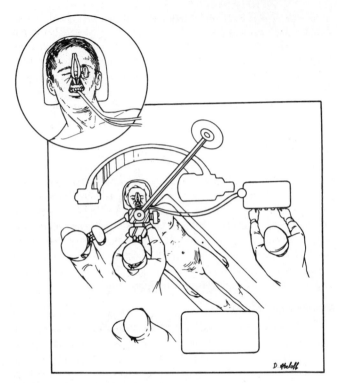

FIG 12-3.
Diagram of typical operating room arrangement for transsphenoidal pituitary surgery. (Courtesy E.R. Laws, Jr., M.D.)

dissection around the optic nerves, optic chiasm, and optic tract. Unfortunately, resection of the tumor often does not restore deficits in the visual field and frequently, in the more difficult dissections, new lesions in the optic tract are produced, which are unavoidable even with careful monitoring. In addition, visual evoked potentials are sensitive to many anesthetic agents that may be used in the management of the patient.

Emergence

Emergence from anesthesia after a transsphenoidal hypophysectomy requires special precautions relative to the airway. First, any throat packs placed intraoperatively should be removed. Before extubation the stomach should be evacuated of blood that might have drained from the posterior pharynx to minimize the tendency to vomit in the postanesthesia care unit. Finally, before the patient awakens and before extubation, an oral airway should be inserted. With the nose packed, postextubation upper airway obstruction frequently occurs despite adequate emergence and reversal of muscle relaxant. The oral airway forces the patient to breathe through the mouth until fully cognizant of the situation.

Caveats

Occasionally the elderly or the hypertensive patient on long-term beta-blocker therapy will become extremely hypertensive when the nasal passages are packed with phenylephrine-soaked pledgets or injected with epinephrine-containing local anesthetics. Alpha-adrenergic receptor activation can be briefly opposed with phentolamine (Regitine), 30 to 70 μg/kg given intravenously.

POSTOPERATIVE CONSIDERATIONS

At our institution we do not routinely monitor all posthypophysectomy patients in the neurosurgical intensive care unit unless specific intraoperative complications indicate such care. The majority of our patients are extubated in the operating room and recover in the postanesthesia care unit before they are discharged to a nursing floor skilled in postoperative neurosurgical care. Surgically induced trauma to the pituitary gland may result in specfic postoperative complications that must be recognized and treated.

HORMONAL SUPPLEMENTATION

Surgery and excision of pituitary tissue may decrease the ability of the remaining pituitary gland to respond to the perioperative stress situation. Most physicians therefore believe that perioperative steroid supplementation is necessary. Steroid coverage can be achieved in many different ways. We usually administer 100 mg of hydrocortisone intravenously 6 to 8 hours before and again on induction of anesthesia, followed by 50 to 100 mg boluses every 6 to 8 hours. Alternatively, a constant infusion of 10 to 15 mg of hydrocortisone/hr (100 mg of hydrocortisone in 500 ml at 50 to 75 ml/hr) can be used. Most patients with microadenomas require steroid replacement only up to the third or fourth postoperative day, after which the dose can be tapered quickly.

Thyroid hormone replacement is rarely indicated in the euthyroid patient while in the operating room because of thyroxin's long half-life of 7 days. Patients with persistent postoperative panhypopituitarism, however, require thyroxin replacement therapy. If needed, 500 μg of L-thyroxine may be given intravenously and continued at 1 to 1.3 μg/kg every 24 hours in patients with severe hypothyroidism. Alternatively, for less severe cases, oral thyroid replacement with 0.1 to 0.15 mg L-thyroxine daily is sufficient. Extreme care should be taken when giving thyroxin to patients with coronary artery disease because it may precipitate cardiac ischemia.

Preexisting diabetes mellitus or perioperative glucocorticoid administration may require perioperative management to maintain serum glucose levels at an acceptable level (<250 mg/dl). Administration of regular insulin given intravenously titrated to desired glucose concentrations provides the most reliable means of serum glucose control.

DIABETES INSIPIDUS

Transient diabetes insipidus, usually lasting <7 days, develops in about 40% of all patients after pituitary surgery. It typically develops as a result of direct surgical trauma or local edema at the surgical site. Diabetes insipidus rarely expresses itself in the operating room but may be seen in the postanesthesia care unit or early postoperative period, typically within the first 12 to 24 hours. The initial manifestation is polyuria, with urine volume typically in the range of 150 to 200 ml/hr but at times up to 2 L/hr. The urine specific gravity and osmolality is low in the face of a high serum osmolality. Once the diagnosis is confirmed, therapy should be initiated as outlined in Chapter 5. Nasal packing in the early postoperative period will usually prevent the administration of intranasal 1-deamino-8-D-arginine vasopressin (DDAVP), and alternative routes (subcutaneous, intramuscular) should be used.

CEREBROSPINAL FLUID RHINORRHEA

Postoperative CSF rhinorrhea is uncommon after transsphenoidal pituitary surgery, but some patients have a transient CSF leak that presents as CSF rhinorrhea. Generally no therapy is necessary; however, in these patients there is a communication of the sub-arachnoid space with the atmosphere and an intracranial infection is more likely to develop. If the leak persists, intermittent CSF drainage through a lumbar subarachnoid catheter or repeated lumbar punctures may decrease the pressure gradient and allow the leak to seal. If surgical closure is required, nitrous oxide should be avoided (because nitrogen is in the subarachnoid space) to prevent the development of tension pneumocephalus.

POSTOPERATIVE PAIN

A common patient complaint after pituitary surgery is headache. The pain is usually transient and is most prominent over the first 24 hours. Nonsteroidal and narcotic analgesics usually provide adequate symptomatic relief. Many patients, however, have minimal or no postoperative pain. The pituitary gland has the highest brain concentrations of beta-endorphins, which may be released during surgical manipulation and may provide some early postoperative endogenous pain control.

Suggested Readings

Fahlbusch R, Honegger J, Buchfelder M: Surgical management of acromegaly, *Endocrinol Metab Clin North Am* 21:669, 1992.

Kammerer WA: The anesthetic management of transsphenoidal pituitary surgery, *Prog Anesth* 7:82, 1993.

Laws E Jr: Functional pituitary tumors: the neurosurgeon and neuroendocrinology, *Clin Neurosurg* 27:3, 1980.

Laws E Jr, Abboud CF, Kern EB: Perioperative management of patients with pituitary microadenoma, *Neurosurgery* 7:566, 1980.

Laws E Jr, Piepgras DG, Randall RV, et al: Neurosurgical management of acromegaly: results in 82 patients treated between 1972 and 1977, *J Neurosurg* 50:454, 1979.

Messick J Jr, Laws E Jr, Abboud CF: Anesthesia for transsphenoidal surgery of the hypophyseal region, *Anesth Analg* 57:206, 1978.

PEDIATRIC NEUROANESTHESIA

13

Terrance A. Yemen

Pediatric neuroanesthesia requires the knowledge and skills of both neuroanesthesia and pediatric anesthesia; children are not small adults. The development of the central nervous system (CNS) is incomplete at birth and undergoes profound maturation during the first year of life. Pediatric anatomy, physiologic features, and pharmacology change significantly until adulthood. These differences are most pronounced in the premature and newborn infant. Successful pediatric neuroanesthesia requires an understanding of the disease processes that affect neonates, infants, and older children. Last, familiarity with the surgical procedures to ameliorate or correct these problems is essential.

ANATOMIC AND PHYSICAL CHARACTERISTICS

The craniospinal compartment is a single continuous space and is well developed to protect the vulnerable neural tissue of the brain and spinal cord. This space is limited by the calvaria and vertebral column and includes the brain parenchyma, which consists of neurons, glial tissue, and interstitial fluid. The parenchyma comprises 70% of the brain by volume, with the cerebrospinal fluid, cerebral blood volume, and extracellular fluids comprising the remaining 30%. An increase in volume of any of one these elements, whether it be caused by tumor growth, hydrocephalus, hemorrhage, or traumatic edema, can result in the compression of vital tissues and the displacement of neural structures. Generally speaking, the cranium functions as a closed box with a fixed volume. A change in volume eventually produces a rise in intracranial pressure (ICP), and this rise is the keystone of neuroanesthesia.

At birth the brain weighs approximately 300 to 400 g and accounts for 10% to 15% of the total body weight. The brain grows rapidly and doubles in weight within 6 months, weighing 900 g at 1 year of age, and reaching its mature weight of 1200 g by age 12 years. By adulthood the brain comprises only 2% of the total body weight.

The calvaria at birth consists of ossified plates separated by fibrous sutures and fontanelles. There are two fontanelles at birth. The posterior fontanelle closes at 2 or 3 months of age, with the anterior fontanelle remaining open until 1 to 1½ years. During the postpubescent years the fontanelles ossify.

There is a mistaken impression that the unossified fontanelles provide the infant with a unique capability to accommodate acute increases in intracranial volume. However, the dura mater in the osteofibrous cranium is not easily distended, offering a high resistance to any acute increase in volume. The ability to accommodate an acute increase in ICP is limited, if not nonexistent. A slow increase in volume can be accommodated by an expansion of fontanelles and separation of the cranial suture lines over a period of weeks or months.

The intracranial space is divided into two compartments by a layer of dura mater called the tentorium cerebelli. The supratentorial compartment is the largest of the two and is occupied by two hemispheres. Each hemisphere consists of three lobes: frontal, temporal, and parietooccipital. The diencephalon forms the center of the supratentorial compartment and includes the thalamus, hypothalamus, epithalamus, and subthalamus. It is particularly vulnerable to involvement by neoplasms or ischemia.

The posterior cranial fossa consists of the cerebellum, pons, and medulla oblongata and is covered by the inferior and anterior segments of the occipital bone. Mass lesions in this area may compromise cardiorespiratory centers or the cranial nerves. Increases in ICP, produced by pathologic disorders in this area, can cause herniation of the cerebellar tonsils, most notably the vermis, through the foramen magnum and produce a "pressure cone" phenomenon.

The spinal cord is the continuation of medulla and occupies a significant fraction of the CNS by volume. The caudal end of the spinal cord reaches its adult position, at the space between intervertebral disk L1 and L2, by 8 years of age. The intradural space is much longer than the spinal cord and ends at approximately S2. This space, from the end of the spinal cord to the end of the dura, represents a reservoir of cerebrospinal fluid (CSF) and serves as a relief mechanism when ICP increases. Because the spinal compartment has greater compliance than the posterior cranial fossa, acute decompression of the spinal compartment may precipitate herniation of the posterior fossa contents through the foramen magnum.

CSF production, and its circulation, begins during the eighth week of intrauterine life. The choroid plexuses, which produce CSF, are located in the temporal horns of the lateral ventricles, the posterior portion of the third ventricle, and the roof of the fourth ventricle. The meningeal and ependymal vessels of the brain and spinal cord contribute a very small amount of CSF. At birth CSF production is approximately 0.35 ml/min and, in the absence of disease states, production and absorption exist in equilibrium. CSF from the ventricular system exits from the fourth ventricle, through the foramina of Magendie and Luschka, and enters the subarachnoid space surrounding the brain and spinal cord. Absorption of CSF occurs in the arachnoid villi that project into the veins and sinuses of the brain. Normally ICP is closely related to cerebral blood flow and cerebral volume, not to CSF production. The reduction of CSF production by one third produces a decrease in ICP by only 1 mm Hg. Obviously, drugs that reduce CSF production will have minimal effects on ICP.

PEDIATRIC NEUROPHYSIOLOGY

To understand neuroanesthesia and its effect on the patient it is necessary to understand the basic principles of neurophysiology.

The human brain represents a complex biologic structure. Inherent in this complexity is a myriad of synaptic connections and intracellular message systems that mediate interneuronal communications. The energy required to maintain this system is considerable. At 8 years of age the brain weighs a mere 2% of total body weight, but it consumes more than 20% of all adenosine triphosphate produced in the body. The primary substrate for cerebral energy production is glucose. Glucose depletion rapidly leads to coma and eventually brain death. The minuscule cerebral stores of glucose and glycogen are incapable of providing more than 3 minutes of adenosine triphosphate consumption. The brain is therefore entirely dependent on the cerebral circulation for glucose. The neonatal brain appears to have greater glycogen stores than the adult, which may explain why they appear more resistant to oxygen deprivation. The cerebral metabolic rate of children is higher than that of adults (5.8 vs 3.5 ml of oxygen/min/100 g brain tissue and 6.8 vs 5.5 mg of glucose/min/100 g of tissue).

Cerebral blood flow (CBF) is readily altered by the anesthesiologist. Because CBF is directly related to cerebral blood volume, control of CBF can be used to alter ICP. Although disease states may alter this relationship, controlling CBF represents the most effective tool the anesthesiologist has to manage ICP.

Values for CBF in premature and newborn infants are 40 ml/100 g/min. In infants and small children between 6 to 40 months old, CBF is approximately 90 ml/100 g/min, and it continues to rise until 11 years of age, at which time CBF is 100 ml/100 g/min. The CBF of gray matter is higher than that of white matter, and areas of predominant brain activity change as children develop. The cerebral metabolic rate of oxygen ($CMRo_2$) of children 3 to 12 years of age is 5.2 ml oxygen/100 g/min, but in newborns and infants it is only 2.3 ml oxygen/100 g/min.

CBF is autoregulated, maintaining a constant oxygen delivery over a wide range of perfusion pressures. Although the values for adults are known, the autoregulatory thresholds for infants and children are not well known. Neonatal animal models suggest the lower limit may be around 40 mm Hg and the upper limit at 90 mm Hg.

Neonates in severe distress have impaired or abolished autoregulation, which may be worsened by hypoxia, vasodilators, or high concentrations of volatile anesthetics. As in adults, hyperventilation is reported to restore autoregulation. Trauma, areas of inflammation surrounding tumors, abscesses, or sites of focal ischemia can also alter autoregulation and lead to intraventricular hemorrhage.

In adults CBF varies linearly with the arterial carbon dioxide partial pressure (Pa_{CO_2}) for values between 20 and 80 mm Hg. A 1 mm Hg fall in Pa_{CO_2} results in a 4% decrease in CBF. These changes are the result of periarteriolar changes in pH. Chronic hyperventilation produces a slow movement of bicarbonate ions out of the CSF, and the pH normalizes within 24 hours. Alternatively, sudden increases in the Pa_{CO_2} can result in cerebral vasodilatation and increased ICP. Recent studies in anesthetized infants and children demonstrated that CBF velocity changes logarithmically and directly with the end-tidal carbon dioxide concentration.

The cerebral vascular responses to hypoxia are not well known in children. In older infants CBF does appear to increase rapidly at arterial oxygen partial pressure (Pa_{O_2}) values below 50 mm Hg. Administration of 100% oxygen in these circumstances can reduce CBF substantially.

Cerebral perfusion pressure is more important than CBF in determining the adequacy of blood flow to the brain. Cerebral perfusion pressure (CPP) is the mean arterial pressure (MAP) minus the central venous pressure (CVP). In the case of the intact cranium, it is the MAP minus the ICP, when ICP exceeds the CVP. Monitoring CPP, especially in a compromised brain, is a valuable guide to the maintenance of adequate cerebral perfusion.

PATHOPHYSIOLOGY OF INCREASED INTRACRANIAL PRESSURE

An increase in ICP constitutes one of the most serious pathophysiologic derangements in pediatric neuroanesthesia. The cranium is a closed space occupied by a relatively incompressible brain mass, with changes in the volume of CSF serving as the primary buffer. When this compensatory mechanism is no longer effective, ICP increases.

The normal ICP of children is between 2 and 4 mm Hg, lower than that measured in adults. Newborns have a positive ICP value on the day of birth but then exhibit a subatmospheric ICP in early life. This is believed to represent the contraction of the intracerebral volume caused by the loss of total body salt and water during the first few days after birth. Unfortunately, this negative ICP can promote intraventricular hemorrhage, especially in the premature infant.

To understand the pathophysiology and management of elevated ICP, it is necessary to be familiar with the intracranial compliance curve (Fig. 13-1). A review of the curve demonstrates that when small volume changes occur in one compartment, compensation is possible, with only a small change in pressure. However, if the increase in volume continues, the noncompliant portion of the curve will be reached. Small changes in volume will then produce large, and potentially dangerous, increases in ICP.

The pressure-volume index (PVI) is an assessment of intracranial compliance, such that $PVI = \Delta V / \log_{10}(P_p/P_o)$. In normal adults a volume change of 25 ml is required to raise the baseline ICP by a factor of 10, but in infants the normal PVI is only 10 ml because PVI is proportional to the neural axis volume. The ICP of infants and children can be expected to rise much faster than in adults. Children can progress from neurologically intact to moribund in a short period of time. The goal of the anesthesiologist in such circumstances is (1) shift the patient's intracranial compliance curve, (2) change the slope of the patient's compliance curve, and (3) move the patient along his/her own curve to a more desirable position.

Hydrocephalus is the result of an increase in CSF within the ventricular system, whether caused by obstruction of CSF circulation or

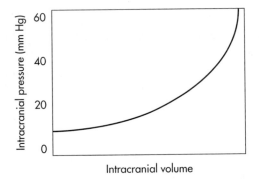

FIG 13-1.
Intracranial compliance curve. Initial changes in volume are accommodated with slight rise in ICP. Further increases result in sharp rise in pressure.

by reduced absorption. In premature and newborn infants hydrocephalus is usually a result of intraventricular hemorrhage, aqueductal stenosis, or Arnold-Chiari malformation. Neonatal hydrocephalus may exist despite a normal ICP. An increase in CSF volume is accommodated by a decrease in brain mass until the compliance limit of the immature calvaria is reached. The Arnold-Chiari malformation results in the brainstem being displaced downward, along with the abnormal vermis, to extend below the foramen magnum and into the cervical canal. The fourth ventricle is subsequently compressed and the foramina obstructed. Other causes of hydrocephalus include the mucopolysaccharidoses, which obliterate the subarachnoid space, and chondroplastic disorders, in which there is alteration of occipital bone growth and impediment of venous outflow. In later childhood brain tumors become the most common cause of hydrocephalus.

The second most common neoplasm in children is a primary brain tumor, which accounts for 20% of all cancers in children and 20% of all childhood cancer deaths. The incidence of intracranial tumors is approximately 3.1 per 100,000 in children <15 years old. Fifty percent of childhood brain tumors occur in the posterior fossa and are frequently associated with an obstructive hydrocephalus. Medulloblastomas comprise about 20% of all CNS tumors in children and usually involve the fourth ventricle. A posterior fossa tumor is suspected in all children who have raised ICP or who have cranial nerve defects. Choroid plexus papillomas are the only known cause of CSF overproduction and hydrocephalus.

Brain tumors are expanding, space-occupying lesions that eventually result in increased ICP and a reduction in CPP. Vessels that grow with these tumors are nonautoregulated. They contribute to peritumoral vascular edema, which aggravates increases in ICP. Administration of dexamethasone, mannitol, hypertonic saline solution, or furosemide may secondarily decrease ICP by reducing the edema surrounding the tumors.

Regarding the complications of elevated ICP, when a mass effect occurs, the brain may be extruded from one compartment to another when the limits of compensation or buffering have been exceeded. For example, as a mass expands in one hemisphere, a cerebral artery in the adjacent hemisphere may be compressed, producing ischemia, more edema, and further increases in ICP. Distortion of posterior fossa contents by a mass effect may obstruct the outflow of CSF and lead to obstructive hydrocephalus. Increases in ICP may also produce global or regional cerebral ischemia. As the ICP approaches the MAP, the CPP falls below critical levels. The result is tissue hypoxia, cell injury or death, and more edema. A vicious cycle ensues, increasing brain volume and ICP. Therefore the treatment of raised ICP may be directed at several points: (1) relieve the obstruction of CSF outflow, (2) reduce CSF production, (3) reduce cerebral ischemia by reducing ICP, (4) reduce vasogenic edema around the tumor, and (5) shrink the volume of the tumor itself. All of these can, singly or additively, be effective in reducing ICP.

NEUROPHARMACOLOGY

Infants, particularly newborns, demonstrate increased sensitivity to sedatives, hypnotics, and narcotics. Concerns regarding the increased sensitivity of infants to intravenous drugs are supported by animal studies that suggest that mean lethal doses for many medications are considerably lower in infants than in adults. The response to these drugs is also extremely variable from one infant to another. Some neonates are very tolerant of a given sedative, whereas others may be very sensitive to the same drug. These medications must be slowly titrated to effect, thereby avoiding life-threatening cardiorespiratory depression. Generalizations regarding narcotic dosages in neonates are best avoided.

The response to volatile agents is also altered and the appropriate use of volatile anesthetic agents is directly related to age. The minimum alveolar concentration (MAC) in neonates is considerably lower than that of infants aged 1 to 6 months. Severely premature infants have a further reduction in MAC values. In contrast, children older than 6 months have an increased MAC value, even compared with adults. To avoid significant cardiovascular depression in the neonate, inspired concentrations of the volatile agents must be reduced, accounting for age-related reductions in MAC. For older infants who have elevated MAC values, increased concentrations of volatile agents must be given. Unfortunately, increased concentrations reduce the therapeutic window of safety with respect to the cardiovascular system. Therefore, similar to the sedatives and narcotics, volatile agents must also be carefully titrated to provide adequate anesthesia without producing cardiovascular collapse.

Clinically, nitrous oxide (N_2O) increases CBF and ICP in both adults and children. Together barbiturates and hypocapnia may prevent this increase. In contrast, volatile agents will further increase CBF. In addition, N_2O can increase cerebral metabolic rates. N_2O, although commonly used in many areas of neuroanesthesia, should be curtailed when dealing with increased ICP or when cerebral perfusion is already reduced.

Halothane is an excellent anesthetic drug for inducing anesthesia in children; however, it is a potent cerebral vasodilator, with increases in CBF occurring in a dose-dependent fashion. In normal children cerebral vascular resistance decreases between 0.5 and 1.0 MAC halothane, without further decreases at 1.5 MAC. The decrease in cerebral vascular resistance results in an increase in CBF and volume and an increase in ICP. Cerebral vascular reactivity to carbon dioxide during halothane anesthesia is preserved between 0.5 and 1.0 MAC, but the vasoconstrictor effect of 20 mm Hg of carbon dioxide is not as strong at 1.0 MAC as it is at 0.5 MAC. Halothane should therefore be avoided in children with raised ICP, or at least until the dura is opened.

The pungency of isoflurane makes it unsuitable for inhalational induction; it is nonetheless the most popular of all the volatile agents in pediatric neuroanesthesia. Isoflurane increases CBF less than halothane at all equivalent MAC doses. In addition, there is some belief that isoflurane may provide cerebral protection. The effect on autoregulation is less with isoflurane than with halothane. In children isoflurane has minimal impact on the cerebral vascular reactivity to arterial pressure of carbon dioxide (Pco_2). Although isoflurane does increase ICP to the same degree as halothane in animal models, it should be used with caution in children with raised ICP, particularly if hypercapnia cannot be achieved.

In adults sevoflurane has the same effect on CBF, $CMRo_2$, and ICP as does isoflurane. However, studies involving children are lacking at this point. In animal models sevoflurane appears to induce smaller increases in ICP than does isoflurane.

Desflurane increases CBF and decreases $CMRo_2$ in animals. Desflurane increases ICP significantly in children with supratentorial mass lesions. This change occurs despite hypocapnia.

Barbiturates decrease CBF and $CMRo_2$ in a dose-dependent manner and they reduce ICP. Barbiturates can be used to prevent increases in ICP during laryngoscopy and intubation. Cerebral autoregulation and cerebral vascular reactivity to Pco_2 are not affected by barbiturates. Barbiturates can significantly reduce myocardial contractility, systemic arterial blood pressures, and CPPs. Therefore they must be used with caution to maximize their beneficial effects while avoiding profound cardiovascular depression. Barbiturates are also effective in controlling epileptiform activities, although methohexital has been shown to activate seizure activity in children with temporal lobe or pychomotor epilepsy. It has not induced seizures in children with generalized seizure disorders, and the use of rectal methohexital as an anesthetic induction agent is not contraindicated in children with generalized seizure disorders.

Etomidate reduces CBF and $CMRo_2$ and directly vasoconstricts cerebral vasculature. Cerebral vascular reactivity to Pco_2 is retained. Its major advantage as an induction agent is the absence of profound cardiovascular depression.

Propofol is a rapidly acting agent that reduces CBF, $CMRo_2$, and ICP. Few data are available regarding its use in pediatric neurosurgery. Like the barbiturates, it should be used with caution because reductions in MAP may jeopardize CPP in patients with raised ICP.

Benzodiazepines produce the effect of decreasing CBF, $CMRo_2$, and ICP.

Opiates have little or no effect on CBF, $CMRo_2$, or ICP. Fentanyl in combination with nitrous oxide decreases CBF, $CMRo_2$, and cerebral autoregulation. Cerebral vascular reactivity to Pco_2 is not affected. In neonates fentanyl has no effect on the cerebral circulation. Fentanyl reduces CSF reabsorption by at least 50%. Alfentanil increases CSF pressures in patients with brain tumors. This increase is less than that observed with sufentanil but is greater than that observed with fentanyl.

Ketamine is a potent cerebral vasodilator that increases CBF by 50% or more in subjects with normocapnia. There is little or no effect on the $CMRo_2$. Because of ketamine's potential to increase ICP, it is contraindicated in all patients at risk of increased ICP.

Muscle relaxants, as a whole, have little or no effect on cerebral circulation. In children with decreased intracranial compliance, succinylcholine can produce an initial fall in ICP followed by a rise. The increase in ICP can be reduced by the prior administration of general anesthesia or by precurarization. Life-threatening hyperkalemia may occur after the administration of succinylcholine to patients with closed head injuries, severe cerebral hypoxia, subarachnoid hemorrhage, and cerebral vascular accidents. Hyperkalemia has occurred in patients without motor deficits. When the use of succinylcholine in children is considered, the benefit of rapid control of the airway must be weighed against the risks of increasing ICP and hyperkalemia.

The nondepolarizing muscle relaxants have little or no effect on cerebral blood volume, $CMRo_2$, or ICP. However, large doses of curare, atracurium, or metocurare cause histamine release and transient cerebral vascular dilation, which results in a slight and transient increase in ICP. Vecuronium is known for its lack of autonomic effects. There is a slight decrease in ICP with its use. In older children the absence of cardiovascular activity combined with its lack of effect on $CMRo_2$, cerebral vascular reactivity, CBF, and a slight decrease in ICP make vecuronium an ideal muscle relaxant for neurosurgery. However, the concomitant use of vecuronium with a potent opioid, such as sufentanil, can result in profound bradycardia in young infants unless a vagolytic agent is given in advance.

PREOPERATIVE ASSESSMENT

The preoperative anesthetic evaluation of the child undergoing neurosurgery includes the following: (1) an assessment of ICP, (2) an assessment of respiratory and cardiovascular centers, and (3) an assessment of specific disturbances in the patient's neurologic function.

Gradual ICP increases in infants may be noted by a history of increased irritability, poor feeding, lethargy, and vomiting. Bulging anterior fontanelles, dilated scalp veins, and motor deficits are not uncommon. Older children will often complain of morning headaches. If the ICP reaches a critical level, a decreased level of consciousness and signs of brainstem herniation are possible. Cervical spinal cord lesions may also affect respiratory and cardiovascular functions.

Laboratory examination is important in assessing electrolyte anomalies that may occur with the syndrome of inappropriate antidiuretic hormone or from protracted vomiting. Diabetes insipidus may result in hypernatremia. In the preoperative assessment drugs the patient is receiving, such as steroids, for increased ICP or antiseizure drugs, especially Dilantin, which profoundly affects the metabolism, and other drugs, including muscle relaxants, should be reviewed.

Premedication that results in marked sedation should be avoided. If sedatives are given, the patient must be closely monitored to prevent respiratory depression, hypercarbia, and increased ICP. A sedative preoperative medication is appropriate in children with intracranial vascular lesions. These children benefit from the sedation by avoiding the crying and distress that might precipitate a preoperative hemorrhage. The most important preoperative medication is the preoperative visit by the anesthesiologist. Providing a thorough explanation of the anesthetic care and answering any concerns comforts both the child and the parents, enabling them to cope with the circumstances.

PATIENT POSITIONING

Patient positioning varies in accordance with the neurosurgical procedure. The principles of positioning the infant and child for neurosurgery are no different than those of the adult. The eyes must be securely taped and protected, particularly if the patient is to be in a prone or sitting position. Vulnerable aspects of the arms, legs, and face, should be adequately protected by padding. Bolsters to decrease compression of the abdomen and thorax should be used and positioned appropriately.

The endotracheal tube must be securely taped in place, particularly in sitting and prone positions, to prevent displacement. The use of an antisialagogue to decrease secretions helps considerably in keeping the tape adhered to the skin. Some anesthesiologists advocate the use of nasal rather than oral endotracheal tubes in the prone position, believing that nasal tubes are easier to secure. When placing an endotracheal tube in children, it is important to know that movement of the head can result in kinking or movement of the endotracheal tube. The tube should be placed in the midtrachea so that extubation will not occur if the head is extended and will not advance into a mainstem bronchi if the head is flexed.

MONITORING

Monitoring children is similar to adults with use of a precordial stethoscope, electrocardiogram, noninvasive blood pressure measuring device, a temperature probe, pulse oximetry, and capnography. For most invasive neurosurgical procedures an indwelling arterial catheter is appropriate and can be inserted in either the radial, femoral, posterior tibial, or dorsalis pedis arteries. Monitoring for air emboli by a precordial Doppler monitor and end-tidal nitrogen is appropriate in sitting or head-up positions.

Peripheral nerve stimulators for monitoring neuromuscular blocks are desirable but not always practical in young infants. The use of traditional peripheral nerve stimulators can result in significant overestimation of the neuromuscular blockade. There may be an absence of the train of four and tetanus at the same time the infant is beginning to breathe and cough. The use of peripheral nerve stimulators in young infants should be viewed with skepticism and caution. Patient movement during intracranial surgery could be disastrous.

FLUID MANAGEMENT

The choice of fluids should be made on the premise that one is trying to maintain an isovolemic, isoosmolar, and relatively isooncotic intravascular volume. Traditional pediatric fluid requirements are 4 ml/kg for the first 10 kg of body weight, 2 ml/kg for the next 10 kg, and then 1 ml/kg for each kilogram of body weight over 40 kg. Balanced salt solutions, such as Ringer's lactate, are preferable to normal saline solution. Normal saline solution has a high chloride content and causes hyperchloremic acidosis, especially in infants. In patients with an intact blood-brain barrier, restricting crystalloid administration will help prevent expansion of extracellular fluid if salt solutions are used and expansion of the intracellular fluid volume if dextrose solutions are infused. However, if the blood-brain barrier is not intact, then both colloid and crystalloid solutions can extravasate into the extracellular fluid and increase ICP.

Blood loss in pediatric neurosurgery is often hard to estimate. Substantial blood loss is concealed by the surgical drapes and floor, making it difficult to measure. Serial hematocrit measurements are the most reliable method to ensure an adequate hemoglobin. It should be kept in mind that normal hemoglobin levels and blood volumes are age dependent. Normal blood volumes are 100 ml/kg in prematures, 90 ml/kg in newborns, 80 ml/kg in infants, and 70 ml/kg in older children. Normal hematocrits are 45% to 60% at birth, falling to 30% to 35% at 3 months of age. There is a gradual increase to adult levels over the next decade of life.

At birth a considerable fraction of the hemoglobin is hemoglobin F. It has a higher affinity for oxygen, which results in a reduced delivery of oxygen to peripheral tissues. By 6 months of age hemoglobin F is not a factor. The lowest safe hematocrit value has not been determined in children; however, values between 30% to 40%

in premature infants and newborns and 20% to 30% in children over 3 months old are used by most anesthesiologists. Blood losses should be replaced at a 3:1 ratio if crystalloid solutions are being used and a 1:1 ratio if colloid solutions are preferred.

Blood glucose levels should be monitored in all patients having prolonged anesthesia but neonates and infants are at particular risk. Although in the past 5% or 10% dextrose solutions were recommended to prevent hypoglycemia, the routine use of these solutions will result in substantial hyperglycemia in many infants and children. I recommend using 1% or 2% dextrose in a balanced salt solution, with frequent monitoring of the serum glucose to maintain normal levels. It should be remembered that normal levels for blood glucose are much lower in infants than adults, measuring 80 to 100 mg/dl in the adult and only 30 to 40 mg/dl in the newborn.

TEMPERATURE MAINTENANCE

Infants have twice the surface area to weight ratio of adults, placing them at greater risk of hypothermia. Heat loss occurs by conduction, convection, radiation, and evaporation. Heat loss is a particular problem in pediatric neurosurgery because 30% of convective heat loss occurs through the head in infants. With the head completely exposed for hours during cranial surgery, heat losses are often high.

Infants < 3 months old do not shiver; rather they rely on stores of brown fat. Hypothermia can result in increased oxygen requirements and may cause infants to become hypoxic, apneic, and produce metabolic acidosis. General anesthesia, intracranial hemorrhage, and prematurity inhibit the metabolic response to cold. Hypothermia reduces surfactant production, impairs coagulation, inhibits hypoxic pulmonary vasoconstriction, and may prolong drug action. Mild hypothermia can reduce $CMRO_2$ and is occasionally used to good effect in selected cases.

Unintentional hypothermia can often be avoided by having the operating room warm and the surgeons ready. Use a warming mattress on the operating bed and an overhead radiant heater during the induction. Warm anesthetic gases and intravenous fluids can all go a long way to prevent hypothermia. Surgeons can help by using warm skin and irrigation solutions.

DRUG THERAPY FOR INCREASED INTRACRANIAL PRESSURE

Osmotic diuretic therapy is common in neurosurgical procedures. Usually a 20% mannitol solution is used to reduce ICP and provide brain relaxation. Small doses of 0.25 to 0.5 g/kg will raise serum osmolality and reduce cerebral edema and ICP. The effect begins 10 to 15 minutes after administration and persists for about 2 hours. Some children show transient hemodynamic instability during the first 1 to 2 minutes after a rapid administration. Therefore mannitol should be given at a rate not to exceed 0.5 g/kg over 20 to 30 minutes. Loop diuretics may reduce brain edema by inducing a systemic diuresis and decreasing CSF production. Furosemide can reduce ICP, but it is not as effective as mannitol. The initial dose of furosemide should be 0.6 to 1 mg/kg. A dose of 0.3 to 0.4 mg/kg is used if combined with mannitol. Steroids can reduce edema around brain tumors, but hours or days may be required to produce an effect. The administration of dexamethasone preoperatively can improve the neurologic status.

HYDROCEPHALUS

Hydrocephalus is either congenital or acquired. It is caused by one of four processes: (1) congenital anomalies, (2) neoplasms, (3) inflammatory conditions, or (4) overproduction of CSF. Three types of ventricular shunts are currently in use: ventriculoperitoneal, ventriculoatrial, and ventriculopleural. Replacement and revision of these shunts is common, especially in severely neurologically impaired children.

Preoperative considerations must take into account the level of consciousness, evidence of vomiting, delayed gastric emptying, coexisting pathologic disorders, and age-related pathophysiologic features.

Induction techniques are chosen depending on the condition of the child. For children with minimally raised ICP and no nausea or vomiting, a mask induction works well. Anesthesia can also be induced with rectal methohexital 30 mg/kg. When there are concerns about a full stomach or clinical signs of elevated ICP, a modified rapid sequence intravenous induction technique is appropriate, by use of thiopental or propofol, lidocaine, a small amount of narcotic, and a nondepolarizing muscle relaxant. In children with increased ICP, placement of the endotracheal tube is a critical event. The increase in ICP that occurs with intubation can be reduced by introducing the tube quickly, avoiding patient bucking or coughing, and by the adjunctive use of thiopental and lidocaine.

Anesthesia is usually maintained with a volatile agent, N_2O, and occasionally a narcotic supplement. Modest controlled hyperventilation is used to maintain a Pco_2 between 25 and 30 mm Hg. The use of narcotics should be curtailed near the end of the procedure, particularly in children with severe neurologic deficits. These children are especially sensitive to narcotics and sedative-hypnotics.

Ventriculoperitoneal shunt placement is usually not associated with significant blood loss or third-space losses. However, the sudden removal of large volumes of CSF may provoke bradycardia and hypotension. Fluid management centers around the maintenance of intravascular volume. Volume losses associated with drug-induced diuresis or with vomiting are replaced with a balanced salt solution.

Effort should be made to prevent inadvertent hypothermia because these children will have the entire head, thorax, and abdomen exposed throughout the surgery.

At the end of the procedure neuromuscular relaxants are reversed. If the patient is hemodynamically stable and has a temperature >35° C, the endotracheal tube is removed once the child responds appropriately. Patients with preexisting nausea and vomiting should be wide awake and have appropriate airway reflexes to prevent aspiration after extubation. Many of the children who require a ventriculoperitoneal shunt already have severely impaired airway reflexes; analgesics should be used with caution. Infiltration of the skin with a local anesthetic before closure can significantly reduce narcotic requirements in the postoperative period.

INTRACRANIAL TUMORS

Intracranial brain tumors are divided according to the site of the tumor. For the purpose of anesthetic management, they are divided into supratentorial, posterior fossa, and craniopharyngiomata.

Supratentorial lesions account for half of all pediatric brain neoplasms. These tumors tend to compress the ventricular system and cause obstructive hydrocephalus. Supratentorial lesions are more common in infants than in children. Anesthetic considerations must particularly address increased ICP, delayed gastric emptying because of raised ICP, and the electrolyte and fluid imbalance seen in children with the syndrome of inappropriate antidiuretic hormone.

Routine neuroanesthesia monitoring is used along with an indwelling arterial catheter. A central venous catheter is inserted when significant blood loss is anticipated or when there is hemodynamic instability. A urinary catheter is required to assess fluid balance and monitor osmotic diuretic therapy.

Intravenous induction of anesthesia is most appropriately followed by rapid securing of the airway and hyperventilation. Induction agents include thiopental, lidocaine, narcotics, and a nondepolarizing muscle relaxant. If the child has a full stomach, then cricoid pressure is applied and the lungs are hyperventilated, maintaining low peak airway pressures until the patient is adequately relaxed for intubation.

Anesthesia is maintained with synthetic narcotics, N_2O, and a benzodiazepine or droperidol. The P_{CO_2} is maintained between 25 and 30 mm Hg. Sub-MAC concentrations of isoflurane can be used if hypocapnia can be maintained. Pancuronium is an appropriate muscle relaxant for neonates and young infants because its vagolytic activity maintains heart rate.

Fluid management depends on the degree of raised ICP. Patients with markedly increased ICP are often dehydrated preoperatively, having received osmotic diuretics. Combined with the significant blood loss that can occur during these procedures, volume expansion is often necessitated. In children without significantly increased ICP or in those patients who have little blood loss during surgery, crystalloid solutions are adequate. Colloid solutions given in a 1:3 ratio with crystalloid solutions are appropriate for children requiring significant fluid resuscitation to maintain an isooncotic circulating volume.

The decision to extubate the child at the end of the procedure is based on the degree of surgical intervention, stability of the intraoperative period, normalization of ICP, and the child's age and temperature. Neonates and infants with coexisting cardiopulmonary problems often require postoperative ventilation. Children who are neurologically impaired often have inadequate airway reflexes and require postoperative intubation until they can protect their own airway. Older children, barring any complication, are often extubated after neuromuscular blockade is reversed and they are awake.

Postoperative pain management is aided by the infiltration of local anesthetics into the wound intraoperatively. The use of narcotics must be balanced with the patient's neurologic status. Obtunded patients should be evaluated for increased ICP or intracranial bleeding. Increased ICP postoperatively is most commonly the result of uncontrolled systemic hypertension. Systemic hypertension should be treated first by making the child adequately comfortable. If the blood pressure remains elevated, vasoactive drugs such as labetalol are used. Seizures may occur in the immediate postoperative period and prophylactic anticonvulsants are useful.

Craniopharyngiomas are histologically benign supracellar tumors, but morbidity results from the local destruction and compression of important structures, notably the hypothalamus, the optic chiasm, and the pituitary gland. Specific considerations include hypopituitarism, diabetes insipidus, altered insulin requirement, hypothermia, and seizures.

Preoperative evaluation should focus on determining the presence of these endocrine abnormalities. Affected children may have symptoms of hypothyroidism, growth hormone deficiency, and adrenocorticotropic hormone deficiency. Hormone therapy may be necessary in the preoperative and postoperative periods. Diabetes insipidus is rarely present preoperatively, occurring several hours after surgery. Significant hydrocephalus with increased ICP may occur and occasionally requires a preoperative ventriculostomy.

The surgical approach in children is a frontal craniotomy. Anesthesia is similar to that for supratentorial tumors. A microscopic surgical technique is common and the procedure is often long.

Postoperative problems are abundant. Diabetes insipidus occurs within hours of surgery. There are large volumes of urinary losses resulting in hypovolemia, hypernatremia, hyperosmolality, and a dilute urine. The diuresis must be replaced by intravenous fluids on a regular basis while serum electrolytes, glucose, and osmolality are maintained. Vasopressin or 1-deamino-8-D-arginine vasopressin (DDAVP) should be administered at the early stages of diabetes insipidus. Intranasal DDAVP, 0.05 to 0.3 mg/kg, can be given in two divided doses. If DDAVP is given intravenously, the dose is one tenth the intranasal dose. A constant infusion of 0.5 µg/kg DDAVP may also be given. Postoperative care also involves the administration of steroids and hormones as necessary. Serum glucose levels must be monitored closely. Seizures may occur in the postoperative period, and anticonvulsant prophylaxis may be prudent. Injury to the hypothalamic thermoregulatory center may result in hypothermia. Obviously these patients require close monitoring in an intensive care setting.

Posterior fossa tumors are more frequent in children than adults, accounting for half of all pediatric brain tumors. The preoperative anesthetic evaluation must include an assessment of ICP. Symptomatic hydrocephalus often requires the placement of an external ventricular drain. Brainstem compression can produce cardiovascular problems, particularly hypertension, loss of protective airway reflexes, and inspiratory stridor. Delayed gastric emptying is common.

Induction of anesthesia centers around the preservation of CPP while avoiding increases in ICP. The anesthetic techniques for this surgery are not unique from those previously described. Usually an intravenous induction combining thiopental or propofol with a nondepolarizing muscle relaxant and a narcotic is adequate. Succinylcholine is not used if there is evidence of increased ICP.

Posterior fossa surgery requires special attention to patient positioning. The prone position is used in approximately 50% of cases, whereas the sitting position and the lateral position are less commonly used. Positioning the child requires that the endotracheal tube be particularly stable. Care should be taken to make sure that the tube is not kinked when the child is placed in the final position for surgery. When the sitting position is used, monitoring to detect air emboli should be used. The detection and treatment of air emboli are discussed elsewhere in this handbook.

Postoperative pain is reduced by the infiltration of local anesthesia into the operative wound during closure. Cranial nerve(s) involvement and brainstem edema requires that most of these patients remain intubated in the immediate postoperative period. Narcotics should be used carefully, and these patients should be monitored for significant respiratory depression.

CEREBROVASCULAR ANOMALIES

Arterial aneurysms are rare in children; however, arteriovenous malformations (AVM) are not. The goal of the anesthesiologist is to minimize the transmural pressure of the vascular malformation to avoid expansion or rupture while preserving CPP. Invasive cardiovascular monitoring and controlled hypotension are common requirements. Vascular anomalies specific to pediatric patients involve the posterior cerebral artery and the great vein of Galen.

These anomalies may be present in the neonatal period with congestive heart failure, but <18% of AVMs are detected before 15 years of age. Cerebral injury may be due to hemorrhage, thrombosis, infarction, compression of adjacent neural structures, or parenchymal ischemia caused by the redistribution of blood flow to the low-resistance network. Many patients with AVMs undergo radiologically controlled embolization of their arterial blood supply or stereotactic radiosurgery as a definitive therapy. Surgical clipping of vessels may be done as either a single or a staged procedure.

Specific anesthetic considerations address increased ICP, congestive heart failure, and massive blood loss.

The low resistance of AVMs results in both pressure and volume overload in infants. Congestive heart failure in these children is similar pathophysiologically to that of persistent fetal circulation. Neonates with severe congestive heart failure may require inotropic support and endotracheal intubation before surgery.

In addition to routine monitors, these patients should have at least two large-bore intravenous catheters inserted. Indwelling arterial catheters and CVP lines are commonly advised for open procedures. An urinary catheter is essential. Surgical interruption of one or more of the large vessels can result in a significant air embolism; therefore monitoring for air emboli is advisable.

The anesthetic technique must take into consideration the compromised cardiovascular system, preventing hypertension at induction, while avoiding significant myocardial depression or cardiovascular collapse. Large doses of thiopental or propofol are avoided, and a gentle induction with a modest amount of thiopental, synthetic narcotic, and a nondepolarizing muscle relaxant is recommended.

The maintenance of anesthesia is similar to that used for supratentorial tumors. In the absence of congestive heart failure, controlled hypotension can be used at the time the AVM is ligated. Maintaining a normal body temperature can be quite difficult, especially when massive transfusions are required. Fortunately, modest hypothermia in the range of 34° C reduces the CMR_{O_2} and may be protective, without increasing postoperative complications.

Although some children without neurologic deficits can be extubated at the end of surgery, most incur a significant neurologic deficit or have had extensive resection of the brain resulting in significant cerebral edema. Children with preoperative congestive heart failure should remain sedated and intubated after surgery. They require several days for improvement and need close observation and treatment in the ICU.

HEAD AND SPINAL CORD INJURY

Head trauma is a major cause of morbidity and mortality in the pediatric population. Head injury can cause several different pathologic events including intracranial hematomas, cerebral edema, and systemic effects. Although adults have more hematomas with head trauma than children, children more commonly have diffuse cerebral edema. Isolated cervical spine injury is uncommon in the pediatric population. Children with cord injury or disruption are commonly seen without respiratory effort and have profound hypotension or cardiac arrest.

Anesthesia for head trauma should first include resuscitation and stabilization of the airway and circulation. Neurologic status can be assessed intermittently with the Glasgow Coma Scale. Associated injuries can occur with pediatric head trauma. These injuries usually involve the neck, chest, and abdominal organs. Although massive head and neck injuries may result in shock, intrathoracic and abdominal bleeding should always be considered in the differential diagnosis of hypotension.

Providing a secure airway is crucial in the management of head trauma. There is a common association between head and neck injury in infants and children. A cervical spine injury is always considered present in children with a head injury until proved otherwise. Intubation must be accomplished with minimal manipulation of the cervical spine; the neck must be stabilized. An assistant should provide in-line neck stabilization to facilitate intubation. An awake intubation is rarely feasible in young children. An effort should therefore be made to provide suitable anesthesia, reducing the hemodynamic stress and rise in ICP that occurs during laryngoscopy and intubation. Ketamine is often popular as an induction agent in children with cardiorespiratory compromise, but it is contraindicated in patients with closed head injuries. Small doses of etomidate are appropriate for children with hemodynamic instability. Pentothal is an acceptable choice if the child has a stable cardiovascular status.

MYELODYSPLASIA

Myelodysplasia is an abnormality in the fusion of the embryonic neural groove during the first month of gestation. Failure of this neural tube to close results in a sac-like herniation of the meninges and neural tissue. The spinal cord is tethered caudally by the sacral roots and results in orthopedic and neurologic problems later in childhood. Myelomeningoceles most frequently involve the lumbosacral region but can occur at any level. Myelodysplasia exposes the CNS tissue, placing the infant at risk of contamination and infection. The risk of infection increases the longer the lesion remains open, but it is minimal if the lesion is repaired within 48 hours of birth. Therefore most infants have surgery within the first 24 to 36 hours of life.

By definition children with a myelomeningocele have an Arnold-Chiari type II malformation, which eventually results in obstructive hydrocephalus. At the time of repair these infants rarely exhibit increased ICP. However, most infants will require a ventriculoperitoneal shunt to prevent or treat hydrocephalus in the days after the primary surgery.

Anesthesia is induced with the infant in either the lateral or supine position. When a large myelomeningocele is encountered, padding may be provided under the head, shoulders, and legs, protecting the neural sac from compression. Anesthesia is then induced in a standard manner with thiopental and a muscle relaxant. Hyperkalemia is not associated with myelomeningocele and the use of succinylcholine.

Closure of the defect is done with the infant in the prone position. Chest and hip rolls are placed carefully to ensure that the abdomen hangs freely, facilitating ventilation, but more important, reducing intraabdominal pressure and decreasing venous distention. Blood loss is often insidious, but serious losses are uncommon unless there is a large sac requiring significant undermining of the skin for wound closure. Blood transfusion is rarely necessary. Infants usually start with a hematocrit of 50% to 55% and can tolerate a considerable loss of red blood cells. Most newborns are at risk for apnea in the first 12 hours after anesthesia. Extubation at the termination of the anesthetic should be followed by apnea monitoring in an appropriate ICU setting.

Infants with spina bifida are particularly prone to have a latex allergy. Care is taken from the time of birth to reduce the exposure of these infants to latex products. Every effort should be made to avoid their use.

Occasionally older myelodysplastic children require decompression of the Arnold-Chiari malformation. This posterior fossa malformation is a complex developmental anomaly characterized by a downward displacement of the inferior cerebellum vermis into the upper cervical spinal canal. Dysplasia and aplasia of the ninth and tenth cranial nerves are common accompaniments. Involvement of the vagus nerve and its division, the recurrent laryngeal nerve, affects vocal cord function and results in stridor or frequent aspirations. The glossopharyngeal nerve innervates the carotid bodies. Dysplasia of this nerve can result in the loss of hypoxic ventilatory drive. The blood supply to the brainstem is also abnormal, resulting in acute and chronic infarcts. As such, this lesion is not static and these patients require careful reevaluation from anesthetic to anesthetic. The anesthetic management for posterior fossa decompressive surgery is similar to that previously outlined for posterior fossa tumors.

Suggested Readings

Berry FA: Perioperative anesthetic management of the pediatric trauma patient, *Crit Care Clin* 6:147, 1990.

Bissonnette B, editor: vol 10, Cerebral protection, resuscitation and monitoring, *Anesthesiology Clinics of North America,* Philadelphia, 1992, WB Saunders.

Crist W, Kun L: Common solid tumors of childhood, *N Engl J Med* 324:461, 1991.

Harris M, Yemen T, Strafford M: Venous air embolism during craniectomy in supine infants, *Anesthesiology* 67:816, 1987.

Holzman RS: Latex allergy: an emerging operating room problem, *Anesth Analg* 76:635, 1993.

Leech R, Biumbaric R, editors: *Hydrocephalus: current clinical concepts,* St Louis, 1991, Mosby.

Leon JE, Bissonnette B: Cerebrovascular responses to carbon dioxide in children anaesthetized with halothane and isoflurane, *Can J Anaesth* 38:817, 1991.

Levin HS: Head trauma, *Curr Opin Neurol* 6:841, 1993.

McLaurin R, Venes J, Schut L, et al, editors: *Pediatric Neurosurgery,* ed 2, Philadelphia, 1989, WB Saunders.

McLeod M, Creighton R, Humphreys R: Anaesthesia for cerebral arteriovenous malformations in children, *Can Anaesth Soc J* 29:299, 1982.

Ogawa A, Sakurai Y, Kayama Y: Regional CBF with age: changes in CBF in childhood, *Neurol Res* 11:173, 1989.

Pilato MA, Bissonnette B, Lerman J: Transcranial Doppler: response of cerebral blood flow velocity to carbon dioxide in anaesthetized children, *Can J Anaesth* 38:37, 1991.

ANESTHESIA FOR CRANIOFACIAL AND CRANIOBASAL SURGERY

14

Terrance A. Yemen
David L. Bogdonoff

Craniofacial and craniobasilar surgery are both specialized fields requiring unique anesthetic skills. In most hospitals these surgeries are rare, and most anesthesiologists are unfamiliar with the complex problems associated with these cases. The goal of this chapter is to provide a fundamental understanding of the anatomy and physiology of these disorders and the surgeries to correct them. A reasonable and commonsense insight into these areas, combined with traditional neuroanesthetic concepts, is the foundation on which sound anesthetic care is derived.

CRANIOFACIAL SURGERY AND ANESTHESIA

The neurocranium (cranial vault) and the viscerocranium (facial skeleton) are highly integrated structures whose development is closely interwoven. The common link between these structures is the cranial base. Its development is important in determining the morphologic features of the entire skull. Craniofacial anomalies result from the abnormal development of one or all of these structures.

Anatomic and Physiologic Considerations

Craniosynostosis is the premature closure of one or more cranial suture(s). Premature fusion results in the arrested growth of the skull perpendicular to the fused suture(s) and compensatory growth in a direction parallel to the suture(s) affected. Craniosynostosis can be the result of a single affected suture or in severe cases involvement of a combination of cranial sutures.

Craniosynostosis can be either an isolated deformity with only a single suture affected or part of a complex craniofacial syndrome. The etiology of craniosynostosis involves multiple factors. Intrauterine, metabolic, and hematologic disorders, along with genetic defects and teratogens, can all cause defective cranial growth.

Isolated craniosynostosis occurs in about 5 per 10,000 live births. The sagittal suture is most commonly affected, accounting for 60% of these cases. Coronal synostosis also occurs, accounting for 25% of patients. Metopic and lambdoidal sutures are infrequently involved.

Over 58 syndromes have been associated with craniosynostosis. Craniosynostosis may represent only one abnormality in what is a widespread malformation involving not only the cranium, cranial base, and facial structures but other organ systems as well.

Apert's syndrome involves all the craniofacial structures. It is characterized by craniosynostosis, midface hypoplasia, and symmetric syndactyly of the hands and feet. The associated craniosynostosis most commonly involves the coronal suture. Midface hypoplasia produces a shortened and narrowed nasal cavity, palate, and maxilla and a predominant proptosis. A significant number of patients are mentally retarded as a result of malformation of the central nervous system. Crouzon's, Carpenter's, and Pfeiffer's syndromes have similar craniofacial features.

Branchial arch anomalies are nonspecific defects in the development of the branchial arches. Microstomia or macrostomia can result from the abnormal merging of the maxillary and mandibular prominences in severe first arch anomalies. Treacher-Collins syndrome involves structures derived from both the first and second branchial arch regions. Characteristically these children have malar deficiencies, microtia, lower lid colobomas, and a retrognathic mandible. Additionally, the hyoid bone is displaced anteriorly and inferiorly.

The Robin sequence is also a branchial arch anomaly in which early mandibular retrognathia is the primary defect. The sequence may be an isolated defect or part of a syndrome. The common feature in either is a failure of mandibular development with a secondary failure of the tongue to descend between the palatal shelves. When the Robin sequence is an isolated anomaly, the mandible is intrinsically normal and will grow at an accelerated rate after birth, eliminating the defect. However, when the Robin sequence is part of a syndrome that includes intrinsic mandibular hypoplasia, the mandible remains small and abnormal throughout life.

The oculoauriculovertebral spectrum includes the hemifacial microsomias and Goldenhar's syndrome. The latter syndrome is the result of defective facial development involving the ear, zygomatic bones, mandible, parotid gland, tongue, and facial muscles. Abnormal development may not be limited to the facial structures. Associated anomalies are common, especially those involving the cardiac, renal, or skeletal systems. Within the oculoauriculovertebral spectrum, maxillary, mandibular, and auricular hypoplasia are the predominant features. Mandibular condyle deformities are significant in all patients. When these deformities are predominantly unilateral, the disorder is called hemifacial microsomia. When similar features are accompanied by epibulbar and vertebral defects, it is called Goldenhar syndrome.

Orbital malposition may occur in any direction and may not affect each orbit similarly. The bones and sutures involved in the walls of the orbit represent a primary defect or may be the result of craniosynostosis or a craniofacial cleft. Isolated orbital hypertelorism is a deformity that consists of lateralization of the bony orbit and enlargement of the ethmoid sinuses. Nasal deformities may be severe and difficult to correct. In addition, there is dysfunction of the upper eyelid and extraocular muscles.

The incidence and severity of intracranial hypertension varies with the suture affected and the associated craniofacial abnormalities. With sagittal synostosis intracranial hypertension is relatively uncommon, occurring in only 5% to 10% of children. When multiple sutures are involved, such as with Apert's or Crouzon's syndrome, more than 25% of patients have intracranial hypertension. With extensive synostosis involving both the coronal and sagittal sutures, more than 50% of patients have elevated intracranial pressure (ICP). The incidence of intracranial hypertension also correlates with the age of the patient, increasing significantly after the first year of age and eventually affecting up to 85% of children.

Clinical signs and symptoms of elevated ICP are uncommon. Intracranial volumes calculated from computed tomography (CT) or cranial ultrasonography do not directly correlate with intracranial pressures. The clinical significance of intracranial hypertension is not well delineated in craniosynostosis patients, but it is nonetheless given as a common indication for surgery.

Surgery

The objective of craniofacial surgery is to remodel the bony and soft tissue deformities of the cranium and face. This objective requires that the malformed tissues be cut, disjoined, mobilized, repositioned, occasionally augmented, and finally fixed into position. Such surgery requires extensive exposure of the skeletal tissues, with both intracranial and extracranial approaches being used.

A clear understanding of the lesion and the proposed surgical procedure is required to plan an appropriate anesthetic. Remodeling may involve an isolated part of the cranium or the entire cranial vault. Complex craniosynostosis often involves the cranial base and face, requiring the surgeon to separate affected sutures and advance the face forward and away from the cranial base, thereby allowing normal cranial growth and proper alignment of the upper and lower dental arches.

Repair of craniosynostosis and supraorbital advancement is generally done during the first 3 to 6 months of life because rapid growth of the cranium occurs during the first year. A frontal craniotomy is made and the frontal bone flap is removed. An osteotomy is extended through the lateral orbital wall, crossing the orbital floor to the nasal bridge, and this segment is contoured, shaped, and advanced. The frontal bone flap is then returned either as a solid piece or in multiple fragments that have been reshaped into a normal-appearing forehead.

Midface advancements, which are usually delayed until patients are 3 to 4 years old, usually require a Le Fort osteotomy. The Le Fort I osteotomy corrects malocclusion caused by underdevelopment of the maxilla. The incision is intraoral and the maxilla is mobilized downward, advanced, and fixed into place. Bone grafts are commonly used.

The Le Fort II osteotomy is used to advance the lower maxilla and entire nose forward, which requires a bicoronal scalp incision and exposure of the midface. An osteotomy is made across the nasal bridge bilaterally down the lateral nasal bones and through the inferior orbital rim and then across the maxilla to the pterygomaxillary junction. These segments are mobilized, advanced, and fixed into place with bone grafts and wires.

A Le Fort III osteotomy is used to repair complete underdevelopment of the midface, as occurs in Apert's or Crouzon's syndrome. It also requires a bicoronal scalp incision and exposure of the midface. After disjunction of the entire midface the nose, maxilla, and orbits are advanced. The osteotomy starts at the frontozygomatic suture, passes through the orbits, below the supraorbital rim, and across the nasal bridge. The pterygomaxillary junctions are separated with an osteotome, and the nasal septum is separated from the base of the skull. This facial segment is then advanced. Spaces between bony segments occur and are filled with bone grafts. The bones are subsequently fixed in position with wires and plates. Surgical correction of the orbital malposition is performed after 4 to 5 years of age.

To correct the hypertelorism, the orbits are freed from the contiguous bone and repositioned. A bicoronal scalp incision is made and an intracranial approach is taken, retracting the frontal lobes of the brain to expose the anterior craniofossa. Intraorbital and extraorbital osteotomies are used to mobilize the orbits. The central block of bone, which includes the frontal, nasal, and ethmoidal tissues, is removed from between the orbits. The orbits are moved medially and fixed into place with bone grafts, wires, and plates. The nose is then rebuilt with bone grafts.

Preoperative Assessment

The preoperative evaluation of craniofacial patients involves understanding (1) the anatomy of the disorder, (2) associated conditions, and (3) the emotional state of the child and parents. Craniosynostosis surgery is often performed in young infants. Parents of affected children experience tremendous stress. In addition to the child having a deformity, there is also the realization that extensive surgery with substantial risk is required to correct these disorders. Emotional and behavioral problems are associated with poor self concept and the negative social experiences so common in pediatric craniofacial patients. Older children and adolescents have tremendous apprehension. They fear the pain and possible complications that may occur as a result of surgery. Efforts must be made to reassure these patients by offering a full, complete explanation of the care and associated risks.

Respiratory, cardiac, and neurologic anomalies occur in many of these patients. Approximately 50% of children with Goldenhar syndrome have a cardiac defect, varying from a simple atrial septal defect to complex heart lesions such as the tetralogy of Fallot. The most common problem in identifying associated conditions with craniofacial syndromes is unfamiliarity with the syndrome itself. It is impossible to become familiar with the 58 relatively uncommon syndromes that are associated with craniofacial malformations. Therefore it is useful to have a textbook of recognizable human malformations to serve as reference. These textbooks are invaluable for identifying potential problems and planning anesthetic management.

Upper airway obstruction is not uncommon in patients with craniofacial malformations. Malformations involving the face and cranial base reduce upper airway dimensions. Commonly the temporomandibular joint is posterior and the mandible is small and retrognathic. The tongue is displaced posteriorly and impinges on the orohypopharynx. Hypoplasia of the midface results in diminished dimensions of the nasal airway. It is therefore not surprising that obstructive sleep apnea is well documented with Treacher-Collins, Stickler's, and Apert's syndromes. At birth airway obstruction with the Robin syndrome can be severe enough to warrant an emergency tracheotomy. The obstruction is primarily the result of posterior displacement of the tongue in the Robin sequence. Placement of nasopharyngeal airway, suturing the tongue to the mandible, or pulling the tongue forward may relieve significant airway obstruction, especially during the first month of life. As these children grow and the airway expands, the problems diminish. In contrast, the obstruction seen in Treacher-Collins and Apert's syndromes does not improve with age and often worsens.

Approximately 50% to 60% of patients with mandibular dysostosis have a difficult airway and require a comprehensive evaluation of the airway before anesthetic induction. Many features of these abnormal airways are grossly evident, but some are not. When the airway is assessed, a careful history is required. Many children with craniofacial anomalies have a history consistent with obstructive sleep apnea. Loud snoring followed by periods of apnea is often noted by the parents. Obstructive sleep apnea may cause irritability, nocturnal enuresis, headaches, daytime somnolence, poor performance at school, and a short attention span in addition to other personality and behavioral changes. Because these patients often have multiple procedures, an anesthetic record of airway problems is often available. An interview of the patient and parents, combined with a review of the medical record, can help to answer questions regarding how these problems were managed previously.

Physical examination should include both the nasal and oral airways. Patients with inadequate nasopharyngeal airways often breathe with their mouths open. The oral airway is commonly inaccessible as a result of mandibular hypoplasia and the common association of abnormal temporomandibular joint movement. These features make direct visualization with a laryngoscope difficult, if not impossible. Additionally, many children have macroglossia, further reducing visualization of the larynx. Neck mobility, especially extension, needs to be assessed. Fusion of the cervical vertebrae is common in Goldenhar's, Apert's, and Crouzon's syndromes.

Laboratory testing consists minimally of hemoglobin, platelets, and tests of coagulation, particularly prothrombin (PT) and partial thromboplastin (PTT) times. Other investigations, including chest x-ray films, electrocardiogram, arterial blood gases, and serum electrolytes are done as necessitated by the patient's coexisting condition(s).

Premedication

The use of preoperative medication requires balancing the need for sedation and relief of anxiety against the presence of coexisting disorders, their physiologic consequences, and associated airway anomalies.

Patients with increased ICP or airway obstruction may not tolerate significant degrees of respiratory depression. Oral premedications such as midazolam are effective anxiolytics and produce little cardiorespiratory depression in the absence of concomitant narcotic administration.

Antisialagogues can be given at the time of induction. Oral atropine or glycopyrrolate at a dose of 10 to 20 µg/kg can be given 20 minutes before induction. Antisialics help prevent or ameliorate the bradycardia that can occur during induction with inhalational agents or with oropharyngeal stimulation. They also reduce the amount of secretions in these potentially difficult airways.

Topical viscous lidocaine can be applied to the posterior one third of the tongue of children with macroglossia. This application allows insertion of an oropharyngeal airway during the early phase of an inhalational induction without evoking coughing, bucking, or laryngospasm. Techniques such as this are particularly useful in patients with either Apert's or Crouzon syndrome.

Monitoring

Standard monitors include electrocardiogram, noninvasive blood pressure cuff, pulse oximetry, end-tidal carbon dioxide and nitrogen, a temperature probe, and a precordial or esophageal stethoscope. Insertion of an arterial line is appropriate for most patients undergoing craniofacial surgery. Arterial lines allow measurement of significant changes in blood pressure that can rapidly occur with massive bleeding. Blood can be sampled to measure hemoglobin levels, electrolytes, glucose, and acid/base values. In some cases of midface surgery hypotensive anesthesia is used. An arterial line is advisable to closely monitor this anesthetic therapy.

Central lines are inserted in children with difficult peripheral intravenous access. In infants a femoral central venous line is easy to place. Central venous lines in the groin seldom kink, even in the prone position, a problem that is common with external or internal jugular venous catheters, especially when head position is changed. Infection rates for jugular or femoral intravenous lines are the same in children.

Venous air embolism is frequent, having been reported as high as 70% in children undergoing craniofacial repair in the supine position. A precordial Doppler monitor should be placed over the right heart position. The proper function and placement of the Doppler probe is verified by rapidly injecting saline solution into a peripheral line and listening for the characteristic "mill wheel" murmur.

Induction of Anesthesia

The choice of anesthetic induction technique in patients with craniofacial anomalies should take into consideration the following: (1) the nature of airway anomalies, (2) coexisting cardiorespiratory disorders, and (3) the preference of the child and parents. Preparation is paramount in managing these patients. The operating room should be supplied with a variety of laryngoscope blades, endotracheal tubes, and ancillary difficult airway equipment. When a critical airway is suspected, a surgeon capable of establishing a surgical airway should be present at induction.

Induction of anesthesia in children with suspected difficult airways or significant cardiorespiratory problems is most appropriately done in the operating room itself and not in an induction room. Mask anesthesia with halothane as an induction agent is reasonable if cardiorespiratory status is normal. The depth of anesthesia can be controlled gradually, ensuring airway obstruction can be managed as the depth of anesthesia increases. Alternatively, an intravenous cannula can be inserted while the child is awake. Induction can then proceed with an inhalational agent with intravenous access already in place for emergency drugs.

Inhalational anesthesia can result in significant cardiorespiratory depression. In a child with a suspected difficult airway and coexisting cardiac disease it is often more appropriate to place an intravenous line in the awake child. Anesthesia can then be induced with intravenous ketamine, avoiding significant cardiorespiratory depression. After induction the airway is topicalized with lidocaine and intubation is attempted. The use of muscle relaxants during induction should be reserved for those children with airways that can be maintained without endotracheal intubation.

The anesthesiologist should be prepared to use a variety of difficult airway techniques. These include direct or indirect visualization, blind nasal or oral intubation, and retrograde wire techniques. The use of a pediatric laryngeal mask airway (sizes 1 or 2) can aid in establishing a patent oral airway or provide a guide to fiberoptic laryngoscopy and intubation. The presence of a second person skilled in airway management is useful in these patients. For example, one pair of hands can be used to visualize the airway while the second pair of hands intubates, the so-called "two person intubation technique."

The choice between an oral or nasal endotracheal tube depends on (1) the child's airway, (2) the preference of the surgeon, and (3) the surgical technique to be used. An oral tube is suitable for most cases. Once the endotracheal tube has been placed, it is carefully secured with tape or by having the surgeon wire the tube in position. Head movement during these cases is common. Flexion of the head advances the tube toward the carina and extension advances the tube cephalad. The endotracheal tube must be placed so that the tube does not become dislodged if the neck is extended and does not become endobronchial when the head is flexed. After intubation the head should be extended and flexed while the anesthesiologist listens to both sides of the chest to demonstrate that the endotracheal tube remains in an appropriate position.

Once the patient is appropriately anesthetized and intubated and vascular access has been established, the patient can be positioned for surgery. Major craniofacial procedures average 5 to 6 hours, with some lasting longer than 12 hours. Therefore meticulous attention must be paid to positioning and protecting vulnerable body parts. Padding should be used to ensure that joints are properly positioned, comfortably flexed, and all peripheral nerves protected. Pressure points, especially those around the head, must be adequately padded. The endotracheal tube and the entire breathing circuit must be carefully positioned and secured, avoiding both pressure points and disconnection during the surgery. The majority of craniofacial surgery is done with the patient in either the supine or prone position. In both positions the head is usually 10 to 20 degrees above the plane of the body. Transducers should be placed at the level of the midhead to measure adequate perfusion to the cranium. All intravenous, arterial, and central venous lines should be checked to ensure that they function as well in their final position as they did at insertion. It is not uncommon for these lines to have worked perfectly after insertion in the supine position, only to find that pressure points and kinking prevent them from functioning in the surgical position.

The induction of anesthesia, placement of lines, and positioning take an extended period of time. The anesthesia, and some aspects of the surgery, requires full body exposure. Efforts should be made to keep the room warm during induction, at least until the patient is covered with surgical drapes. Infrared heating lamps significantly cut down conductive and convection heat loss during induction. A warming blanket or forced air warmer significantly reduces heat loss during surgery. Intravenous and irrigation fluids should be warmed. Inspired gases should be heated and humidified. Remember that in babies the head represents 30% of the body surface area. The head is exposed for the vast majority of the surgery, acting as a radiator, and causing significant heat loss by convection.

Maintenance of Anesthesia

Craniofacial surgery involves extensive fluid loss and requires meticulous intravenous fluid management. The fluid management of these patients can be divided into two categories: (1) the management of maintenance and third-space fluids and (2) blood replacement. Maintenance fluids are calculated on the basis of standard pediatric formulas.

Third-space losses in these children are commonly high. Crystalloid fluids are given at a rate of 6 to 10 ml/kg. Ringer's lactate is a reasonable solution for this use. In children the use of large volumes of normal saline solution should be avoided, thereby preventing the production of hyperchloremic acidosis. During prolonged procedures a non-glucose-containing solution is used. However, blood glucose levels should be measured hourly. Hypoglycemia in babies is not common but occasionally occurs. If blood glucose levels fall below 80 mg/dl, add enough glucose to Ringer's lactate to generate a 1% glucose solution. In our experience this has been more than adequate to prevent hypoglycemia. Hyperglycemia should be avoided because neurologic deficits have been reported to be worse when hyperglycemia is associated with hypoxemia.

Although there is no objective evidence to support the use of colloid over crystalloid solutions, it has been our opinion that total crystalloid usage should not exceed 100 ml/kg of body weight for the entire operation. Use of crystalloid solutions in excess of this volume are associated with excessive edema formation, particularly affecting the cerebrum and airway. In addition, rapid administration of crystalloid solutions can result in a dilutional coagulopathy. The use of 5% albumin reduces total fluid administration and the resultant edema.

The degree of blood loss is related to the extent and duration of the surgical procedure. For simple strip craniectomies blood loss is usually low and rarely requires transfusion. Hematocrits usually fall to 20% to 25% by the end of the procedure. When remodeling is combined with the crainiectomy, an average of 50% to 60% of the blood volume is lost. However, blood losses of three to five blood volumes is not uncommon with complex synostosis and midface involvement. In these procedures blood loss starts with the initial scalp incision. It is a good idea to have one or two units of packed red blood cells in the operating room before the start of surgery. Bleeding from the skin and bone is continuous throughout the procedure and is often unpredictable in major craniofacial reconstruction. A laceration in the dural sinuses can result in rapid, massive blood loss. With Le Fort I or II procedures arteries may be severed and result in extensive blood loss. Blood loss should be replaced with packed red blood cells from the beginning of major craniofacial reconstruction. This is particularly true in children 2 or 3 months old. These children have reached their physiologic nadir and have hematocrits of approximately 30% at the start of surgery.

The goal of blood replacement is to maintain an intraoperative hematocrit of approximately 25%. Remember, packed red blood cells have a hematocrit of 70%, so for every milliliter of blood loss only 0.3 to 0.5 ml of packed red blood cells is necessary to maintain a resonable hematocrit. Packed red blood cell replacement is best monitored by measuring serial hematocrits. Samples are taken on a half-hour to hourly basis and adjustments made accordingly. Although traditional teaching states that fresh-frozen plasma is not required until at least one blood volume of blood is lost, in our experience this has not been true. Serial measurements of PT and PTT have been prolonged after loss of only one third of the blood volume in these cases. Platelet counts have rarely fallen below 100,000/ml even after one or two blood volumes have been lost. We commonly add fresh-frozen plasma in equal volumes to the packed red blood cells as a fluid replacement once one half to two thirds of the blood volume has been lost and more is expected.

Blood loss is not easily measured. It is obscured by the surgical field and drapes. Care must be taken to monitor the blood volume as assessed by heart rate, intraarterial pressure and waveform, central venous pressure, and serial hematocrits.

The rapid transfusion of blood products can produce significant hypocalcemia, particularly when fresh-frozen plasma is given. Serum calcium should be monitored if blood replacement is rapid, and the threshold for calcium replacement should be low, especially if blood pressure falls.

Massive blood transfusion can result in life-threatening hyperkalemia. This is characterized by peaked T waves and widened QRS complexes and ultimately leads to cardiovascular collapse, if left untreated. This complication can be reduced by three methods: (1) use blood that is either fresh or at worst, a week or two old, (2) infuse the blood through a peripheral intravenous line rather than through a central line, allowing some dilution of the hyperkalemic blood to occur before it reaches the heart, and (3) use washed red blood cells.

Induced hypotension is used in some centers to reduce blood loss. Although some craniofacial teams believe this is effective, there is no consensus. Currently there are no objective data supporting this technique. We do not use hypotensive anesthetic techniques for these surgeries.

Intracranial hypertension present preoperatively may continue in the operative and postoperative periods. Additionally, the cerebrum is often manipulated and retracted to provide adequate exposure to the anterior cranial fossa and facial bones. Cerebral edema should be anticipated in these situations. Anesthetic agents that can increase intracranial volume should be avoided once the cranium is closed. We traditionally use a narcotic relaxant technique in combination with hyperventilation, maintaining a carbon dioxide pressure of 25 to 30 mm Hg. When intracranial hypertension is noted after closure of the cranium, mannitol and controlled hyperventilation may be required to reduce cerebral edema. At the end of the surgery an ICP monitor may be placed by the surgeon, and it is helpful in monitoring therapy for intracranial hypertension.

Postoperative Concerns

Ideally, the decision to extubate or transport the patient to an intensive care unit with the endotracheal tube in place is made before the surgery and discussed with the parents at that time. Children are usually suitable for extubation when the surgery is a simple strip craniectomy. With complex craniofacial surgery we usually leave the endotracheal tube in place, extubating the patient only after there is demonstrated cardiovascular stability, the patient is warm, and airway edema is resolving. Caution must be used when deciding to extubate these patients. It should be done in an appropriate environment with a care team capable of providing an emergency airway nearby. The reintubation of patients with massive facial swelling and airway edema can be difficult, if not impossible.

Postoperatively, significant concealed blood loss can occur. Fatalities have occurred when, despite adequate blood product replacement in the operating room, extensive hemorrhage in the intensive care unit was not followed by adequate replacement. Intravascular volume assessment must be continued into the immediate postoperative period. Serial blood sampling should continue as a guide to blood product replacement. Prolongation of the PT and PTT is not uncommon even 24 to 48 hours after surgery. In our experience knowledge of the fluid management in the immediate postoperative period significantly reduces serious complications with this surgery.

CRANIOBASAL SURGERY AND ANESTHESIA

Craniobasal surgery is a highly complex and specialized area of neurosurgery that has emerged in the last two decades. This subspecialty, also known as skull base surgery, involves procedures at the base of the skull involving both brain and basicranium. Caring for patients requires teamwork with input from multiple disciplines including interventional radiology, otorhinolaryngology, plastic and reconstructive surgery, and, of course, anesthesiology.

Most cases involve tumors of which approximately one fourth are malignant. Benign tumors are no less problematic because their cranial base anatomic location is sufficiently "malignant." The region is extraordinarily complex with its confluence of blood vessels and cranial nerves and irregular bony topography. Exposure of lesions may involve transgression of sinuses, division of major blood vessels or cranial nerves, extensive brain retraction, or removal of large pieces of bone and dura.

Advances in microvascular techniques, neural anastomosis, subtleties in the complex anatomy, microvascular free flap reconstruction, and preoperative localization and embolization of tumors have all contributed to increasing success. In addition, anesthetic advances, particularly with regard to sophisticated neurophysiologic monitors, have contributed to the overall success of the few centers involved with these complicated cases.

Preoperative Assessment

The approach to the patient for cranial base surgery begins with contemplation of the specific region that will be involved. The cranial base may be split into regions that correspond to the anterior, middle, or posterior fossae. Some surgeons group the middle and posterior divisions into three sections on the basis of the bony anatomy: the sphenoid base, petrous portion of temporal bone, and clivus. The relevant aspects of the location revolve around what structures are present within the affected region and what approach to exposure will be taken.

Posterior fossa surgeries are usually performed with the patient in a lateral or prone position, whereas surgery in other parts of the skull base is done with the patient supine with varying amounts of head rotation. Potential involvement of a major intracranial blood vessel is evaluated by preoperative neuroradiologic procedures. Documented involvement or proximity will demand an evaluation of the potential consequences of injury or sacrifice of the vessel because of a planned or unplanned surgical intervention. Balloon occlusion tests may be used to address these issues.

It is important to note any symptoms that develop during the test occlusion of the internal carotid artery and also, in the absence of symptoms, to note the levels of blood pressure that exist during the procedure. Preoperative embolization of the tumor may significantly decrease intraoperative bleeding and thereby enhance surgical visibility and patient stability. Patients with tumors near the sella should have endocrinologic evaluations with appropriate hormone replacement. Metastatic workups are likewise relevant for those patients with known malignant lesions.

As with all neurosurgical patients, an assessment of the degree of any elevation of ICP should be made. Even in the absence of elevated pressure symptoms, there should be concern for the potential presence of increased intracranial elastance because tumor mass or blockage of cerebrospinal fluid (CSF) outflow.

A thorough neurologic examination is necessary to identify and further document the preoperative status of the patient. Preoperative neurophysiologic studies such as evoked potentials and electroencephalograms may be useful as baselines, especially given the high level of dependence on these studies intraoperatively.

Premedication

Premedication is often avoided, facilitated by a thoughtful, unhurried preoperative visit. Highly anxious individuals are treated effectively with benzodiazepines or diphenhydramine. Narcotics are best avoided except in individuals without intracranial mass lesions or when given under the direct supervision of the anesthesiologist in the operating room or holding area.

Monitoring

Hemodynamic preparation for the anesthetic begins with consideration of the monitors that will be necessary during the procedure. Arterial catheterization for blood sampling and pressure monitoring is uniformly used and almost always is accomplished before induction. Central venous or pulmonary artery catheterization may also be used but is accomplished after induction.

Determination of volume status and the potential need for rapid and central injection of vasopressor or antihypertensive medications serves as the primary indication for this central monitoring. An antecubital or external jugular venous site is our first choice for central monitoring. We will use subclavian access if necessary but will always radiographically confirm the absence of a pneumothorax because the patient will be anesthetized for several hours after the line insertion. Internal jugular venous catheterization is best avoided to minimize any potential for blockage of cranial venous return, which could aggravate blood loss and cerebral edema.

Respiratory end-tidal carbon dioxide monitoring is routine and essential and is complemented by end-tidal nitrogen monitoring, which may be useful when the question of air embolism is entertained.

Neurophysiologic monitors are an integral component of the multidisciplinary approach to these cases and will involve a dedicated team of monitoring technicians and possibly neurologists or neurophysiologists as well. Monitors of cortical, brainstem, and cranial nerve function may all be necessary. The cortex is analyzed using information from raw and processed electroencephalography, somatosensory evoked potentials (SSEPs), or visual evoked potentials. Brainstem function is assessed with brainstem auditory evoked potentials and SSEPs. Electromyograms (EMG) may be used to evaluate almost all the cranial nerves that are not assessable by the previous techniques. Preoperative baseline values for these studies are helpful.

Sophisticated monitoring provides the operating team with the capability of identification of neural structures and warns them of impending damage to structures by surgical encroachment or interruption of blood supply. The need for immediate feedback to the surgeon necessitates a dedicated team of neurophysiologists, and it is imperative that the anesthesiologist be intimately involved with the monitoring plans so that the anesthetic will not interfere with the set goals. Therapeutic manipulations such as barbiturate-induced burst suppression or blood flow manipulation by intracranial or blood pressure manipulation will be aided by the available monitoring.

The anesthesiologist must be aware of potential effects that various anesthetics and physiologic manipulations have on neurophysiologic monitoring. In general, it is best to use a balanced technique with infusions to minimize potent inhalational agents that have the most profound effects, particularly on cortical functions. EMG, however, requires an intact neuromuscular junction that may at times interfere with the choice of the balanced technique. The anesthetic technique may therefore need to be modified at different times during the same case depending on the specific monitoring needs of the surgeon.

Cortical function is most highly affected by inhalational agents and intravenous sedatives. Cortical responses of SSEPs are similarly sensitive. Brainstem auditory evoked responses and EMGs are highly resistant to anesthetic agents. It is also important to recognize that cerebral perfusion pressure, arterial carbon dioxide tension, and temperature may have profound effects and should be kept relatively constant. Changes in any of these latter variables may be necessary during the course of the anesthetic and should always be communicated to the monitoring personnel so that they may use the information to better understand any resultant changes in their signals. Even subtle interventions such as localized temperature changes caused by surgical irrigation solutions can have effects on neurophysiologic monitoring. Attention to detail and communication between all members of the operating room team are obviously required.

Induction of Anesthesia

The anesthetic approach to the patient depends in large part on the particulars of the patient and whether elevated ICP symptoms predominate. Many patients do not have large masses but have symptoms related to the encroachment of small tumors on specific vital structures. Such patients do not require aggressive ICP control during induction, but it may be required later in the course of the anesthetic to facilitate exposure.

Induction of anesthesia requires meticulous attention to control of arterial blood pressure and ICP. Thiopental is almost universally chosen, although etomidate may be considered for potentially unstable patients. Patients with large masses or tight brains should not be premedicated with narcotics, although moderate doses are administered during induction because of their beneficial effects on hemodynamic control before and particularly during intubation. Voluntary hyperventilation should be instituted before induction and continued by the anesthetist once unconsciousness is achieved. Lidocaine 1.5 mg/kg may be given 3 minutes before intubation to further diminish ICP responses to intubation. Additional doses of thiopental are effective toward this goal as well. Succinylcholine may be used for intubation if not otherwise contraindicated, but we almost uniformly use a nondepolarizing muscle relaxant.

The choice of relaxant will be determined by the need for prolonged relaxation (or the desire to avoid it) and the potential for risk from any adverse hemodynamic effects from specific relaxants. We commonly use vecuronium 0.2 mg/kg or rocuronium 0.6 mg/kg for induction and change to a longer-acting, less-expensive agent for maintenance of relaxation. Reversal of blockade is possible, if necessary, by the time the procedure is actually underway because of the time involved in positioning, draping, and subsequent surgical exposure of the involved region.

The airway is usually not problematic, but previous surgical procedures may have compromised relevant structures such as the upper airway, the temporomandibular joint, or the cervical spine.

Maintenance of Anesthesia

The choice of maintenance anesthetic is determined largely on the basis of surgical needs. Surgical exposure, control of blood pressure (low, normal, or high), and requirements for monitoring all influence the anesthetic choice. If motor monitoring of cranial nerves will be required, relaxants are avoided. This generally demands that a deeper level of inhalational anesthesia be used to ensure a still surgical field. Deep inhalational anesthesia, unfortunately, interferes with other electrophysiologic monitoring, as previously discussed.

Surgical exposure may be facilitated as it is during aneurysm surgery with judicious use of mannitol, CSF drainage, and mild hyperventilation. CSF drainage is often continued postoperatively to decrease the likelihood of the persistent CSF leaks that plague this patient population.

Blood pressure manipulation is commonly required and is guided by surgical needs. Hypotension may be helpful during resection of vascular tumors to both decrease blood loss and facilitate visualization by the surgeon. Hypertension may be necessary to help increase collateral blood flow and alleviate hypoperfusion from temporary clipping of major vessels. Preoperative studies will guide temporary clipping or sacrifice of these arteries.

Cerebral ischemia or seizure activity resulting from the surgical manipulations is readily detected by appropriate neurophysiologic monitoring, although the activity may be otherwise completely asymptomatic. The use of barbiturate boluses may be considered in an effort to decrease cerebral oxygen needs for a short time or to stop seizure activity. Manipulation of carbon dioxide tension during temporary clamping is a potential therapeutic option, but the direction of blood flow change is not always known.

Hypercarbia will theoretically increase flow to the brain, which could be helpful. Hypercarbia may be used for extracranial-intracranial bypasses to bring the brain surface closer to the craniotomy site. These may be required to allow for necessary occlusion of blood vessels for complete resection. Conversely, hypocarbia could potentially result in vasoconstriction of vessels in normally perfused brain, allowing the remaining available cerebral blood flow to be shunted to the ischemic brain, which resulted from the temporary clipping. The latter is called *inverse steal*. With feedback on cerebral function from neurophysiologic monitors, the appropriate manipulation of ventilation may be selected to achieve the desired carbon dioxide tension. In the absence of feedback, neutral stance of normocarbia may have to be adopted. Infusions of low doses of barbiturates and fentanyl and the use of low doses of isoflurane (<0.4%) and nitrous oxide are usually combined to form the basis for a stable anesthetic. After the initial scalp and dural incisions, surgical stimulation is less and anesthetic requirements are low. Certain surgical manipulations may, however, result in significant changes and the need to modify anesthetic depth. Cranial nerve stimulation is one such example that may produce unpredictable changes in heart rate, cardiac conduction, and blood pressure. The trigeminal or vagus nerves are commonly implicated, and the resultant changes are usually self-limited. Positioning is important to facilitate venous drainage and surgical exposure. Both the beneficial and adverse results of head elevation must be considered. Additional elevation decreases venous bleeding while at the same time increasing the risk of venous air embolism and slightly decreasing arterial blood pressure in the brain.

Careful monitoring for venous air is indicated and is best done with a precordial Doppler monitor with supplementation by respiratory gas monitoring. Blood pressure should always be measured at the level of the circle of Willis, thereby allowing closer determination of cerebral perfusion pressure.

Certain neurosurgical maneuvers may require an extremely still field, such as during the performance of extracranial-intracranial bypasses. This may be facilitated by considering low tidal volumes with high frequencies in an effort to minimize respiratory-induced movement of the cerebral contents.

Fluid shifts are not uncommon and will need to be addressed carefully. Mannitol will result in a large diuresis and will require replacement of much of the urine output. Blood loss can be acute and massive and will often require transfusion therapy. Colloids may be effectively used for volume replacement and offer the advantage of less postoperative fluid overload. The length of these cases requires that fluids be carefully administered in a manner that does not result in overhydration and brain swelling. Use of central venous pressure monitoring or determination of respiratory-induced arterial blood pressure waveform changes will help guide this therapy.

Completion of the anesthetic will depend on surgical preferences as well. Many surgeons desire that patients be awake immediately after the procedure to allow a neurologic examination. Others prefer the theoretic safety of continued intubation and sedation to allow airway protection, return to normal temperature, and stabilization of vital signs. Postoperative CT scans may be obtained immediately after the procedure.

When extubation is contemplated, anesthetic agents with short half-lives or easy reversibility should be chosen during closure. Alfentanil may be substituted for fentanyl, propofol, for thiopental or a total inhalation technique may be instituted. The ability of the patient to maintain an airway must be carefully assessed, especially when the surgical procedure involved those cranial nerves necessary for these functions.

Postoperative Concerns

Postoperatively, these patients are at risk from the same complications as other intracranial procedures. Postoperative intracranial bleeding is certainly a concern and can result in sudden increases in ICP or localized increases in vital areas near the brainstem, such as the posterior fossa. An awake or minimally sedated patient allows for use of the neurologic examination as a monitor and decreases the need for radiographic determinations. When patients are expected to be sedated for long periods, use of prophylactic postoperative CT scans is not unusual and at the least establishes a postsurgical baseline study.

Significant blood loss and replacement and large fluid loads associated with prolonged surgical procedures places these patients for increased risk of cerebral swelling in the postoperative period. Additionally, any brain rendered ischemic or with mild injury from retraction or temporary clipping will likely add to swelling. Fluid replacement and maintenance fluid needs should be minimized, and the use of hypertonic or colloid solutions may be considered.

CSF leaks are common when large dural openings are made or when large defects are left after extensive excisions. Lumbar CSF drainage may be continued into the postoperative period to minimize complications and promote dural healing. Continued drainage may require reexploration of the craniotomy site and may prove to be quite problematic.

Suggested Readings

Broennle MA, Teller L. Anesthesia for craniofacial procedures, *Clin Plast Surg* 14:17, 1987.

Fok H, Jones BM, Gault DG, et al: Relationship between intracranial pressure and intracranial volume in craniosynostosis, *Br J Plast Surg* 45:394, 1992.

Gault DT, Renier D, Marchac D, et al: Intracranial pressure and intracranial volume in children with craniosynostosis, *Plast Reconstr Surg* 90:377, 1992.

Gonzalez RM: Special anesthetic considerations in cranial base tumor surgery. In Sekhar LN, Janecka IP, editors: *Surgery of cranial base tumors,* New York, 1993, Raven Press.

Harris MM, Strafford MA, Rowe RW: Venous air embolism and cardiac arrest during craniectomy in a supine infant, *Anesthesiology* 65:547, 1986.

Harris MM, Yemen TA, Davidson A: Venous embolism during craniectomy in supine infants, *Anesthesiology* 67:816, 1987.

Imberti R, Locatelli D, Fanzio M, et al: Intra- and postoperative management of craniosynostosis, *Can J Anaesth* 37:948, 1990.

Kapp-Simon KA, Figueroa A, Jocher CA, et al: Longitudinal assessment of mental development in infants with nonsyndromic craniosynostosis with and without cranial release and reconstruction, *Plast Reconstr Surg* 92:831, 1993.

Kearney RA, Rosales IK, Howes WJ: Craniosynostosis: assessment of blood loss and transfusion practices, *Can J Anaesth* 36:473, 1989.

Meyer P, Renier D, Arnoud E, et al: Blood loss during repair of craniosynostosis, *Br J Anaesth* 1:854, 1993.

Palmisano BW: Anesthesia for plastic surgery. In Gregory GA, editor: *Pediatric anesthesia,* New York, 1994, Churchill Livingstone.

Sclabassi RJ, Krieger DN, Weisz D, et al: Methods of neurophysiological monitoring during cranial base tumor resection. In Sekhar LN, Janecka IP, editors: *Surgery of cranial base tumors,* New York, 1993, Raven Press.

Sekhar LN, Goel A, Sen C: General neurosurgical operative techniques and instrumentation in cranial base surgery. In Sekhar LN, Janecka IP, editors: *Surgery of cranial base tumors,* New York, 1993, Raven Press.

Shillito J: A plea for early operation for craniosynostosis, *Surg Neurol* 37:182, 1992.

ANESTHESIA AND NEURORADIOLOGY

15

Robert S. Holzman

Advances in diagnostic and interventional radiology, enlarging populations of patients requiring sophisticated imaging as an adjunct to diagnosis, availability of radiation therapy with increasingly precise delivery, and requests from our colleagues for anesthesia support during prolonged or risky procedures further our involvement with patients outside the operating room compared with previous years.

Minimally invasive techniques such as stereotaxy have reduced surgical trauma by allowing surgeons to plan the least damaging route to operative sites and obtain brain biopsies from sites, such as the brainstem, that were rarely sampled before. Solid intracranial lesions may be removed by computerized image processing under stereotactic conditions. For superficial lesions located near eloquent areas, local anesthesia may be administered, and removal is performed by loupe magnification, bipolar coagulation, and ultrasonic aspiration of the neodymium: yttrium-aluminum-garnet (Nd:YAG) laser fiber. In deep-seated lesions a surgical "corridor" is established and kept by means of retractors adapted for use with the stereotactic apparatus. Microsurgical techniques and the CO_2 laser are used in solid lesions; in vascular lesions bipolar coagulation or the Nd:YAG laser can be used. Stereotactic radiosurgery under local anesthesia with the Leksell Gamma Knife can effectively treat some patients with recurrent tic douloureux after unsuccessful medical-surgical procedures. Brain tumors can be treated by interstitial radiotherapy (stereotactic insertion of catheters into the lesion for loading of radioactive iodine) or radiosurgery (focusing of intense beams of radiation on lesions without needing surgical incisions). With interventional neuroradiology fine catheters can be introduced into most vessels in the cranium for embolization or dilatation. Pediatric anesthesiologists have become involved with these procedures. Current methods of neuroimaging can confirm the clinical assessment of dementia and further refine the diagnosis, prognosis, and treatment evaluation. Future developments will probably include frameless stereotaxy (when the rigid attachment of the stereotactic apparatus to the patient's head can be dispensed with) and at least partial automation of procedures such brain biopsy, the imaging and localization portion of which may take place outside the operating room.

From the anesthesiologist's perspective the potential hazards of neuroradiologic care outside the operating room are multiple. Equipment may consist of operating room "leftovers" and undesirables. Scheduling typically does not reflect similar considerations given to operating room scheduling such as induction, emergence, transport, and room turnover times before the next case. Medical, nursing, and support personnel working in nonsurgical areas usually have little experience with the requirements of an anesthesiologist; furthermore, they may be unable to anticipate specific needs during emergencies. Although most anesthesiologists gain considerable knowledge about surgical procedures during their training and beyond, few are familiar with the specific procedures or needs for a variety of diagnostic or interventional radiologic or radiation treatment procedures. Finally, some physicians question whether adults or even children require the involvement of an anesthesiologist for these procedures simply to provide comfort and analgesia. Such an attitude may promote antagonism rather than understanding and cooperation between medical and administrative personnel and insurers and should be addressed early in the involvement of an anesthesia department with anesthetizing locations outside of the operating room.

So as not to constrain the breadth of choices that are important to have available in these varying situations, we will first review some general issues of administering anesthesia outside the operating room, second examine some of the anesthetic options available, and finally look at the specific areas in which neurosurgical and neurologically impaired patients may require care.

EXTRAMURAL LOCATIONS: DESIGN

Few extramural locations are designed to deliver anesthetics. Floor space is given to imaging equipment or special needs of the radiologist or radiation oncologist. Although most newer facilities have pipeline sources of oxygen and suction, these may be in an area far away from the patient's head. Extra room that can be used as a preoperative holding or recovery area is relatively rare, let alone space to meet the clinical and logistic needs of an anesthesiologist. Anesthesiologists should be involved early with other specialists, engineers, and architects in the planning of an extramural location, to help direct and justify the reasons for placing equipment and oxygen risers in certain locations or to plan extra space if it potentially involves anesthetic induction and emergence.

The rooms themselves are often dark, small, and crowded. Supplemental lighting for record keeping and label verification is critical. Monitoring by simple direct observation becomes difficult. Special equipment, such as the magnetic resonance imager (MRI), the computed tomography (CT) scan, and the ionizing radiation accelerator, imposes additional requirements such as remote television monitoring or hard-wiring through reinforced walls.

Extramural anesthetizing locations are often located far from the operating room both in horizontal and vertical distance. Preplanned travel routes are needed, and assured elevator access with emergency key-controlled overrides is a must. Oxygen and monitoring for transport needs to be available. In some circumstances patients will remain anesthetized during or even after transport (if, for example, they are returning for another procedure several hours later, such as stereotactic radiosurgery).

Personnel, Support, and Logistics

Equipment in extramural anesthetizing locations tends to be less frequently used and ocasionally is incompatible with operating room equipment; it therefore must be rigorously examined before use. Missing or faulty anesthetizing or monitoring equipment must be repaired or replaced, which involves close coordination with the anesthesia technicians and biomedical engineers. Piped gases may not be available, and tanks may be in use. Although electrical outlets are generally grounded and hospital grade, if explosion-proof plugs are still present on operating room equipment used in non–operating room locations, plug incompatibility occurs. A cart should be suitably stocked for routine and emergency use, identical to the cart used in the operating room so that confusion is minimized for clinicians.

Clean-up, turnover, and restocking plans have to be specific for proper support by anesthesia technicians. A storage area large enough to stock resupply materials must be readily available on-site and a routine established for surveillance of adequate stock and supplies. This is even more important for extramural locations, because short supply items outside the operating room are not as readily obtained. Redundancy of nondisposable supplies is another issue; are two laryngoscopes enough, or should there be a third? Is one electrocardiographic (ECG) monitor enough, or should there be a battery-operated monitor for back-up and transport? Drugs should be checked according to the usual operating room routine and outdated drugs replaced. Gas cylinder supplies must be reliable for areas designed without piped oxygen. The anesthesia machine can be supplied from an H cylinder (6600 L) with E cylinders (659 L) as a reserve supply. If pipeline oxygen is not available, wall suction typically is not either, and a reliable source of portable suction is needed. The absence of wall suction will often mean that scavenging of waste anesthetic gases is impossible; alternative anesthetic techniques should be considered, such as total intravenous anesthesia.

Support and medical personnel in nonsurgical areas usually have little experience with the routine and emergency requirements of an anesthesiologist. The help we receive in the operating room from experienced circulating nurses and surgeons—during intubation, rapid sequence induction, intravenous insertion—may all be absent outside of the operating room. Periodic, short in-service programs conducted by the anesthesia department serve the purpose of training for non–operating room personnel.

Although it is not a job requirement, talent for improvisation is frequently helpful. Modifications to anesthetic circuits and intravenous tubing and creative positioning of equipment (and the anesthesiologist!) are often called for. Although most nonanesthetizing locations were not designed so that an observer could conveniently stand at the patient's head and see the procedure at the same time, things can often be altered with enough notice and the understanding of the radiologist and radiology technicians, once it is made clear what is needed.

Organization and Administration

Special additional considerations for those working in extramural locations include the need for familiarization with strange surroundings. There is no substitute for time; it is unrealistic to expect anyone to administer an anesthetic for a procedure scheduled at 11 AM by arriving at 10:50 AM. Checklists are invaluable when working in strange surroundings. It is crucial to know who to call for assistance if a problem arises, such as an episode of malignant hyperthermia, bleeding, or a cardiac arrest. We use a speed-dial system from all of our extramural anesthetizing location sites—just picking up the "hot line" will speed-dial the caller to the front desk of the operating room.

Appropriate planning for an anesthetic begins with knowledge of where and when the procedure will take place. Scheduling for procedures outside the operating room is a task of the requesting service, typically the department of radiology or radiation oncology, which communicates with the operating room booking coordinator to plan for staffing allocations. Radiologists recognize that involvement with anesthesia will often lengthen their total time commitment to a patient and potentially limit the number of procedures they may accomplish in a day. To justify our involvement for what might otherwise be construed as an unnecessary additional charge, we use a form to request the presence of an anesthesiologist to provide services outside the operating room; suitable justification for reimbursement from third-party payers can then be provided. This form accompanies the booking.

A well-coordinated system of patient arrival is a must, with adequately experienced personnel assigned to take initial vital signs and make the family and patient comfortable while waiting for the procedure. Because most of our patients are scheduled through our Day Surgery Unit, they pass through this unit for the initial work-up. Patients undergoing daily radiation therapy go directly to that department, where they are seen by a nurse for admission vital signs and a short-interval history.

Standards of Practice

The practice standards, adopted by the American Society of Anesthesiologists in 1986 for basic intraoperative monitoring, also apply to extramural locations. Practice standards promulgated by the American Academy of Pediatrics (Box 15-1) are exceeded by established practice standards in anesthesiology, but significant variances may exist when nonanesthesiologists sedate.

BOX 15-1.
Guidelines For Monitoring and Management of Pediatric Patients During and After Sedation for Diagnostic and Therapeutic Procedures (Synopsis)

Facilities

The practitioner who uses any type of sedation medication or general anesthetic agent must have available the proper facilities, personnel, and equipment to manage any reasonably foreseeable emergency situation experienced by the patient and as mandated by state law.

Back-up Emergency Services

Back-up emergency services should be identified with a protocol outlining necessary procedures for their immediate employment. For nonhospital facilities an emergency-assist system should be established with the nearest hospital emergency facility, and ready access to ambulance service must be assured.

Equipment

A positive-pressure oxygen delivery system that is capable of administering >90% oxygen at a 5 L/min flow for at least 60 minutes must be available. All equipment must be able to accommodate children of all ages and sizes.

BOX 15-1—*cont'd*

Equipment—cont'd

Inhalation sedation equipment must (1) provide a maximum of 100% and never <20% oxygen concentration at a flow rate appropriate to the child's size and (2) have a fail-safe system that is checked and calibrated annually.

Equipment that is appropriate for the technique being used and that can monitor the physiologic state of the patient before, during, and after the procedure must be present.

An emergency cart or kit must be readily accessible and should include the necessary drugs and equipment to resuscitate a nonbreathing and unconscious patient, and provide continuous support while that patient is being transported to a medical facility.

There must be documentation that all emergency equipment and drugs are checked and maintained on a scheduled basis.

Informed Consent

Each family is entitled to be informed and to give consent regarding risks of conscious sedation, deep sedation, and general anesthesia. Written consent should be obtained according to the procedure outlined by individual state laws.

Responsible Adult

The pediatric patient shall be accompanied to and from the office by a parent, legal guardian, or responsible adult who shall be required to remain at the office for the entire treatment period.

Documentation

Prior to Treatment: The practitioner must document each sedation and general anesthetic procedure in the patient's chart. Documentation shall include instructions to parents, dietary precautions, vital statistics (weight and age), preoperative health evaluation (including risk assessment, health history, review of systems with a statement as to airway patency, vital signs, and physical examination), child's physician, and rationale for sedation.

During Treatment: Including vital signs at specific intervals before, during and after procedure, and medications given.

After Treatment: The time and condition of the child on discharge should be documented.

• • •

Specific guidelines are provided for conscious sedation, deep sedation, and general anesthesia.

From Committee on Drugs, American Academy of Pediatrics, Elk Grove Village, IL, 1992, The Academy.

Preparation of Patients

In contrast with ambulatory surgery patients who are generally healthy, many neurologic or neurosurgical patients scheduled for evaluations or procedures outside the operating room are acutely or chronically ill, neurologically or nutritionally impaired, and have a history of multiple prior procedures and concurrent pharmacotherapy, including chemotherapy. There is often urgency in going ahead with diagnostic or therapeutic procedures despite an upper respiratory tract infection or obvious poor tolerance of the therapy (i.e., nausea, vomiting, diarrhea), and this urgency must be a part of the anesthetic plan; many of these patients cannot wait or come back when they are better. The potential for hypoglycemia and hypovolemia, particularly for immobile adults and chronically ill children, must be remembered. Of particular importance is recent chemotherapy that may influence the use of potent inhalational agents or certain levels of the fraction of inspired oxygen. If indicated by history, laboratory investigations including echocardiography need to be performed before the administration of anesthesia. We obtain separate consent for the administration of anesthesia, although for fractionated treatments such as radiation therapy we consider the entire treatment course as "one procedure" and therefore obtain a consent for multiple administrations of an anesthetic to accomplish "a course of radiation therapy."

Many neurologically impaired patients will be unable to give a history. Care must be taken to cull information from all available sources (old charts, nursing home transfer records, family members) and examine for signs and symptoms of elevated intracranial pressure (ICP). The Glasgow Coma Score should be recorded as a baseline. Neurologically impaired patients can be subject to a variety of arrythhmias, abnormal ventilatory responses to anesthetics, and altered reactions to anesthetic medications such as succinylcholine and nondepolarizing neuromuscular blocking agents. They are also frequently receiving short-term steroid therapy for elevated ICP and must be covered with additional doses and anticonvulsants when required. Neurologic injuries occurring in conjunction with trauma may be accompanied by disorders of other organ systems and injury to other elements of the neuraxis such as the cervical spine.

SELECTION OF AGENTS AND TECHNIQUES

The selection of an anesthetic technique depends on a variety of considerations. The patient's age, condition, and requirements of the procedure, such as duration, position, and the possibility of pain are all important. The assistance of the department of anesthesia is frequently sought when other methods, such as basal sedation administered by a nonanesthesiologist, have already failed; the anesthesiologist may then be (realistically or unrealistically!) expected to provide ideal conditions to accomplish the originally scheduled procedure. Techniques for accomplishing these ideal conditions vary, and it is important to remain versatile with the options outside the operating room. Monitored anesthesia care, light to deep sedation, general anesthesia, regional anesthesia, and hypnosis have all been used.

Premedication should be considered during this evaluation. Premedication has many purposes: relief of anxiety, sedation with easy arousability, analgesia, amnesia, reduction of salivary and gastric secretions, elevation of gastric pH, and decreased cardiac vagal activity. Neurologically impaired patients may be at increased risk because of impaired handling of secretions, presence of a tracheostomy, or diminution or absence of a gag reflex. Medications should be adjusted to the psychologic and physiologic condition of the patient and should not be ruled out because of the diagnostic or outpatient nature of the procedure. There may be cogent reasons to consider having a parent present for induction in children.

Barbiturates have the advantage of sedation with minimal respiratory and circulatory depression and rarely cause nausea and vomiting. However, they lack analgesia, can be antalgesic and disorienting, and a specific antagonist is not available. Intravenous pentobarbital by titration has been used successfully by radiologists while monitoring oral and nasal air flow, transcutaneous oxygen saturation, and cardiac rate and rhythm, with transient decreases in arterial oxygen saturation in 7.5% of patients; interventions included stimulation and head repositioning. Recently sodium thiopental in a mean induction dose of 6 mg/kg (with a mean total dose of 8.5 ± 3 mg/kg) was reported as a sole anesthetic for CT and MRI in 200 children from 1 month to 12 years of age. Methohexital has a shorter recovery time than thiopental and is more efficacious than oral chloral hydrate. Although rare, methohexital-induced seizures in children with temporal lobe epilepsy have been reported, and thiopental is an alternative for these patients. For patients on anticonvulsant medications, the higher dose limit is generally more successful. Methohexital has also been used intramuscularly for radiotherapy in children, in doses of 8 to 10 mg/kg, although the onset time is often twofold to threefold longer than rectally administered methohexital.

Narcotics reduce total anesthetic requirements and preprocedure and postprocedure analgesic requirements; they are furthermore reversible with naloxone. Although narcotics may be unnecessary for purely nonpainful diagnostic procedures, they may be very useful for therapeutic interventions, especially those with postprocedural pain, such as ethanol injection or other endovascular procedures. They are also useful when patients may be intolerant of volatile anesthetics, such as after anthracycline chemotherapy with documented impaired myocardial performance. Narcotics depress the medullary respiratory center by shifting the responsiveness to carbon dioxide. This fact may be of particular concern for patients with intracranial tumors receiving fractionated radiation therapy. Narcotics may also worsen preexisting nausea and vomiting.

Tranquilizers and sedative-hypnotics consist of three subgroups. *Benzodiazepines* have the advantage of anxiolysis with minimal vomiting and cardiorespiratory depression. Diazepam (Valium) is painful during intravenous injection and may lead to thrombophlebitis; midazolam (Versed) is water soluble and therefore may be more suitable intravenously or intramuscularly. The elimination half-life of midazolam averages 2.5 hours, compared with 20 to 70 hours for diazepam without the presence of active metabolites causing a "second peak" effect. Patients at extremes of age or with significant liver disease may be particularly sensitive to the duration of effect of the benzodiazepines. *Droperidol,* a butyrophenone, has the advantage of profound sedation, a potent antiemetic effect, and mild alpha-adrenergic blockade. There is occasionally acute anxiety after administration. The dopaminergic receptor blockade centrally may produce extrapyramidal symptoms. *Hydroxyzine* (Vistaril) and *promethazine* (Phenergan) are antihistaminic, antiemetic, and sedative. There can be some mild anticholinergic and extrapyramidal side effects.

Anticholinergics have been a component of routine pediatric premedication for decades. *Atropine* and *scopolamine* are tertiary amines and can therefore cross lipid barriers; *glycopyrrolate* is a quarternary ammonium compound, which acts on peripheral cholinergic receptors without crossing lipid membranes. The antisialagogue effect is particularly important for patients with glossopharyngeal nerve dysfunction and difficulty handling secretions because of brainstem disease. Anticholinergics decrease gastric $[H]^+$ secretion to variable degrees, but the amount and predictability of gastric pH elevation cannot be relied on as the sole method for chemoprophylaxis of aspiration. Anticholinergics have a considerable spectrum of side effects in addition to their normal effects on chronotropy and secretions, the most disturbing of which in the recovery period is the central anticholinergic syndrome, characterized by restlessness, agitation, stupor, and possibly convulsions or coma. Atropine and scopolamine are associated with central nervous system (CNS) symptoms much more frequently than is glycopyrrolate. *Physostigmine* (Antilirium) is a specific antidote, in doses of 25 μg/kg. Other anticholinergic side effects include relaxation of lower esophageal sphincter tone potentially increasing the risk of gastroesophageal reflux, heart rate changes (increased or decreased, mediated through central vagal stimulation), mydriasis, and cycloplegia. Because of suppression of cholinergically mediated portions of the peripheral sympathetic nervous system, sweat mechanisms are interfered with, and body temperature may become elevated. Physiologic dead space may increase after the administration of anticholinergics by as much as 20% to 25%; although this dead space is compensated for by an increase in spontaneous minute ventilation in healthy patients or controlled minute ventilation in anesthetized patients, the patient with a marginal respiratory or cardiac status may be adversely affected.

Preparation of the stomach and aspiration prophylaxis with histamine receptor antagonists (cimetidine, ranitidine) is frequently used to depress histamine-mediated gastric $[H]^+$ secretion. Short-term side effects may include headache, dizziness, fatigue, fever, and constipation, with neurologic dysfunction in prolonged therapy. Bradycardia, hypotension, and cardiac arrest have all been reported after intravenous use. Bronchospasm may occur in asthmatic patients because of the relative increased availability of H^1 receptors. H^2 blockers may also inhibit metabolism of other concurrently administered medications. Intravenous metaclopramide (children <6 years, 0.1 mg/kg; 6 to 14 years, 2.5-5 mg; adults, 10 mg) accelerates gastric emptying and increases tone in the lower esophageal sphincter but is associated with a significant incidence of extrapyramidal side effects in children when administered in doses >2 mg/kg/day or even less. Ondansetron is also an effective agent because it works synergistically with other agents through its vagal blocking actions in the gastrointestinal tract and through inhibition of the chemoreceptor trigger zone by serotonin receptor antagonism, particularly for patients undergoing radiation therapy with pulses of chemotherapy.

Ketamine has enjoyed great popularity for over 20 years for sedation or anesthesia outside the operating room because of its support of the cardiovascular and respiratory systems and excellent analgesia and achievement of unconsciousness. Care must be taken, however, in patients with known or strongly suspected elevated ICP. Tolerance often develops after several administrations, and the potential remains for complete or partial airway obstruction, copious oral secretions, and hyperactive airway reflexes. There is also a significant association, even in children, with unpleasant dreams. Moreover, daily intramuscular injections in patients without central or peripheral lines are painful and unpleasant.

Propofol (Diprivan) has only recently been approved for pediatric use but has been used for several years in many institutions as a means of providing sedation or anesthesia for diagnostic, therapeutic, and interventional procedures. Propofol sedation by bolus and continuous infusion for cranial MRI, with a total dose of 5 mg/kg/hr, left patients fit to return to the ward after 20 minutes. Total intravenous anesthesia with propofol has been described in children, and propofol has been used for long-term sedation of adults and children in the intensive care unit. However, fatal metabolic acidosis and myocardial failure associated with lipemic serum have been reported in five children admitted to the intensive care unit for respiratory support for upper respiratory tract infections while being sedated with continuous infusion propofol. In small sedative doses (0.3 to 0.6 mg/kg) in adults, propofol has been found to not have any significant effects on respiratory rate, minute volume, tidal volume, inspiratory and expiratory time, total expiratory cycle, $P_{0.1}$ (a measure of pressure generated against a temporarily occluded airway), end-tidal carbon dioxide, or arterial blood gas analysis. We have used propofol undiluted for infusions through an existing central venous line or diluted with lidocaine for peripheral vein infusion delivered by syringe pump calibrated in milliliters per hour (IVAC model 710). We then begin with the syringe pump set at 99 ml/hr until the patients fall asleep, from 60 to 180 seconds later, then gradually decrease the infusion rate during treatment until it is shut off at the end. Patients are typically awake, alert, and taking at least clear liquids 20 minutes later. Our average doses were a mean induction dose of 1600 μg/kg/min and a mean infusion dose of 200 to 250 μg/kg/min (Fig. 15-1).

Although specific antagonists for benzodiazepines and opioids exist and should always be available, such availability should not

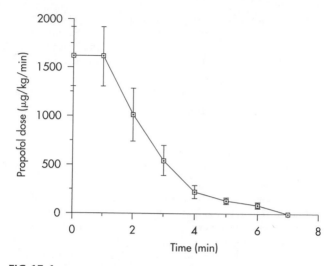

FIG 15-1.
Propofol dosing by continuous infusion. A total of 693 doses for radiation therapy were given to 28 patients.

encourage the cavalier use of their respective agonists. Efficacy notwithstanding, administration of an antagonist does not alter the requirement to monitor vital functions where depression of these has occurred. Flumazenil may take several minutes to completely reverse benzodiazepine-induced respiratory depression. The duration of the effect of opioid and benzodiazepine antagonists is less than that of their agonists, and reversal may be short lived.

Volatile agents and general endotracheal anesthesia should not be ruled out in this patient population strictly because of traditional neuroanesthesia concerns; the clinical significance of anesthetic choice still remains unclear despite the state of knowledge of underlying pathophysiologic features. Some patients will require general endotracheal anesthesia because of previous failures, the need for motionlessness or a secure airway, or a prolonged procedure. Newer, less soluble anesthetic agents such as desflurane and sevoflurane, which have pharmacokinetic profiles consistent with more rapid recovery, compare favorably with propofol in adults and may provide good alternatives for neuroanesthesia in equal minimum alveolar concentrations with isoflurane.

The output of a Fortec II vaporizer (Fraser Harlake, Orchard Park, N.Y.) was found to be variable according to the vaporizer's location and the orientation of the vaporizer's bimetallic strip within the magnetic field of an MRI. The movements of the bimetallic ferromagnetic temperature compensator altered vaporizer output by as much as 91% of the dialed output concentration. Several other vaporizers examined were incompatible with the MRI environment because of stronger ferromagnetic internal component content or the location of a ferromagnetic spring within the temperature compensator. It may be important to retain the capability of measuring inspired and end-tidal levels of volatile agents through an aspiration line extending outside the MRI suite to the analyzer.

Anesthetics may potentially affect the neuroradiologic treatment plan as well. The area of inorganic phosphate resonance was greater under pentobarbital (PB) anesthesia in mice, suggesting that the hypoxic fraction of the tumor increased after PB anesthesia. Near-infrared laser spectroscopy in vivo directly demonstrated that tumor oxyhemoglobin was reduced by >20% and total hemoglobin (tumor blood volume) was reduced by 11% after PB anesthesia. Tumor growth delay induced by gamma irradiation was shorter when tumors were irradiated under PB anesthesia, showing that PB anesthesia had a radioprotective effect.

A recent alternative for airway maintenance is the laryngeal mask airway (LMA). This device has been used successfully for radiotherapy in children, even those in the prone position. The LMA is manufactured in four sizes to fit patients from neonates to large adults. Certain features of pediatric airway anatomy have prompted an insertion technique different from adults (rotation through 180 degrees with the LMA initially open to the palate, then with rotation, sealing at the laryngeal inlet). Airway maintenance with an LMA may be less stimulating than with an endotracheal tube, as reflected by intraocular pressure measurements, and may be a consideration for those with elevated ICP.

Standard monitoring includes ECG, blood pressure cuff, and pulse oximetry. Quantitative capnography may be more difficult to accomplish in nonintubated patients, although qualitative capnography is easy; transcutaneous carbon dioxide analysis should be considered. Monitoring techniques include creative ways of incorporating remote monitoring into the anesthetic management plan. Remote cardiorespiratory monitoring during radiation therapy has been accomplished by electronically amplified esophageal stethoscopy. Other aspects of remote monitoring include television cameras mounted in strategic locations: one to see the patient's chest, one to see the monitors, which can be conveniently located on an arm mounted on the anesthesia machine. All monitors should have the capability of remote zoom and focus.

Smoothness of emergence may be particularly important for angiographic procedures because of the risk of dislodging a clot and bleeding at the puncture site, because control of bleeding after puncture is usually achieved by local pressure and keeping the patient quiet.

A final word—the best choice may be no medication. Occasionally the loss of control with the administration of sedation produces a bad result, and some patients may be capable of doing much better if they are completely awake; children may have a parent read a story to them, even over a microphone while they are undergoing treatment.

POSTANESTHETIC CARE

Adequate space and personnel are necessary for the proper recovery of the patient who had just been anesthetized several moments ago. In addition, prolonged repeated fasting, particularly in children with poor appetites undergoing radiation therapy, remains a concern with regard to hypoglycemia and decreased intravascular volume. Requirements of the postanesthetic area include the availability of routine monitors such as ECG, blood pressure, pulse oximetry, a means of delivering positive pressure 100% oxygen by bag-mask-valve, and an appropriately equipped resuscitation cart.

RESUSCITATION

A careful inspection of extramural anesthetizing locations must be conducted with regard to the potential for resuscitation. Each environment is unique with a specific set of problems that should be anticipated. Redundancy of monitoring devices is important, and if at all possible, the anesthesiologist should not be left with single items that can become critical at the time of resuscitation. One stationary physiologic monitor, for example, bolted onto the anesthesia machine should be capable of multichannel (e.g., lead II and modified V5) monitoring, along with at least two pressure channels and temperature. Other standard monitors should be available and placed securely (i.e., bolted) onto the anesthesia machine because cannibalization of equipment in extramural locations is not uncommon. Equipment such as defibrillation units and pacemakers may fail in high-energy magnetic fields.

Allergy should have a high index of suspicion when contrast material is used, and pharmaceuticals available to quickly treat anaphylaxis should be handy. For restricted access areas during diagnostic study such as CT or MRI the ability to quickly wheel a patient out of the scanner and into a readily available monitored area with oxygen and suction should be preserved. A Laerdal self-inflating silicone bag (no ferromagnetic working parts) can be kept inside the MRI room.

SPECIFIC SITES

Computed Tomography

CT scan is frequently the best method of assessment in trauma, particularly for the CNS, spinal cord, neck, chest, and abdomen. These patients will often be intubated in the emergency department and require care in the CT scanner continuing on to the operating room. Initial treatment may include hyperventilation to treat elevated ICP. The patient with concomitant cardiovascular deterioration and head injury presents a treatment conundrum; the support of the circulation with volume and vasoactive agents may worsen elevated ICP. Management of blood glucose level is critical because hyperglycemia appears to be related to adverse outcome. Cautious analgesia and minimal sedation may be required until further resuscitation, monitoring, and surgical procedures can be performed after diagnostic scanning.

Interventional Radiology

Interventional neuroradiologic techniques have advanced in recent years to the point where a wide variety of diseases affecting the CNS and head and neck can be treated using refined imaging, vastly improved catheter techniques, and new embolic agents. These procedures may be an adjunct to other neurologic or neurosurgical therapy, palliative or curative. Diseases for which interventional neuroradiologic techniques provide major advances in treatment include cerebral aneurysms, vasospasm after subarachnoid hemorrhage, cerebral arteriovenous malformations (AVM), dural arteriovenous fistulas, dural sinus thrombosis, atherosclerosis, scalp arteriovenous fistulas, carotid-cavernous fistulas, and stroke. The benefits of endarterectomy for severe symptomatic carotid stenosis have been supported by recent trials; percutaneous transluminal angioplasty may provide an alternative treatment. Recent advances in the management of cerebral aneurysm include new treatments for cerebral vasospasm and the use of endovascular occlusion to treat inoperable aneurysms. Endovascular embolization for AVMs also looks promising. Trials for new approaches to tumor embolization and local fibrinolytic therapy in the treatment of acute intracranial arterial or venous sinus thrombosis are under way. The survival rate and subsequent quality of life has improved significantly for neonates with cerebral AVM associated with ectasia of the vein of Galen. Good results are seen primarily in institutions with a large experience in treating this rare type of congenital malformation. Although more randomized trials are required to establish the benefit of these interventional procedures, it is clear that anesthesiologists will be asked to participate in more of these interventions in the foreseeable future.

Endovascular Interventional Neuroradiology

Interventional techniques include nonvascular and vascular intervention (Box 15-2). In vascular interventional radiologic procedures, embolization has become an important technique for treat-

---

BOX 15-2.
Interventional Radiology Procedures

Endovascular approaches are the treatment of choice for
  Cerebral vasospasm
  Carotid cavernous fistulas
  Vertebral artery origin stenosis
  Subclavian artery stenosis
  Innominate and left carotid origin stenosis
  Giant intracranial aneurysms
Endovascular treatment is developmental and should be restricted to centers performing formal trials in the treatment of
  Cerebral AVMs
  Internal carotid artery and intracranial stenosis

ing vascular malformations and hemorrhage. Percutaneous transluminal angioplasty and fibrinolytic therapy are gaining popularity even in pediatric institutions. Great success is being reported even in the smallest babies, and the important contribution that adequate sedation and analgesia can make to the ultimate outcome has been recognized.

Cerebral angiography requires motionlessness and exquisite control of ventilation. Positive pressure ventilatory excursions may affect the quality of the angiographic image. Anesthetic technique, both in choice of agent and control of arterial carbon dioxide tension, may affect cerebral blood flow (CBF) and hence the quality of the scan. Bucrylate glue (isobutyl-2-cyanoacrylate) injected into the nidus of a cerebral AVM remains an experimental technique. Anesthetic considerations include preoperative administration of a calcium channel blocking agent such as nimodipine for vasospasm prophylaxis caused by catheter manipulation and induction of systemic arterial hypotension to reduce transit time so that more AVM vessels will occlude and the bucrylate will not pass into the venous drainage system or to normal cortical tissue. Occlusion of the venous portion of the AVM without complete occlusion of the arterial inflow vessels could result in acute swelling and bleeding. Vascularity reduction through occlusion of major feeder vessels is the goal of embolizing large AVMs before planned surgical excision, which may be accomplished as a staged procedure over several days involving repeat anesthetics or sedation sessions.

Angiographic imaging may be enhanced through the use of vasodilators. We currently administer glucagon intravenously when needed in divided doses of 0.25 mg to a maximum of 1.0 mg. Glucagon has been found efficacious for digital subtraction angiography. Risks include glucagon-induced hyperglycemia, vomiting (particularly when given rapidly), gastric hypotonia, and provocation signs of pheochromocytoma.

Embolization or balloon occlusion of AVMs, vascular tumors, and intracranial aneurysms and fistulas carries considerable risk of catastrophic results, including sudden intracranial bleeding, acute cerebral ischemia, or catheter or balloon migration. If sedated, the patient may require urgent airway management. Cases with a long operative time often require a Foley catheter, especially if contrast material is used, with an obligatory osmotic diuresis expected. Angiography, digital subtraction angiography, and surgery may be combined, as in the surgical treatment of basilar trunk aneurysms. Patients may be treated with temporary balloon occlusion and intraoperative digital subtraction angiography. A silicone balloon catheter may be introduced through an angiography catheter in the basilar artery just proximal to the aneurysm. After the aneurysm is exposed, the occlusion balloon can be advanced and inflated temporarily within the basilar artery to prevent premature rupture and facilitate dissection of the aneurysm.

Embolization Procedures

The basic indications for embolization are occlusion of vascular malformations, management of uncontrollable hemorrhage, and presurgical embolization of hypervascular masses. The prognosis for patients with aneurysms has improved with the introduction of detachable coils, which may even be retrievable. Parent vessel occlusion is a good alternative for treating dysplastic aneurysms at the circle of Willis after functional testing. Vein of Galen malformations of the mural type are usually treated by the arterial route; the venous route is useful for treating choroidal forms when treatment by the arterial approach fails. AVM embolization with either particles or glue has about a 10% permanent complication rate and, when combined with radiosurgery or surgical resection, is successful in curing 74% of patients. Carotid cavernous fistulas are now also treated by a microcatheter and coils through the arterial or venous routes. Angioplasty in the neck and intracranially results in improved cortical perfusion. Gelfoam sponge, alcohol, stainless steel minicoils, detachable silicone balloons, or cyanoacrylate glue have all been used. There is a risk of stroke and damage to surrounding organs and tissues. In one series of 136 patients undergoing 310 procedures, the complication rate was 16%. In most of these cases embolization was followed by either operative removal of the AVM or by radiosurgery. Ethanol produces a coagulum of blood and causes endothelial necrosis, typically resulting in pain at the time of injection, and pain and edema from tissue injury for the following 48 to 72 hours.

Sedation allows neurologic assessment at all points of the procedure, and such close monitoring of the neurologic condition can give an early warning of adverse neurologic events, whereas general anesthesia permits easier control of blood pressure and respiration and eliminates concern about patient movement. For children general anesthesia is typically used. Preprocedural assessment should include any history of transient ischemic attacks or evidence of cerebrovascular occlusion, which would not favor aggressive use of controlled hypotension. Because these patients are anticoagulated during the procedure, a preoperative coagulation profile should be obtained. Adequate venous access is critical, as is arterial access for continuous monitoring during controlled hypotension and use of a urinary catheter (prolonged procedure, use of contrast agents). Cerebral function monitoring may aid interpretation of neurologic effects, particularly during controlled hypotension.

Procedural considerations involve sedation and motionlessness. Vasodilator agents (calcium channel blockers) or nitrate derivatives may need to be administered after embolization. A variety of anticoagulants may have to be on hand for prophylaxis of thrombosis. The anesthesiologist may be asked to participate in the perioperative care of patients undergoing embolization because they have pain crises after the procedure. The degree of pain depends on the extent of embolization, postembolic swelling, and amount of tissue necrosis but may begin as early as hours after the procedure and may last for weeks. A variety of analgesic techniques are available, and the use of steroids perioperatively, although not decreasing pain, may be of benefit in reducing edema and postembolic neuritis.

Magnetic Resonance Imaging

MRI has become an essential part of the diagnostic evaluation of the CNS. Atoms having an odd number of protons or neutrons are capable of acting as magnets. When they are aligned in a static magnetic field, they can be subjected to radiofrequency energy that alters their original orientation. With removal of the radiofrequency pulse, the nuclei rotate into their original alignment (relaxation), and the energy released can be detected and transformed into an image. Hydrogen is the atom most often used for imaging because it is present in most tissues as water and long-chain triglycerides. The most common cause of image degradation in MRI scans of children or uncooperative adults is patient movement. Techniques for monitoring anesthetized or critically ill patients during MRI have been described in several papers.

It is important to decide at the outset whether the anesthesia support should be within the magnetic field or outside it because the site will determine the configuration and composition of the equipment. A standard anesthesia machine can be situated outside the magnetic field (e.g., outside the 30 to 50 Gauss line) with a long breathing circuit and gas aspiration tubing. The risks are related to disconnection and impaired direct contact monitoring. When close to the magnet, the anesthesia machine and its components must be nonferrous, with power supplied by filtered sources. The characteristics of internal compression volume and respiratory minute volume in a 9-meter mechanical ventilation circuit in children and infants have been studied, and effective nomograms have been established to provide "long-distance" mechanical ventilatory support for patients undergoing MRI. Breathing circuits should be extra long (e.g., 18 to 20 foot Mapleson D, Jackson-Rees modification of Ayre's T-piece, Bain circuit, or circle absorption system) to provide continuity of the circuit during movement of the gantry in and out of the scanner bore. A ventilator specifically designed for MRI (225/SIMV ventilator, Monaghan Medical Corp., Plattsburg, N.Y.) has become available, which may be particularly important for patients who would be adversely affected by the length of circuit needed in the above circumstance.

All battery-operated equipment must be securely fixed in position. None of this equipment can be moved when the examination is in progress, lest the repositioning of this metallic mass influence the homogenity of the magnetic field and degrade the diagnostic images. Most intravenous needles and catheters with metallic hubs are composed of high-grade stainless steel, which is not ferromagnetic. Continuous infusion pumps can be located outside of the magnetic field as well, because the pump itself may malfunction under the influence of the strong magnetic field. When located outside the magnetic field, extra-length tubing of small bore is required for infusion. Intravenous or inhalation general anesthesia may be used effectively; there is some suggestion that the MRI signal may be altered under the influence of general inhalation anesthetics, although the clinical significance is unclear. Sedation can be problematic in the MRI environment when so little of the patient is directly visible.

Temperature monitoring can be accomplished by liquid crystal display (skin temperature). Anesthesia providers must be aware of many personal items taken for granted—clipboards, pens (use a pencil if necessary for record keeping), watches (digital acceptable; hands will not move in field), scissors, clamps, credit cards, eyeglasses, and paper clips. Laryngoscopes and blades are not ferromagnetic, but the batteries contained within the handle are. As an alternative, a plastic laryngoscope can be modified to be powered by a single paper-covered nonmagnetic 3 V lithium battery, or a direct-current light source can be used to power the laryngoscope. Conventional ECG monitoring is not possible because image degradation occurs as the lead wires traverse the magnetic fields. ECG by telemetry is often chosen. Nonferrous pulse oximeters are becoming available, and in some circumstances fiberoptically cabled pulse oximeters may be shielded by aluminum foil to minimize magnetic field degradation. Burns have resulted from pulse oximetry monitoring in the MRI. Any wire in the magnet bore that is a sizable portion of a wavelength may absorb a considerable amount of energy from the transmitting coil, and large voltages may build up on the surface of the wire with no discharge path other than free space; if the wire is poorly insulated or partly exposed, the voltage may discharge through space into the skin, causing significant local burns. Precordial stethoscopes made of nonferrous materials are acceptable, but the amount of noise generated during radiofrequency pulsing and the length of tubing required usually prohibits adequate auscultation. Average noise levels of 95 db have been measured in a 1.5 T MRI, comparable to noise levels of very heavy traffic (92 db) or light road work (90 to 110 db). Infrared transmission of breath and heart sounds with a special microphone has been described.

There are important nonmagnetic considerations as well. Some patients have claustrophobia and have difficulty cooperating during the study because of the small bore of the magnet. Anxiety-related reactions (distress, panic, claustrophobia) have been estimated to occur in 4% to 30% of patients. Some obese patients or those with skeletal abnormalities such as advanced scoliosis or cerebral palsy with flexion contractures cannot be examined. The strong static magnetic field may interfere with the proper function of life-support equipment, and the small bore of the magnet may make it difficult or impossible to examine some critically ill patients.

In our MRI for pediatric patients, anesthetic induction is typically accomplished with parents present, usually in the holding anteroom just outside the scanner. The airway is controlled by one anesthesiologist, and the anesthesia machine by another, through the long breathing circuit passing into the scanning room and then out the entry door. After intubation, the patient is positioned in the scanner, with the pulse oximeter and any other monitors kept as far away from the bore of the magnet as possible so as not to become missiles. The pulse oximeter probe is placed on a toe, with the wire leading to the oximeter box on the window ledge and the digital reading displayed toward the viewing room. A qualitative end-tidal carbon dioxide analyzer is positioned in our 56-foot modified Mapleson D circuit. ECG wires are braided to reduce looping and minimize the generation of potential differences and placed in a cluster centrally on the chest (magnetic gradients change least at the center of the magnet bore), and personnel leave the room. The ECG is hard-wired to a slave monitor in the control room that displays ECG; systolic, diastolic, and calculated mean blood pressure; and a respiratory rate detected by impedance pneumography. T wave changes on the ECG may be due to reading leads in line with blood flow perpendicular to the magnetic field, such as blood flow in the aortic arch. The pulse oximeter (Microspan 1040A pulse oximeter, Biochem International, Waukesha, Wisc.) and qualitative end-tidal carbon dioxide monitor (Biochem respiration monitor No. 525, Biochem International) are turned to face the window and therefore the observers.

In addition to diagnostic studies, magnetic resonance guidance has been used for bilateral radiofrequency cingulotomy for intractable cancer and noncancer pain. Stereotaxis with magnetic resonance guidance and local anesthesia was used to place a radiofrequency lesion (75 degrees, 60 s) in 10 patients with metastatic lesions, with good overall results.

Radiation Oncology

Radiation therapy uses ionizing photons to destroy tumors of the CNS as well as other malignancies. Short, repeat sessions of 10 minutes are typical, requiring reliable motionlessness and remote monitoring with the patient in isolation to precisely aim the beam at malignant cells while sparing healthy cells. A planning session in a simulator is usually scheduled before the initiation of radiation therapy so that fields to be irradiated can be plotted and marked. This procedure usually lasts 30 to 45 minutes.

Fractionated radiation therapy divides the total radiation therapy course into discrete daily sessions, allowing normal tissue repair between sessions while the tumor burden is destroyed or lessened. Hyperfractionated, or multiple-session daily, radiation therapy is a modality reported primarily in adults for head and neck cancer to minimize the frequency of radiation-induced side effects. The rationale for twice-daily fractionation in children is based on the observation that fractionation to growing bone in rats reduces the growth deficit by 25% to 30%, with the hope that other normal tissues may be similarly spared during growth.

Radiation therapy is usually brief and nonpainful and may be approached with a variety of plans for rendering the patient temporarily motionless. The key issue is the anesthesologist's limited access to the patient. Remote video monitoring and ECG and pulse oximeter use is crucial, and we use two, or in some locations three, video cameras to look at the monitors, the chest, and the face of the patient. A central venous line in young children undergoing a long course of radiation therapy helps immensely. It is important to remember that babies undergoing radiation therapy after a prolonged fast are at risk for hypoglycemia; delayed awakening or tremulousness should prompt a Dextrostix check.

Stereotactic radiosurgery differs from external beam radiotherapy in several important ways. A single large fraction of radiation is used as opposed to smaller daily fractions. In pediatric and adult patients most radiosurgery originally concentrated on treatment of small histologically benign lesions such as vascular malformations, acoustic neuromas, and pituitary adenomas. This has more recently been expanded to include malignant tumors such as solitary metastases, ependymomas, glioblastomas, and several other tissue types; tumor volume ideally has to be small (≤ 14 cm^3) for optimal results. Radiation outside the target structures is minimized principally through the sophisticated stereotactic technique used, allowing for accuracy of treatment to within a few millimeters of the target.

Although the actual radiosurgery lasts about an hour, the duration of imaging, computer calculations, and anesthetic or sedation often totals 4 to 6 hours. A stereotactic frame is fixed in position to the patient's head with the target determined by CT scan for tumors or angiography for AVMs. The physical characteristics of the frame and the length of time of the procedure influence anesthetic management. Pediatric patients (including most teenagers) typically require a general anesthetic induced before placement of the head frame. For airway security we place a transnasal endotracheal tube, secured with tape and tincture of benzoin, before placement of the head frame, which crosses over the tip of the nose making mask fit or reintubation in an emergency difficult or impossible. The key for removal of the head frame is taped to the frame itself. A nasogastric tube is placed for the day's anesthetic.

Calculations for dose and the three-dimensional coordinates for the beam take several hours to compute after the initial radiologic study and head frame placement. A variety of anesthetic techniques are used, from continuous infusion sedation medications to volatile anesthetic techniques and combinations of both. Some patients do well with sedation and spontaneous breathing; however, younger patients are usually mechanically ventilated. An initial CT scan is followed by several hours in the postanesthesia care unit while computer calculations are being completed, followed by 45 minutes to 1 hour in the radiosurgery suite, removal of the head frame, emergence from anesthesia, monitoring in the postanesthesia care unit, and overnight admission to the hospital. The most common perioperative problem is nausea and vomiting, probably from sensitivity of chemoreceptor trigger zone centers to radiation. For large radiation doses to brainstem structures with significant concern about brainstem swelling, patients have remained intubated in the intensive care unit up to several days, lest vital center compromise result from radiation-induced edema.

Stereotactic radiation therapy provides more precise localization of the fractionated radiation dose over the same duration as conventional radiation therapy, with the adjunctive use of a head frame. Anesthetic considerations for the headframe include ease of daily application, reliability, ability to deliver supplemental oxygen and support the airway with a face mask if needed, and rapid removal of the facial restraint should it become necessary. The head frame should hold the head immobile for the radiation treatment. Frames have been used before.

FUNCTIONAL EVALUATION IN NEURORADIOLOGY
Dominance and Lateralization

The carotid Amytal test was introduced in 1948 by Wada to localize speech function before temporal lobectomy in patients with medically refractory epilepsy, and it remains the standard for that purpose. Preoperative evaluation for epilepsy surgery is typically carried out in two phases: noninvasive studies (electroencephalogram and videomonitoring, brain imaging, psychometrics) and invasive techniques (videomonitoring with intracranial electrodes, angiography, Wada test, functional mapping). However, the specificity of the Wada test has been called into question as a predictor of involved areas of the brain. In one series 88 patients underwent Wada testing and unilateral extraoperative cortical electrical stimulation with subdural electrode arrays. In none of the patients with left dominance by Wada testing were language areas found with right-sided stimulation, but two patients with right dominance by Wada testing had language areas mapped on the left side. These findings suggested that left dominance by Wada testing is strong evidence for lateralization of language function in the left hemisphere, but there is concern about the ability of the Wada test to exclude the possibility of some left-sided language function despite apparent right-sided dominance. The authors concluded that patients with right or bilateral dominance on Wada testing should have cortical stimulation for localization of language areas if extensive left or right temporal or frontal resection is planned. State-of-the-art techniques include a "superselective" Wada test performed under wake-up anesthesia, before transcatheter embolization with a mixture of acrylic glue and iodized oil for intracerebral AVMs.

Rapid-rate transcranial magnetic stimulation may be a noninvasive method for determining lateralization of speech arrest, as has been suggested by its correlation with Wada test results. Other newer techniques for functional mapping of the brain in conjunction with neurosurgical care are emerging, including optical imaging, functional positron emission tomography (PET) studies, transcranial magnetic stimulation, and magnetoencephalography. Studies have used these new techniques, and the potential for these procedures to replace the established but more invasive techniques is being considered.

Magnetic Resonance Angiography

Magnetic resonance angiography (MRA) is a novel technique that uses gradient echo pulse sequences and computer postprocessing techniques to create vascular flow images. The technique is easy to apply, noninvasive, and frequently yields information not available by other noninvasive means. MRA may be particularly useful for lesions such as aberrant arteries, AVMs, and ischemic disease. The noninvasive nature of MRA makes it particularly appealing in the evaluation of the neurovasculature, and this techique has already led to a reduction in conventional angiographic and duplex Doppler ultrasound procedures.

Magnetic Resonance Spectroscopy

In vivo magnetic resonance spectroscopy provides biochemical information on living organisms in a noninvasive manner and has recently been used to study neonatal brain energy metabolism. High-energy phosphate metabolism and phospholipid metabolism can be evaluated in this manner; clinical correlations can be made regarding seizures or long-term neurologic sequelae associated with a decreased phosphocreatine/orthophosphate ratio. Future trends in neonatal MRS may provide further information on morphologic and metabolic brain development.

Positron Emission Tomography

Functional PET scanning has been used to precisely localize a structural brain lesion to the precentral gyrus, confirmed by intraoperative cortical mapping, by first obtaining a resting PET scan identifying the AVM followed by a second PET scan performed during vibrotactile stimulation to identify a particular somatosensory area and to localize the AVM to that part of the precentral gyrus immediately in front of it. The relationship and localization were confirmed by cortical mapping at the time of craniotomy under local anesthesia.

Localized Hyperthermia

Localized hyperthermia is becoming a potent therapeutic method for malignant brain tumors, either alone or in combination with radiation therapy. The heat response of organized tissues includes other factors besides cellular thermosensitivity; tissue pH, partial pressure of oxygen, and nutrient supply are largely influenced by tissue blood flow. In an experimental model, regional CBF (rCBF) changes in monkeys' brains during hyperthermia were investigated; under general anesthesia and controlled respiration a parietooccipital craniectomy, 4 x 4 cm, was performed, and brain tissue was heated with 2450 MHz microwave irradiation. During hyperthermia the rCBF linearly increased at a rate of 10% per 1° C temperature rise. Above 45° C the rCBF transiently increased and then started to decline during heating. No consistent results were obtained with heating at 43° C. These results show that normal monkey brain tissues respond to hyperthermia by an rCBF increase so long as the threshold values of tissue temperature (43° C) and exposure time (40 to 60 minutes) are not exceeded. Excessive heating may lead to irreversible damages to normal tissue and vasculature.

Awake Discography

MRI is a static test and discography the only available dynamic test for disc evaluation; awake discography can determine which abnormal discs are symptomatic by the patient's pain response. In a study undertaken to determine the correlation between awake discography findings and MRI, MRI was performed before discography in 164 symptomatic patients. Discography was performed with patients minimally sedated and under local anesthesia. MRI and discography correlated in 90 cases (55%) and differed in 74 (45%). There were 172 normal discs and 199 abnormal discs. Of the abnormal discs 151 (76%) reproduced symptoms. In 60 discs (13%) MRI showed abnormal findings and the discogram normal findings. Disc levels classified as abnormal on MRI demonstrated that 108 discs (37%) were asymptomatic. MRI showed normal findings and the discogram abnormal findings in 34 discs (7%), of which 21 (5%) recreated exact symptoms and 13 (2%) caused no pain. "Awake" discography therefore remains part of the diagnostic armamentarium that complements noninvasive neuroradiologic evaluation.

SAFETY ISSUES

Because anesthesiologists find themselves participating in the care of patients requiring increasingly sophisticated imaging techniques, it is appropriate to examine the risks for patients and staff when they are exposed to the types of high energies and contrast agents used to obtain images.

Use of Intravascular Contrast Media

In a comprehensive review Goldberg noted that approximately 5% of radiologic exams with contrast media are complicated by adverse reactions, with one third of these severe enough to require immediate treatment. In the presence of a history of atopy or allergy, the risk of a reaction is increased from 1.5 to 10-fold. The amount of iodine in contrast media seems to be important because fewer reactions tend to occur with <20 gm of iodine. Reactions vary from mild, subjective sensations of restlessness, nausea, and vomiting to a rapidly evolving, angioedema-like picture accompanied by bronchospasm, arrythmias, and cardiac arrest. Agents with a high osmolar concentration should be administered with caution in patients who have a limited cardiovascular reserve (e.g., congestive heart failure or cardiomyopathy). In addition, volume depleted young children who have been given nothing by mouth for prolonged intervals or who have had bowel preparation would do well to be prehydrated before injection of contrast. Those patients dependent on a relatively full intravascular volume status should be monitored carefully for the usual initial rise in filling pressures and intravascular volume, followed by diuresis and volume depletion. Patients with impaired excretory mechanisms such as those in renal failure must be followed closely with regard to elimination of high osmotic contrast agents. Treatment of contrast media reactions may include epinephrine, circulatory support with other inotropes, anticholinergics, ventilatory support with endotracheal intubation, administration of steroids, and possibly diphenhydramine.

Gadolinium diethylenetriaminepentaacetic acid is a low osmolar ionic contrast medium used for MRI, with a slower clearance in neonates and young infants than adults, yielding longer windows for imaging. Gadolinium is a paramagnetic substance that enhances proton relaxation and thereby enhances diseased tissue imaging on MRI. Newer low osmolar nonionic contrast agents such as gadodiamide (Omniscan) are becoming available as well. In adults subjective sensations of lightheadedness, dizziness, and alterations of taste or smell have been reported, as well as transient elevations in serum iron. Adverse reactions to MRI contrast agents are reported as 2.4%. Of particular concern for children are the rare reports of anaphylactoid reactions (<1:100,000 doses) and mild elevations in serum bilirubin levels. Mild hemolysis may be associated with this drug. One theoretic concern in patients with sickle cell disease is sickle crisis and vascular occlusion. Sickled cells are known to align with external magnetic fields to which they are exposed; it is unknown how this theoretic concern compares, for example, with the normal forces of deformation imposed on red blood cells in their normal course through the vascular tree in patients with sickle cell disease.

Ionizing Radiation

The radiation exposure of pediatric anesthesia fellows during a 2-month period has been reported. Fellows assigned to the cardiac catheterization laboratory had fluoroscopy exposure time of 14 to 85 minutes per case, typically for two to three cases per day. For these anesthesiologists badge readings ranged from 20 to 180 mrem/month; all noncardiac anesthesia fellows received undetectable (<10 mrem/month) levels. With the maximum permissible dose limit for nonradiation workers (including anesthesiologists) set at 42 mrem/month, anesthesiologists would do well to become aware of principles of radiation safety in clinical practice and remember that exposure is directly proportional to the duration of the procedure and inversely proportional to the square of the distance from the source.

High-Intensity Magnetic Fields

MRI exposes the patient (and the health care workers surrounding the patient) to a static magnetic field, a rapid switched spatial gradient magnetic field, and radiofrequency magnetic fields. The static magnetic field, which causes alignment of unpaired tissue protons, may cause movement of ferromagnetic devices such as vascular clips, ventricular shunt connectors, casings for pacemakers, and control devices for pacemakers (potentially converting them from demand to fixed mode). Metallic devices in other areas, particularly when invested with fibrous tissue are less problematic.

The gradient magnetic field generates electrical current, typically of a density two to three orders of magnitude less than a defibrillator (10 mA/m^2, compared with 1000 to $10,000$ mA/m^2). This current strength, however, may reprogram a programmable pacemaker and therefore interfere with its function. Patients with implantable defibrillators or cardioverters are also considered at risk, as are patients with implantable infusion pumps (e.g., insulin pumps), cochlear implants, and neurostimulators. Excellent reviews of monitoring considerations and equipment choices in the MRI environment and patient safety principles are available.

MRI and spectroscopy do not use ionizing radiation. However, secondary harmful effects, such as magnetic objects becoming projectiles within the magnetic field as they approach the bore of the magnet and potentially causing injury, are a consideration. Implants such as vascular clamps, hemostatic clips, dental devices, heart valve prostheses, intravascular coils, filters and stents, ocular implants, orthopedic implants, otologic implants, shrapnel, penile implants, and vascular access ports have been reviewed with regard to the specific object tested, the material used for construction, whether the object was deflected or moved during exposure to the static magnetic field, and the highest static magnetic field strength used for testing the object. Each patient or medical staff member must be individually evaluated for these risks when present in the area of a MRI.

Increased permeability of the blood-brain barrier has been found in rats after exposure to the various electromagnetic field components of proton MRI. Although the clinical significance is unclear, Evans blue–labeled proteins and tagged albumin, normally not passing the blood-brain barrier of rats, have been found after exposure to MRI.

As with patient precautions, equipment precautions should be taken for all potentially ferromagnetic objects such as stands used for intravenous delivery, oxygen and nitrous oxide cylinders, and monitoring equipment. The anesthesia machine, if used in the scanning room, should be outfitted with aluminum gas cylinders and kept in the corner of the room. An anesthesia machine especially designed to be MRI compatible is now commercially available (Excel 210, Ohmeda, Madison, Wis.). Although laryngoscopes made of plastic have been fashioned, the batteries in the handle mitigate against its use.

● ● ●

We have considered some general issues and some specific situations for anesthesia for neuroradiology and the neurologic patient outside the operating room. There is no "correct technique" for anesthetics in these areas; thorough familiarity with the pathophysiologic features of the neurologically impaired and neurosurgical patient and clinical versatility must be maintained to adapt to specific situations in different institutions while preserving the working relationships between anesthesiologists and their medical colleagues. Rather, this discussion has been a broad review of issues and concerns that influence anesthetic choice and method that have worked well at a variety of institutions, including our own, over the past 10 years. Because of the evolution of specialized equipment for diagnostic radiology and radiation therapy and the lack of need for an operating room setting for these procedures, it is likely that anesthesiologists' involvement in caring for these patients outside of the operating room will increase in years to come.

Suggested Readings

American Society of Anesthesiologists: *Standards for Basic Anesthetic Monitoring,* 1994.

Benati A: Interventional neuroradiology for the treatment of inaccessible arterio-venous malformations, *Acta Neurochir* 118:76, 1992.

Bloomfield EL, Masaryk TJ, Caplin A, et al: Intravenous sedation for MR imaging of the brain and spine in children: pentobarbital versus propofol, *Radiology* 186:93, 1993.

Brown TR, Goldstein B, Little J: Severe burns resulting from magnetic resonance imaging with cardiopulmonary monitoring: risks and relevant safety precautions, *Am J Phys Med Rehabil* 72:166, 1993.

Chernish SM, Maglinte DD: Glucagon: common untoward reactions—review and recommendations, *Radiology* 177:145, 1990.

Committee on Drugs, American Academy of Pediatrics: Guidelines for monitoring and management of pediatric patients during and after sedation for diagnostic and therapeutic procedures, *Pediatrics* 89:1110, 1992.

Cremin BJ: Sedation for CT examinations in children, *Br J Radiol* 63:316, 1990.

Erlebacher JA, Cahill PT, Pannizzo F, et al: Effect of magnetic resonance imaging on DDD pacemakers, *Am J Cardiol* 57:437, 1986.

Harpur ES, Worah D, Hals PA, et al: Preclinical safety assessment and pharmacokinetics of gadodiamide injection, a new magnetic resonance imaging contrast agent, *Invest Radiol* 28:S28, 1993.

Henderson KH, Lu JK, Strauss KJ, et al: Radiation exposure of anesthesiologists, *J Clin Anesth* 6:37, 1994.

Hubbard AM, Markowitz RI, Kimmel B, et al: Sedation for pediatric patients undergoing CT and MRI, *J Comput Assist Tomogr* 16:3, 1992.

Kanal E, Shellock FG, Talagala L: Safety considerations in MR imaging, *Radiology* 176:593, 1990.

Keeter S, Benator RM, Weinberg SM, et al: Sedation in pediatric CT: national survey of current practice, *Radiology* 175:745, 1990.

Manuli MA, Davies L: Rectal methohexital for sedation of children during imaging procedures, *AJR Am J Roentgenol* 160:577, 1993.

Martin LD, Pasternak LR, Pudimat MA: Total intravenous anesthesia with propofol in pediatric patients outside the operating room, *Anesth Analg* 74:609, 1992.

Menon DK, Peden CJ, Hall AS, et al: Magnetic resonance for the anaesthetist, I: physical principles, applications, safety aspects, *Anaesthesia* 47:240, 1992.

O'Mahony BJ, Bolsin, SNC: Anaesthesia for closed embolisation of cerebral arteriovenous malformations, *Anaesth Intens Care* 16:318, 1988.

Pandya PB, Martin JT: Improved remote cardiorespiratory monitoring during radiation therapy, *Anesth Analg* 65:529, 1986.

Patteson SK, Chesney JT: Anesthetic management for magnetic resonance imaging: problems and solutions, *Anesth Analg* 74:121, 1992.

Peden CJ, Menon DK, Hall AS, et al: Magnetic resonance for the anaesthetist, II: anaesthesia and monitoring in MR units, *Anaesthesia* 47:508, 1992.

Shellock FG: Biological effects and safety aspects of magnetic resonance imaging, *Magn Reson Q* 5:243, 1989.

Spear RM, Waldman JY, Canada ED, et al: Intravenous thiopentone for CT and MRI in children, *Paediatr Anaesth* 3:29, 1993.

Steen RG, Wilson DA, Bowser C, et al: 31P NMR spectroscopic and near infrared spectrophotometric studies of effects of anesthetics on in vivo RIF-1 tumors: relationship to tumor radiosensitivity, *NMR Biomed* 2:87, 1989.

Strain JD, Campbell JB, Harvey LA, et al: IV nembutal: safe sedation for children undergoing CT, *AJR Am J Roentgenol* 151:975, 1988.

Thomas DG, Kitchen ND: Minimally invasive surgery: neurosurgery, *BMJ* 308:126, 1994.

Vangerven M, Van Hemelrijck J, Wouters P, et al: Light anaesthesia with propofol for paediatric MRI, *Anaesthesia* 47:706, 1992.

Young WL, Pile-Spellman J: Anesthetic considerations for interventional neuroradiology, *Anesthesiology* 80:427, 1994.

ANESTHESIA FOR INTRACRANIAL VASCULAR SURGERY

16

David J. Stone
David L. Bogdonoff

PREOPERATIVE ASSESSMENT

Cardiovascular Assessment

VOLUME STATUS

The battle with neurosurgeons who are attempting to keep their patients as "dry as a chip" is over. Clinicians realize that hypovolemia is an inefficient and ineffective means of blood pressure control and, in fact, makes precise control even more difficult as the peaks and valleys of blood pressure are exacerbated. Furthermore, the hypovolemic patient may be more likely to display undesirable symptoms from vasospasm. However, the laws of nature must still be considered. More than half of patients with a ruptured aneurysm have a significant (>10%) decrease in plasma volume. The patient with a recent subarachnoid hemorrhage (SAH) may be vasoconstricted because of high catecholamine levels and may be hypovolemic because of the influence of atrial natriuretic factor. Therefore the volume status of each patient should be carefully reviewed by the usual clinical means before anesthesia is induced. This may include a review of weight changes; fluid ins and outs; serum sodium level; hematocrit; blood urea nitrogen; pulse rate; blood pressure, including orthostatic changes; and, probably most important, the appearance of the patient. The anesthesiologist must then decide whether a significant intravascular volume deficit is present and the extent to which it should be corrected before anesthesia can be safely induced without the risk of excessive hypotension or hypertension. We generally use glucose-free crystalloids such as normal saline solution alternated with Ringer's lactate while checking blood sugar levels to avoid hypoglycemia or hyperglycemia. Awareness of the possibility of hypovolemia is half the battle, with the other half consisting of clinical judgment, which comes from clinical experience (which is a result of clinical mistakes). If in doubt, give a little extra fluid before starting the case: the patient may require more volume to maintain blood pressure after the institution of mechanical ventilation, especially in the presence of hyperventilation.

HYPERTENSION

Many patients with aneurysmal disease are basically healthy adults who may or may not have essential hypertension. Other patients may have hypertension from the previously noted elevated catecholamine state or from the awareness that they are about to undergo major neurologic surgery for a life- and brain-threatening process. Hypertension may also represent a proper physiologic response, an attempt to maintain cerebral perfusion in the face of increased intracranial pressure (ICP) resulting from blood, edema, or hydrocephalus. In the latter instance it is essential to ensure that the clinician's reflex treatment of blood pressure does not result in the ischemia that the organism is (wisely) trying to avoid. Clearly, it is important to avoid severe spikes of hypertension, especially in the patient with a freshly ruptured aneurysm. If vasospasm is also present, the treatment becomes a tightrope walk between adequate perfusion by hypervolemia and hypertension and rerupture of the aneurysm.

The precise drugs used are dictated by availability (e.g., the recent disappearance and reappearance of hydralazine), familiarity, ICP, and concurrent medical problems. For example, nitroprusside, nitroglycerin, calcium channel blockers, and even hydralazine should be used with caution in the patient with elevated ICP. On the other hand, nitroglycerin might be the drug of choice in the patient with clinically significant coronary artery disease. The ability to discontinue a nitroprusside, esmolol, or nitroglycerin infusion is an advantage not afforded by most other means of treating hypertension. Intravenous calcium channel blockers such as nicardipine, when available, may be preferred if hypertension is to be treated in the presence of vasospasm. Drugs that are alpha$_2$-receptor agonists, such as clonidine, may have the theoretic advantage of providing some element of brain protection but are not currently available in a parenteral form that allows for intraoperative supplementation.

The current favorite in our institution and others is labetalol, a combined alpha- and beta-receptor antagonist. In the hypertensive adult patient a dose of 10 to 20 mg given intravenously (IV) before the induction of anesthesia often helps minimize the blood pressure spike of laryngoscopy and intubation without producing severe hypotension during the subsequent long period of neurosurgical preparation. In the anesthetized patient it is prudent to administer a small labetalol dose, such as 2.5 to 5 mg, and to wait about 5 minutes before a doubled dose is administered (unless the blood pressure requires a very quick and extensive reduction; thiopental is an excellent and often-forgotten hypotensive agent in this event but obviously requires the institution of airway management). Other clinicians favor esmolol (0.5 to 1.0 mg/kg bolus), which has the advantage of an extremely short half-life and can be used continuously as an infusion (vide infra). Preoperative administration of an angiotensin-converting enzyme (ACE) inhibitor such as captopril can also be used, but with clonidine it may be a struggle to keep blood pressure acceptably high after induction and before significant surgical stimulation. ACE inhibitors can now be administered IV (enalapril 1.25 to 5.0 mg), and we are only now gaining experience in their use and usefulness.

The overall goal in this setting is to avoid blood pressure elevations that might cause or contribute to rupture or rerupture of the aneurysm. Often we tolerate lower blood pressures (i.e., mean blood pressures of 50 to 60 mm Hg) that we would treat with fluids, ephedrine, etc., during a nonneurovascular case, for example. However, concurrent neurologic (vasospasm, elevated ICP, cerebrovascular occlusive disease) or nonneurologic disease (coronary artery disease, renal insufficiency, valvular heart disease) may dictate modifications in care on the basis of individual patient physiologic characteristics.

CARDIAC ABNORMALITIES

It has been observed for many years that electrocardiographic (ECG) changes occur in a large percentage of patients with SAH, including changes that can be confused with myocardial ischemia such as ST segment and T-wave changes and even, rarely, Q-waves. These changes may be the result of hypothalamic ischemia leading to increased catecholamine production and a resulting microscopic myocarditis. It has been postulated that beta-blockers may be particularly beneficial in this setting for treatment of tachycardia or hypertension. Although wall motion abnormalities have been demonstrated echocardiographically, it is important that cardiologists and other consultants involved in the patient's care realize that the cardiac pathophysiologic processes involved are much more likely to be due to SAH than to coronary artery disease and that, in most cases, neurosurgical treatment of the problem at hand should proceed. Other ECG abnormalities are reported to include changes in QT interval and serious ventricular arrhythmias. We have not had clinical difficulties with ventricular function or intractable arrhythmias. If acute ECG changes occur in the operating room in conjunction with hypertension or tachycardia and require treatment, it is probably appropriate to use beta-blockers as first-line therapy, with nitroglycerin reserved for those cases in which clinical judgement dictates that myocardial ischemia is resulting from coronary artery disease. Although we have not had to use them in this setting, diltiazem or verapamil may also be reasonable choices if heart rate is an issue and beta-blockers are unavailable, contraindicated, or ineffective.

Neurologic Evaluation
DIAGNOSIS

The classic description of a patient who complains of the worst headache of his/her life often holds true. Consciousness may be lost temporarily (or longer) because of the acute rise in ICP, followed by a headache and stiff neck as a result of subarachnoid blood. Mild and repeated warning leaks may occur, so the diagnosis that may seem obvious to those in the operating room with a computed tomographic (CT) scan and angiogram hanging on the wall may not be quite so obvious to the busy primary-care practitioner with an office full of patients with functional complaints. The diagnosis is made from the CT scan in most cases, with lumbar puncture reserved for the suspicious case with a negative scan. Lumbar puncture is used with caution when indicated because the decrease in ICP can theoretically cause rupture of an unstable aneurysm by increasing pressure across the aneurysm wall:

Transmural pressure = Mean arterial blood pressure [MAP] − ICP

Furthermore, herniation through the foramen magnum could also occur if a large intracranial mass effect exists from blood, edema, or hydrocephalus. The definitive diagnostic test is angiography, with current intraarterial digital methods allowing for the use of smaller dye volumes than previously.

Aneurysms do not appear to be congenital and certainly do not cause pathologic features in the pediatric population. Patients with SAH are often in the 40- to 60-year age group. Aneurysms often occur at branch points of vessels around the circle of Willis and the bifurcation of the middle cerebral artery. Local symptoms may be produced by aneurysms acting as mass lesions in their neuroanatomic neighborhood. Most aneurysms are 6 to 15 mm in diameter, and aneurysms >25 mm are referred to as "giant aneurysms."

Those who enjoy numbering systems for clinical situations have come to the right place; there are several "quantitative" scales that classify the clinical status of patients with ruptured aneurysms on a scale of 0 or 1 to 4 or 5. The lowest numbers represent the intact patient, the highest numbers the comatose, and the numbers in between varying stages of neurologic misery. It is important to remember that patients who start with less neurologic disability do better than those who start with minimal or no neurologic function. Focal or generalized neurologic deficits may be the result of hematoma, edema, or vasospasm. Communicating hydrocephalus caused by blood clots in the cerebrospinal fluid (CSF) ventricular system may require ventriculostomy for drainage and monitoring. In patients with problems involving ICP increases above or below the tentorium or with ischemia from vasospasm, anesthesia is conducted with consideration of all the physiologic trespass that is present and attempts to minimize further injury by application of compromises in the "usual" care of these patients, as judged appropriate. For example, if ICP is severely elevated, controlled hypotension should not be administered to the extent that cerebral perfusion is further compromised.

Although vasospasm can be angiographically demonstrated in the majority of patients with SAH, it has functional significance in a minority. The time for peak incidence of vasospasm is from about day 4 to day 14 after the bleeding. This peak incidence does not mean that vasospasm cannot occur at other times. The etiology of vasospasm is under intense investigation and nitric oxide–endothelin and the inflammatory response appear to be intimately involved in its pathogenesis. Effective treatments now include nicardipine, which has recently become available, intraarterial papaverine, and most high-tech of all, cerebral angioplasty. Vasospasm will be further considered in the chapter on the intensive care unit (see Chapter 20).

TIMING OF SURGERY AND SURGICAL CONSIDERATIONS

In addition to the above, rebleeding is an obvious and serious cause of morbidity and mortality in the population with SAH. Rebleeding is most likely to occur soon after the initial rupture. Because early surgery poses unique problems, the timing of aneurysm surgery has been a matter of some controversy in the neurovascular literature. In the past, surgeons were more likely to wait several weeks before surgery, encountered better operating conditions than possible in early surgery, and reported that surgical mortality was reduced by waiting. Unfortunately, this finding was a result of operating on a diminished and highly selected population that had survived the demons of rebleeding, vasospasm, and medical complications such as pneumonia and pulmonary embolism, which inevitably occur in sick patients lying in hospital beds. Technical advances in anesthesia and neurosurgery now make the conditions of early surgery more tolerable and more tenable. In anesthesia this is primarily due to increased knowledge of the physiologic impact of anesthetics, carbon dioxide, and blood pressure on the acutely angry and swollen brain. Surgically this increased knowledge results in the routine use of the operating microscope, constantly improving equipment such as vascular clips, and the development of a specialty within neurosurgery devoted to vascular problems. Many surgeons now advocate "early" (within 72 hours) surgery before rebleeding, vasospasm, and other complications occur. Early surgery removes blood that may contribute to the production of vasospasm and allows for more aggressive treatment of vasospasm. An international study performed several years ago found no difference in outcome between early and late (11 to 14 days after bleeding) surgery, but analysis of the results of North American surgeons found that early surgery had the advantage. In any case, early surgery has become more common in our institution.

The position of the patient depends on the location of the aneurysm and the implications for optimal surgical approach. We take special care to avoid extremes of neck movement, whether lateral turning, flexion, or extension. This appears to reduce the severity of postextubation stridor caused by excessive pressure of an endotracheal tube on the larynx at an extreme angle. After we encountered several cases of swelling of the posterior part of the tongue with cases done with the patient in the prone position, we abandoned the use of the oral airway and extreme neck flexion in prone cases, which seems to have eliminated this complication. Care must also be taken to avoid neck positions that can kink the internal jugular vein, inhibit venous cerebral blood flow, and seriously interfere with operating conditions. See Chapter 6 on positioning and Chapter 1 on anatomy for further details.

The majority of aneurysms are currently treated by a metal clip placed on the aneurysm base, although technically difficult situations may challenge surgical creativity or require the wise surgeon to abandon the attempt on occasion. Although the delicate approach to the aneurysmal sac has been most often facilitated by controlled hypotension in the recent past, the use of temporary clips to isolate the aneurysm from the surrounding circulation is now used in the majority of cases at the University of Virginia (see later discussion of controlled hypotension). Cerebrovascular neurologic surgery is a demanding and exacting specialty generally performed with the aid of an operating microscope. Movement in the operative field is therefore amplified and should be minimized. Stable hemodynamics also aid the security of the surgery and the surgeon because the experienced operator can detect blood pressure changes as transmitted to him/her by the "feel" of the cerebral vasculature.

Pulmonary Evaluation

The obtunded patient with an SAH may have retention of secretions with subsequent atelectasis and propensity to airway hyperirritability. Chest physical therapy and vigorous coughing are probably not to be encouraged in a patient with fresh clot in a ruptured aneurysm, but deep breathing and gentle clearing of accumulated pulmonary secretions are reasonable. Although anticholinergics are not required, we advocate their perioperative use in this situation to minimize the further impact of secretions. In addition to making atelectasis more likely, secretions may predispose to a longer period of laryngoscopy while suction is accomplished, as well as to laryngospasm, bronchospasm, and continued outpouring of saliva that can potentially loosen the securement even of a carefully taped endotracheal tube. The dislodgement of the airway in a prone patient with a pinned head and an exposed posterior fossa is a true neuroanesthetic nightmare. If oxygenation appears to be impaired by secretions or atelectasis, the old-fashioned use of several large "sigh" volumes (two times the usual tidal volumes) followed by a reasonably large tidal volume (12 to 15 ml/kg) along with appropriate suction is generally curative. In fact, the majority of the problems we have encountered with oxygenation and ventilation have occurred in heavy smokers, rather than problems related to neurogenic pulmonary edema or $\dot{V}/\dot{Q}$ abnormalities that have been mythically related to SAH.

Premedications and Preoperative Visit

In the patient who is neurologically intact, the preoperative visit is an especially important component of anesthetic care. These patients and their families are justifiably upset and anxious and a satisfactory meeting with a calm, well-informed anesthesiologist is important in producing a patient with a controllable blood pressure and psyche the next morning. The use of medications to aid sleep and specific premedications is, of course, up to the individual anesthesiologist, and this is one situation in modern anesthesiology where the use of an anxiolytic as a premedication is reasonable. As noted, we favor the use of an anticholinergic, which is given IV in the operating room, preferably at least 10 minutes before induction. Often we give nonsmokers 0.2 mg of glycopyrrolate IV, smokers without a notable history of bronchospasm 0.4 mg, and higher doses (up to 1.0 mg) to bronchospastic patients, depending on severity of disease, accompanying coronary disease, and body habitus. It is a good idea to have midazolam in hand to give in 0.5 to 1.0 mg IV increments as dictated by the patient's emotional state. In fragile or older patients, diphenhydramine 12.5 to 25 mg IV may provide very good, rapid sedation. In the tachycardic patient without contraindications, IV propranolol in 1.0 mg increments can produce surprisingly good anxiolysis.

The morbidity and mortality of this kind of neurosurgery has been drastically lowered since its beginnings. However, it is still a high-risk enterprise, especially for patients who already have neurologic impairment, significant coexistent medical problems, or especially technically difficult lesions. Although this risk should not be emphasized to a patient with a thin layer of fibrin and platelets plugging the dam from the leakage of the entire cerebral blood flow, it is reasonable to ensure that family or responsible significant others are aware of the magnitude of the problem.

MONITORING

Cardiovascular Monitoring
BLOOD PRESSURE

It is especially critical to have intraarterial monitoring of blood pressure because the systemic pressures are the same as the pressures distending the aneurysm wall. Some clinicians prefer to place the arterial catheter after induction to avoid the possibility of aneurysmal rerupture from pain and subsequent hypertension. We have not found the latter to be a problem and strongly urge the placement of the cannula in the awake patient. We have also noted that the gods of neuroanesthesia seem to frown on delayed placement and that difficulties in successful placement appear to multiply in the anesthetized patient surrounded by nurses with Foley catheters, attendants with pads, and neurosurgeons with head-pinning devices. Seriously, the risk of preinduction placement is more than made up for by the availability of beat-to-beat pressures during the period of induction, laryngoscopy, and intubation. Of course, there are unusual occasions when a sensitive or uncooperative patient or extreme difficulty in awake placement justifies induction of anesthesia with an automated oscillometer, preferably set to the "stat" mode to obtain frequent blood pressures.

CENTRAL LINES AND VENOUS ACCESS

We believe that central venous or pulmonary artery catheters are not necessary in the majority of patients. We attempt to insert an antecubital central venous catheter if the patient is to be operated on in the seated position or the appropriate catheter (central venous pressure [CVP] or pulmonary artery) as dictated by underlying cardiovascular abnormalities. If unsuccessful, we will proceed without the "benefit" of a CVP catheter. If a pulmonary artery catheter is required for optimal cardiac care, we use an internal jugular approach, but have had to do so rarely. In contrast to our opinion, North American anesthetists insert CVP catheters in 59% of patients (A. Gelb, M.D., personal communication). Those clinicians who insert CVPs routinely in their patients do so to monitor intravascular volume status and to have central venous access for drug administration. Many of these clinicians use internal jugular or even subclavian approaches to catheterization, but we are not convinced that any potential benefit outweighs the admittedly small risk. We have not found central venous access, per se, to be necessary for drug or fluid administration, but it is essential to have at least two functional intravenous cannulas of adequate size (18-gauge or greater) to provide access for rapid infusion of blood and fluids. More often, it is useful to have two lines so that one can be used for infusions and the other as a utility line for fluid maintenance and bolus drug administration. As far as evaluation of intravascular volume is concerned, we have found that analysis of the "cycling" of the arterial pulse pressure waveform is at least as useful as a CVP. In brief, there is a normal, so-called "delta-up" and "delta-down" of 4 to 5 mm Hg of the arterial systolic pressure with mechanical inspiration and expiration, respectively. With volume depletion, the "delta-up" is reduced or absent and the "delta-down" magnitude is augmented; the opposite occurs with volume overload. This situation is only useful in the paralyzed, mechanically ventilated patient who can be made temporarily apneic to establish a pressure baseline. However, we have found it adequate for our needs in assessing and treating fluid status in patients with reasonably normal or close-to-normal hearts and kidneys.

Respiratory Monitoring

The capnograph has become a virtually indispensable monitor for confirming tracheal intubation and providing continuous information on the state of the respiratory system throughout the case.

Once a gradient between arterial and end-tidal carbon dioxide has been established, the need for further arterial blood gases is diminished (in conjunction with the pulse oximeter, of course). In our experience the provision of hypotension to mean blood pressures of 50 to 60 mm Hg does not significantly (in a clinical sense) increase the gradient. This is probably because cardiac output and therefore $\dot{V}/\dot{Q}$ ratios are not much altered by hypotension achieved with isoflurane, nitroprusside, or other means that produce reductions in blood pressure primarily by decreases in systemic vascular resistance rather than decreases in cardiac output. To optimize surgical exposure in early aneurysm surgery, we provide hyperventilation (arterial partial pressure of carbon dioxide [$Paco_2$] $\cong$ 24 to 28 range) in spite of theoretical concerns that this might provide a fertile substrate for cerebral ischemia. In the normal brain hyperventilation probably does not produce ischemia in blood pressure ranges above the lower limit for autoregulation. The use of hyperventilation in the not-so-normal brain may carry some risk, especially in the presence of vasospasm, but it also provides an essential improvement in operating conditions, which appears to justify its use.

Neurologic Monitoring

There are no "routine" intraoperative monitors of cerebral function for these operations. Different institutions may monitor a variety of evoked potentials or selected electroencephalograms by surface or cortical electrodes, but the clinical role of this information is by no means certain to us. In theory, these monitors should allow anesthesiologists to use drugs, blood pressure levels, and hyperventilation in a fashion that will not exacerbate ischemia. Furthermore, they should be even more important in the detection of undue pressure from brain retraction, clip misplacement, or surgical elimination of essential perforating vessels. We believe, however, that there is still a large gap between these hopes and clinical reality. We would encourage the (expensive) use of these monitors primarily in a research setting where there can be quantitative analysis and correlation of the clinical outcome with the electrical signals.

INDUCTION OF ANESTHESIA

Anesthesia can be induced after the placement of the arterial cannula (usually) and at least one secure IV line (always). This is not a situation to begin a case with a tenuous 22-gauge cannula that infiltrates after half the thiopental is administered. We generally use thiopental in 4 to 5 mg/kg doses unless the patient is hypovolemic or has cardiac dysfunction. Other clinicians may prefer propofol, but we would not advocate the use of etomidate in this setting because marked hypertension sometimes results. Hypovolemia should be corrected before induction. This may require a delay of 5 to 10 minutes in a 4- to 6-hour case. The patient with notable cardiac dysfunction should receive a careful induction as for any anesthetic but the anesthesiologist should watch for hypertension from inadequate anesthesia. Clinicians may choose from some combination of a reduced dose of thiopental, narcotic, and lidocaine or even a pure narcotic "cardiac" induction if ejection fraction is low. If possible, huge doses of narcotics that will delay resumption of spontaneous ventilation and wake-up should be avoided. We no longer make up an infusion of nitroprusside for every case but have the components of the infusion immediately available. It is also a good idea to check on the availability of adequate blood for transfusion before induction and to have extra thiopental in the room ($\cong 1$ g).

After the patient loses the eyelash reflex, mask ventilation is assured and an intubating dose of nondepolarizing muscle relaxant is then given. We have generally preferred vecuronium because of the stable hemodynamics produced and the reasonably fast onset in large doses. We administer double doses to patients receiving phenytoin or carbamazepine because of the increased pharmacokinetic and pharmacodynamic requirement for nondepolarizers when these anticonvulsants are present. Succinylcholine is probably best avoided after SAH even if neurologic function is intact; however, it may be used for rapid sequence induction if it is judged that the risks of aspiration justify it. It may also be used in the neurologically intact patient if the clinician does not wish to use a nondepolarizer because of airway anatomy and does not feel comfortable in conscious intubation in this setting. If the airway appears to be difficult, even a recent SAH does not contraindicate conscious intubation because excellent blood pressure control is meaningless in the absence of oxygenation.

After the relaxant begins to work, anesthesia is usually supplemented with a dose of narcotic. The narcotic administration is best delayed to avoid the chest rigidity sometimes produced that makes the efficacy of mask ventilation difficult to evaluate. Sufentanil is most commonly used in our institution because it appears to provide the best hemodynamic control in low doses. The dose ranges from 0.25 to 2.0 μg/kg depending on the patient's blood pressure response to the induction agents. It is best to start with low doses and then supplement as needed; the patient left with a large sufentanil burden may become hypotensive during the sometimes long period of neurosurgical preparation. Whether sufentanil or fentanyl is chosen for this purpose, it is important to recall that low-dose narcotics may take several minutes to take effect. If more immediate narcotic effect is desired, alfentanil is a reasonable choice. However, if laryngoscopy or intubation is prolonged, the alfentanil effect may wear off before the endotracheal tube cuff is finally inflated. Before and during laryngoscopy additional small doses of thiopental, propofol, or alfentanil are used to keep blood pressure at the desired level.

The patient with a full stomach for aneurysm clipping does not present a true clinical problem because this operation can be delayed until 6 to 8 hours have gone by after eating. However, the patient may require emergency ventriculostomy or hematoma drainage and have a full stomach. In this setting, it is reasonable to pretreat with metoclopramide, H_2 blocker, or nonparticulate antacid as is customary and to proceed with a modified rapid-sequence induction in which careful cricoid pressure is continuously applied, the patient is very gently mask ventilated to keep peak pressures below 20 cm H_2O, and intubation is accomplished as quickly as possible without causing an unacceptable rise in systemic blood pressure. In this setting, as in the more routine setting, it is useful to have an assistant to monitor blood pressure and quickly administer indicated drugs.

Obviously the goal is to avoid rupture or rerupture of the aneurysm, which is of course disastrous. Rupture during induction should be suspected if the patient has signs of severely elevated ICP with hypertension and bradycardia (or sometimes tachycardia). Blood pressure should then be carefully controlled with thiopental or nitroprusside with care not to lower pressure so severely that cerebral perfusion is jeopardized. It is a good idea to have a capable neurosurgeon immediately available when anesthesia is induced in these patients. The patient may require emergency neuroradiologic evaluation with continued anesthesia care. Hematoma evacuation may then be required, but clipping of the aneurysm may be technically impossible at this time.

MAINTENANCE OF ANESTHESIA

Anesthetic Considerations

Once anesthesia has been induced and the airway secured, special concerns in aneurysm surgery include continued prevention of aneurysm rupture (from a stimulus such as pinning or incision) and provision of optimal surgical conditions. The nature of neurologic surgery involves long periods of low-level stimulation (preparation period, intracranial surgery after dura opened) punctuated by brief, intense stimuli including those named above plus turning of bone flaps, dural incision, and reflex cardiovascular stimulation resulting from manipulation of brainstem, blood vessels (on occasion), and cerebellar tentorium. Our general approach is to provide a reasonable and stable anesthetic base of isoflurane, nitrous oxide (N_2O), and narcotic, and to supplement prophylactically for the intense stimuli with small boluses of thiopental, propofol, or alfentanil. Painful stimuli can also be ameliorated by application of lidocaine to the sites of stimulation, such as for head pinning. It is essential for surgeon and anesthesiologist to communicate so that the patient is adequately anesthetized before painful stimuli are applied and so that unexpectedly high resultant blood pressures can be treated. Communication is also important during patient movement for pinning, insertion of spinal drains, and head or body positioning so that hard-won vascular cannulas and intratracheal tubes are not inadvertently dislodged.

As noted, the usual anesthetic regimen includes isoflurane, N_2O, and a narcotic, usually sufentanil. Isoflurane is generally used in adults because of the remote possibilities of halothane hepatitis and the epileptogenicity of enflurane when the patient is hypoventilated. Desflurane may be a reasonable option for those who have it available; we have used it on a preliminary basis without difficulty. We do not use isoflurane because we have no delusions that it provides better brain protection (vide infra) or operating conditions than the other potent agents. The primary advantage may be that it can provide controlled hypotension without marked reduction of cardiac output, cerebral blood flow or uterine blood flow. As we have noted, we generally use sufentanil as our narcotic and attempt to limit the total dose to 3 μg/kg to allow for faster reawakening. The sufentanil can be given in boluses or as an infusion. Fentanyl can also be similarly administered, but alfentanil must be given as an infusion and can become expensive if used for an entire case. Anesthesia can also be administered by the total IV approach with a propofol infusion and sufentanil or alfentanil.

The controversy concerning the use of N_2O is a bit of a tempest in a teapot, but there are some genuine physiologic concerns that preclude its thoughtless routine use or nonuse. We use 50% N_2O unless there is preoperative evidence of a problem with ICP, which is not generally the case with aneurysm surgery. It is useful in providing some degree of an anesthetic state during periods of extremely low stimulation when hypotension rather than hypertension is often the problem. We have not abandoned its use for the theoretic concern of a negative effect on brain protection. Studies from the Mayo Clinic have shown that the effect of N_2O on seated cases (i.e., venous air embolism and tension pneumocephalus) is neither particularly helpful nor harmful.

If the patient has a tight, swollen brain that is interfering with surgical exposure, N_2O is discontinued, the position of the patient's head is checked for the possibility of a kinked jugular vein, and the $Paco_2$ rechecked. Our initial dose of mannitol is generally so large (200 g) that more mannitol is not likely to be helpful, but an additional bag may be sacrificed to the gods of brain exposure. At this point, a lidocaine infusion of 1 to 4 mg/min can be begun after a bolus of 1.0 to 1.5 mg/kg: This provides almost one third the maximum allowable concentration (MAC) of anesthetic contribution and a salutary effect on ICP. If exposure continues to be a problem, the isoflurane is discontinued and a continuous infusion of thiopental 1.0 to 10.0 mg/min after a small bolus (25 to 100 mg) is begun. The anesthetic contribution of the thiopental depends on the precise serum level produced but is likely to provide 0.4 to 0.5 MAC in accordance with the results of our laboratory studies. At this point the anesthetic provided by lidocaine and thiopental with residual narcotic is likely to be adequate because there are virtually no painful stimuli and the patient's temperature is 33° to 34° C, reducing anesthetic requirement by 20% to 30%. If possible, it may be best to avoid further narcotic in view of recent studies claiming increases in ICP with alfentanil, fentanyl, and sufentanil. If further narcotic is indicated, the first-choice in this situation would be low doses of fentanyl because it has been least implicated in this problem. It may also be reasonable to ensure that mean systemic blood pressure is at a "middle of the road" level because either low pressure (with autoregulation intact) or high pressure (with autoregulation impaired) may increase cerebral blood volume and ICP.

The following sections discuss those special techniques and considerations used in aneurysm surgery to improve patient safety and facilitate successful clipping.

Controlled Hypotension and Hypertension

Controlled hypotension, otherwise known as hypotensive anesthesia, has been the special province of the neuroanesthetist and has been used to decrease the likelihood of rupture by decreasing aneurysmal transmural pressure, mechanically improving the approach to, handling, and actual clipping of the aneurysm, and reducing bleeding should it occur. In the patient who has intact cerebral autoregulation, hypotension within the lowest autoregulatory limits may increase cerebral blood volume and ICP, as noted. Oral pretreatment with clonidine (0.05 mg/kg) or captopril (3 mg/kg) will facilitate the provision of desired levels of hypotension but may also result in excessive hypotension in some anesthetized patients. Efficacy and effect on outcome has not been comparatively studied but the alpha$_2$-agonists contribute to anesthesia and may provide some degree of brain protection. When these drugs are used, the anesthesiologist should be able to modify the anesthetic so that less isoflurane +/or narcotic total dose is administered.

When hypotensive anesthesia is required, our basic technique involves the manipulation of isoflurane levels on top of a narcotic base. A mean blood pressure of 50 mm Hg is generally achieved by this means, although some robust patients may require just a touch of labetalol (2.5 to 5.0 mg boluses to effect) to avoid the use of an inordinate amount of anesthetic. An additional small dose of sufentanil (10 to 25 µg) may also be helpful. Other clinicians use a basic nitrous or narcotic anesthetic with nitroprusside for hypotension with equally good effects. We have mostly abandoned this drug as a result of its adverse effect on ICP, which can be a problem with early aneurysm surgery and because our surgeons prefer not to work on blood vessels dilated by nitroprusside. Furthermore, Lam has shown that when isoflurane is used to produce hypotensive anesthesia to the lower limits of cerebrovascular autoregulation (i.e., 50 mm Hg, cardiac output and cerebral blood flow are relatively well-preserved making isoflurane at least theoretically advantageous). On the other hand, nitroglycerin might be a reasonable choice if mild hypotension is absolutely required in a patient with known significant coronary artery disease. As with the "tight brain" situation, a thiopental infusion can be used to provide hypotension with excellent operating conditions. If doses >30 mg/kg are used, awakening is likely to be significantly delayed. Hydralazine has become somewhat elusive in its pharmaceutic availability. It can be used to provide hypotension but is slow in onset and can also raise ICP. It is essential to have some idea of cerebrovascular stenotic disease, coronary disease, renal function, chronic blood pressure levels, etc., so that an appropriate and safe level of hypotension can be applied to each patient. On infrequent occasions the surgeons may request even lower blood pressure levels briefly for technically difficult situations. Judgment must be used in determining the level and duration of severe levels of controlled hypotension but must consider that the aneurysm itself is a life-threatening lesion.

In the earlier book on which this handbook is based, it was noted that hypotensive anesthesia was used for aneurysm surgery in "the vast majority of cases." Currently the "vast majority" of cases do not require hypotensive anesthesia at the levels formerly used. In a recent survey North American anesthesiologists reported the use of hypotension in 28% of patients (A. Gelb, M.D., personal communication). We do use a mild degree of hypotension (i.e., mean blood pressure of perhaps 60 to 70 mm Hg but do not usually maintain the mean blood pressure at 50 mm Hg throughout the period of approach to and clipping of the aneurysm as previously). As noted, isoflurane is still used for this purpose. However, in view of recent studies it is unlikely that isoflurane is providing any clinically significant degree of brain protection (vide infra).

Our practice has been continuously modified as more aneurysms are approached with the help of so-called temporary clips. Well over half our aneurysms are managed in this fashion, which basically involves control of the afferent and efferent vessels with temporary clip placement. In some instances a balloon guided by a neuroradiologist serves as the proximal or afferent blood flow controller. During the period of temporary clipping blood pressure is kept at normal or slightly increased levels to optimize collateral blood flow. This can usually be done with small boluses of phenylephrine (25 to 50 μg) and appropriate modification of the inhaled or continuous IV anesthetic level but may require use of a phenylephrine infusion (start at 20 to 40 μg/min and titrate upward) to maintain the desired blood pressure. An adequate but not excessive level of anesthesia is desirable so that the blood pressure goal is facilitated.

Some clinicians administer a bolus of a "brain protective" agent such as thiopental, etomidate, lidocaine, or mannitol before the clips are applied, but we rely primarily on the underlying mild hypothermia, which allows for less resultant injury after a period of controlled ischemia such as temporary clipping. Other clinicians will discontinue N_2O at this time to avoid a possible negative brain protectant effect, but we do not believe this is necessary. If N_2O is discontinued, it is probably a good idea to leave it off to decrease the risk of enlarging an already-present pneumocephalus. Care must be taken not to seriously overshoot the blood pressure level, especially before the temporary clips are in place. In short, the neuroanesthesiologist today must be ready to provide controlled hypertension as well as controlled hypotension.

In addition to the example of temporary clipping, various levels of controlled hypertension may be required for the patient with known vasospasm or concurrent cerebrovascular occlusive disease. Patients with unusual cardiac problems such as asymmetric septal hypertrophy or valvular stenosis may require careful maintenance of normotension. Notably, continuous infusions of calcium channel blockers such as nicardipine may prove to be the optimal blood pressure controllers in vasospastic patients or in early surgery in general.

Whether hypotension or hypertension has been administered, resumption of normotension is the goal after the aneurysm itself has been successfully clipped. This is important so that bleeders can be detected before the dura is closed. This can usually be achieved by lightening the isoflurane level in the case of hypotension or discontinuing phenylephrine and deepening the anesthetic after hypertension.

Cerebrospinal Fluid Drains

The surgeon may choose to place a lumbar subarachnoid drain to remove CSF to improve surgical exposure by producing a slacker brain. This drain may not be placed for middle cerebral artery aneurysms because drainage may obscure the sulcus in which the aneurysm lies. In our institution the surgeon places the drain, which is probably just as well from a liability standpoint (CSF leaks, headaches, nerve injuries, infections, etc.). In theory, an acute removal of CSF may increase the aneurysmal transmural pressure (MAP-ICP) and provoke a rupture, but this does not seem to be the case in practice. As previously noted, the lumbar puncture was long used to diagnose SAH and may still be used when CT scan is non-diagnostic.

The actual technique resembles that used for continuous sub-arachnoid anesthesia in which a catheter is threaded into the sub-arachnoid space. After it is confirmed that the catheter is function-ing initially and then again after final patient positioning, the stopcock is closed until the surgeon requests that a specific amount of CSF be removed. It is important to be familiar with the mecha-nism of the stopcock before this happens. It is essential to clearly la-bel the catheter so that undesirable substances are not inadvertently injected into the central nervous system. At times the surgeon will request that a volume of crystalloid be reinfused into the catheter to help keep the brain up. Preservative-free saline solution is a reason-able choice, but we prefer not to reinject anything into the catheter if possible.

Mannitol

Mannitol is used in aneurysm surgery primarily to improve op-erating conditions but may improve cerebral rheologic processes and provide some degree of brain protection as well. We administer a relatively large total dose of 200 g given as half before incision and half after. This dose is 2 to 4 g/kg depending on patient size but is only given once and does not produce undue dehydration or meta-bolic disarray. On occasion a rapid mannitol infusion will result in hypotension, possibly from hyperosmolarity-related vasodilation. The optimal dosing and pharmacologic analysis of mannitol is cur-rently under clinical investigation. It is wasteful to undertake a ma-jor laboratory reevaluation of the patient (arterial blood gases are fine) right after a huge dose of mannitol because values such as sodium and hematocrit will be falsely low and potassium may be somewhat high.

Hyperventilation

As noted, we use hyperventilation in spite of the risk of isch-emia, especially in conjunction with vasospasm, controlled hy-potension, retractor pressure, or temporary clips. The primary pur-pose of hyperventilation is to improve surgical exposure so that

$Paco_2$ should be titrated to this end point rather than to an arbitrary number. When early surgery is performed, at least moderate hyperventilation ($Paco_2$ 25 to 30 mm Hg) is likely to be required simply because the recent hemorrhage has left the brain angry and swollen. This hyperventilation also is indicated if ICP is elevated by the previously discussed causes. The hyperventilated brain seems to make the task of the vascular neurosurgeon substantially more feasible without an undue cost.

Hypothermia

There is now an extensive experimental literature that supports the efficacy of mild hypothermia (33° to 35° C) in the provision of brain protection. A decrease in the cerebral metabolic rate of oxygen consumption ($CMRo_2$) may account for a substantial proportion of this protection because the decrease in $CMRo_2$ in humans at 34° may be closer to 40% rather than the often quoted 15% to 20%. In addition, a decrease in the release of excitatory amino acid neurotransmitters such as glutamate may contribute. A controlled multicenter trial of hypothermia is now planned, but the laboratory efficacy in conjunction with the clinically benign nature of mild hypothermia has led our group and others to apply it rather routinely in aneurysm surgery. The preliminary survey for the study found that about two thirds of North American anesthesiologists are using mild hypothermia for these cases (A. Gelb, M.D., personal communication).

We administer mild hypothermia with a simple cooling-warming blanket and aim for esophageal temperatures of 32.5° to 33° C because brain temperatures are probably about 0.5° higher. Temperatures <32° C are avoided because problems may theoretically begin with coagulation and arrhythmias. Doses of narcotics and relaxants should be appropriately reduced. Anesthetic requirement and drug metabolism will be significantly reduced with mild hypothermia. It is important to begin the rewarming process sufficiently early so that excessive hypothermia does not occur. In addition, care must be taken to avoid skin burns and hyperthermic overshoot, which may have a deleterious effect on brain protection. Recent work indicates that the small degree of protection afforded by isoflurane may lie in prevention of a hyperthermic response to ischemia. Often the patient is not quite ready for awakening and extubation at the end of the case, and it may be best to first reachieve normothermia to avoid a miserable, shivering patient who may be hemodynamically unstable.

The patient is then brought to the intensive care unit intubated (and ventilated, if necessary) and is usually ready for extubation in 30 to 90 minutes. In our experience the reawakening process is delayed slightly even after mild hypothermia, and a few additional patients have received neuroradiologic intervention because they were slow to awake but had no mechanical insult.

Deep hypothermia with circulatory arrest is a complex procedure requiring expert consultation with a team of nurses, technicians, and physicians familiar with the process, which includes cardiopulmonary bypass. It probably should be undertaken in only a few tertiary research centers, and each case should be analyzed and studied because the risk-benefit ratio of this event remains to be seen. Patient selection is key because only those patients who cannot be treated conventionally should be candidates for this major undertaking.

Anesthetics and Brain Protection

Our belief in the ability to provide an important degree of cerebral protection with anesthetics has undergone a revision in the past several years. Currently it is believed that even what we considered our most valuable protectants such as isoflurane and thiopental are not really terribly effective. Recent experimental work indicates that the suppression of $CMRO_2$ achieved with many anesthetics is not synonymous with an equal brain-protective effect. The notion that the production of pharmacologic EEG isoelectricity is a marker for brain protection is under similar question. Although the presence of a volatile agent or a bolus of an appropriate IV agent may provide from seconds to a minute or two of additional time before injury becomes irreversible, they are not effective at preventing injury from the kind of prolonged and severe insult that occurs when a noncollateralized, perforating vessel is inadvertently or knowingly ligated during surgery. It is not clear to us that additional protection is afforded when mild hypothermia has already been provided. Our point is that we should not smugly assume that we have done something truly effective for brain protection when a bolus of etomidate or thiopental is given before temporary clipping, for example.

Intraoperative Aneurysm Rupture

Although aneurysm rupture during induction or before craniectomy is a disaster, as noted, it is fortunately rare. More often the aneurysm ruptures during the approach to or handling of the aneurysm by the surgeon. In fact, this occurs to some degree in 15% to 40% of cases, but if the anesthesiologist is inattentive the surgeon may well have dealt with a controllable rupture before the anesthesiologist is aware of the problem. More serious ruptures are less common and require our input to lower blood pressure to reduce bleeding and improve surgical exposure and to replace blood loss, if necessary. The surgeon may request pressure on both carotids to reduce the blood in the field and may have to clip a major proximal artery to get control. Although uncontrolled hypotension may result from severe blood loss, it is critical to attempt to maintain intravascular volume status and control blood pressure pharmacologically so that the situation does not deteriorate into a cardiac arrest. MAP <50 mm Hg may be requested in this life-threatening situation and may be provided by thiopental, propofol, esmolol, nitroprusside, or isoflurane, among the more common choices. It is a good idea to have skilled help in the room when this sort of major problem occurs.

PREGNANT PATIENT

The pregnant patient presents a variety of special clinical problems for aneurysm surgery. If aneurysm clipping is to be performed before delivery, the usual physiologic implications should be considered, including awareness of a full stomach, increased likelihood of a difficult airway, potential drug toxicities, and the effects of everything done on uterine blood flow and fetal outcome. If a cesarean section is to be performed before aneurysm clipping, anesthesia and blood pressure control must be adequate to prevent rupture. This may require a depth of anesthesia and use of drugs that will produce a transient fetal depression that the pediatricians must expect and be capable of treating.

These patients should receive some form of prophylaxis for aspiration, which may be simply a dose of nonparticulate antacid. The airway must be carefully evaluated and a decision made on the acceptability of succinylcholine and the possible need for conscious intubation. The use of new rapid-onset nondepolarizing relaxants such as rocuronium may prove efficacious. If a rapid-sequence intubation is chosen, special care must be paid to the immediate treatment of hypertension. This can be done with a preinduction dose of fentanyl 2 to 5 μg/kg, use of rapid-acting drugs such as nitroprusside or esmolol in a bolus, and an adequate but not excessive induction dose of thiopental. Even if the classic rapid sequence is not performed, careful cricoid pressure should be maintained and mask ventilation kept at the lowest inspiratory pressures that produce acceptable ventilation. An assistant who can redose thiopental, propofol, or alfentanil to quickly deepen the anesthetic is desirable, in addition to an assistant who can maintain cricoid pressure throughout.

The fetus can theoretically sustain damage from many of the standard care procedures in aneurysm surgery. The obstetrics service should be fully involved in the case and provide fetal monitoring if they believe it is indicated. Drugs that are potentially toxic include nitroprusside, beta-blockers, and mannitol. Although nitroprusside may decrease uterine blood flow and cause fetal cyanide toxicity, one or two boluses of 25 to 100 μg may be extremely useful during laryngoscopy and intubation. Beta-blockers can theoretically contribute to neonatal bradycardia, hypoglycemia, apnea, and acidosis, but again, a bolus of esmolol (0.5 to 1.0 mg/kg) may be critical in preventing aneurysm rupture. Both drugs, given briefly in bolus form before delivery, are unlikely to produce fetal problems that cannot be dealt with by the neonatologist who is aware of their presence. We would be careful to reduce our usual dose of mannitol and, in fact, avoid it entirely unless required for exposure. In doses of $\leq$1.0 g/kg it is unlikely to create severe fluid and electrolyte abnormalities in the fetus, and we would start at 0.25 g/kg and titrate as required.

Hypotension is required less often than in recent years, as noted. If absolutely necessary, isoflurane seems a good choice because it maintains uterine blood flow in experimental animals at levels of 1.5 MAC. It is probably advisable to avoid drugs such as captopril and clonidine because of a lack of accumulated experience. In general, we try to stay with older, proved agents in this setting. Fetal heart monitoring should provide some help in achieving a desirable but not excessive level of hypotension. Severe hyperventilation (pressure of carbon dioxide <30 mm Hg) should be avoided because it can markedly reduce uterine blood flow.

EMERGENCE

After the aneurysm has been clipped, the blood pressure is allowed to rise to normal or high normal levels so that the security of the clip and excessive bleeding can be evaluated before the dura is closed. If mild hypothermia has been used, the thermal blanket is turned up to 39° to 40° C to begin rewarming. The level of isoflurane is reduced as tolerated. Blood pressure control can usually be obtained with labetalol given in incremental doses of 5, 10, 20, and 40 mg boluses (total 75 mg), which can be supplemented by additional 20 mg boluses if bradycardia is not excessive and blood pressure control is inadequate. A small additional dose of sufentanil or hydralazine (5 to 20 mg) will usually produce reasonable blood pressure control, but the occasional patient still requires nitroprusside. If temperature returns to 35° C, the patient was not severely impaired before surgery, and surgery has proceeded without difficulty, it is ideal to attempt to awaken and extubate the patient in the operating room at the end of the procedure. Other considerations that may call for continued ventilation and sedation include complicated posterior fossa surgery, significant concomitant medical illness, extreme lability in hemodynamics, intraoperative difficulties such as aneurysm rupture, prolonged thiopental infusion, known inadvertent occlusion of a blood vessel that may result in significant ischemia, or a swollen, angry brain throughout. Often in our current practice the patient is not quite warm enough to wake up in the operating room but is ready within 30 to 120 minutes after arrival in the intensive care unit. Although the price for this slight delay may be an increase in postoperative radiograms, it is better to be a little patient than to thrash with a hypertensive, shivering, uncooperative patient. Blood pressure should be carefully monitored during transport or in radiology.

ARTERIOVENOUS MALFORMATIONS

The pathologic process of arteriovenous malformations (AVMs) is complicated and controversial; this handbook will not go into the neuropathologic details. The classic AVM is a congenital lesion forming a high-flow, low-resistance shunt because of a vascular anatomy in which arteries flow directly into veins. They are usually superficial and supratentorial. Patients most often have bleeding but can have seizures, headaches, or even neuroischemia because of a shunting of blood flow away from normal areas. These patients often undergo preoperative embolization, which may alter volume and neurologic status. The good news about AVMs is that they are high-flow, low-resistance anomalies and therefore not as prone to rupture as a result of hypertension as are aneurysms, but blood pressure should still be carefully controlled during induction. These procedures are generally long and may involve extensive blood loss for which the anesthesiologist must be prepared. Controlled hypotension is selectively used as required with the knowledge that it can produce ischemia in areas that are not well perfused because of steal and may even contribute to postoperative edema and hemorrhage by venous occlusion. We generally provide mild hypothermia for these cases. The wake-up period is particularly difficult in AVMs because of the risk of bleeding and hemorrhage, which have been previously attributed to normal perfusion pressure breakthrough in which areas that receive a low blood flow preoperatively dilate chronically and lose the ability to autoregulate. When a normal flow is restored, the relative increase in local flow may result in the above problems. Recently, the pathophysiologic processes of normal perfusion pressure breakthrough have come into question, but it is clear that patients with large high-flow lesions are at particular risk. Because of the need to control blood pressure and ventilation carefully in these patients, who are often hypothermic, we tend to go with a particularly slow wake-up period for AVM patients so that they may remain intubated and sedated for several hours after arrival to the intensive care unit. Continued intubation also allows for the use of thiopental as a hypotensive agent that produces cerebral vasoconstriction.

Suggested Readings

Archer DP et al: Haemodynamic considerations in the management of patients with subarachnoid haemorrhage, *Can J Anaesth* 38:454, 1991.

Chong KY, Gelb AW: Management of intracranial aneurysms and subarachnoid hemorrhage, *Curr Opin Anesth* 5:620, 1992.

Coriat P et al: A comparison of systolic blood pressure variations and echocardiographic estimates of end-diastolic left ventricular size in patients after aortic surgery, *Anesth Analg* 78:46, 1994.

Dodson BA: Interventional neuroradiology and the anesthetic management of patients with arteriovenous malformations. In Cottrell JE, Smith DS, editors: *Anesthesia and neurosurgery,* ed 3, St Louis, 1994, Mosby.

Drummond JC: Brain protection during anesthesia—a reader's guide, *Anesthesiology* 79:877, 1993.

Eng CC, Lam AM: Cerebral aneurysms: anesthetic considerations. In Cottrell JE, Smith DS, editors: *Anesthesia and neurosurgery,* St Louis, 1994, Mosby.

Himes RS et al: Effects of lidocaine on the anesthetic requirements for nitrous oxide and halothane, *Anesthesiology* 47:437, 1977.

Kinkor RD, Warner DS: Unexpected myocardial complications after controlled hypotension, *J Neurosurg Anesth* 3:136, 1991.

Lagerkranser M: Controlled hypotension in neurosurgery PRO, *J Neurosurg Anesth* 3:150, 1991.

Lam AM et al: Cardiovascular effects of isoflurane-induced hypotension for cerebral aneurysm surgery, *Anesth Analg* 62:742, 1983.

Milde LN: Clinical use of mild hypothermia for brain protection: a dream revisited, *J Neurosurg Anesth* 4:211, 1992.

Newman B et al: The effect of isoflurane-induced hypotension on cerebral blood flow and cerebral metabolic rate for oxygen in humans, *Anesthesiology* 64:307, 1986.

Ornstein E et al: Deliberate hypotension in patients with intracranial arteriovenous malformations: esmolol compared with isoflurane and sodium nitroprusside, *Anesth Analg* 72:639, 1991.

Perel A: Cardiovascular assessment by pressure waveform analysis, *ASA refresher course lecture,* no. 264, 1991.

Ruta TS, Mutch WAC: Controlled hypotension for cerebral aneurysm surgery: are the risks worth the benefits? *J Neurosurg Anesth* 3:153, 1991.

Stone DJ et al: Thiopental reduces halothane MAC in rats, *Anesth Analg* 74:542, 1992.

Szabo MD et al: Hypertension does not cause spontaneous hemorrhage of intracranial arteriovenous malformations, *Anesthesiology* 70:761, 1989.

Todd MM, Warner DS: A comfortable hypothesis reevaluated— cerebral metabolic depression and brain protection during ischemia, *Anesthesiology* 76:161, 1992.

Wijdicks EFM et al: Atrial natriuretic factor and salt wasting after aneurysmal subarachnoid hemorrhage, *Stroke* 22:1519, 1991.

Young WL et al: Pressure autoregulation is intact after arteriovenous malformation resection, *Neurosurgery* 32:491, 1993.

ANESTHESIA FOR EXTRACRANIAL VASCULAR SURGERY

17

David J. Stone
Cosmo A. DiFazio
David L. Bogdonoff

PREOPERATIVE ASSESSMENT

The preoperative assessment of the patient undergoing carotid endarterectomy is especially important because so many of these patients have the common illnesses seen in older patients, such as coronary artery disease (CAD), congestive heart failure (CHF), hypertension, stroke, chronic obstructive pulmonary disease (COPD), diabetes, and renal dysfunction. More than any other group of neurosurgical patients the carotid endarterectomy population is likely to have significant disease outside the nervous system that can have an impact on the course of an anesthetic.

Cardiovascular System

The patient with carotid artery stenosis of sufficient magnitude to justify endarterectomy possesses a cardiovascular risk that is probably unique among neurosurgical patients. There is approximately a 60% incidence of significant CAD in this population. Cardiac problems are as likely to cause significant perioperative morbidity and mortality as neurologic problems are. In evaluating a patient who is likely to have the ischemic-hypertensive heart disease so prevalent in this population, the important questions are:

1. Is the myocardium at risk for ischemia?
2. How well does the myocardium function?

CORONARY ARTERY DISEASE

Although the answer to the first question may be answered by a clinical history of myocardial infarction (MI) or angina, it is just as likely that a picture of ambiguous chest pain, silent ischemia, non-Q wave MI, and lack of exercise tolerance make the question difficult to deal with adequately by the usual clinical means of history, physical examination, and resting electrocardiogram (ECG). Furthermore, clinical risk indices such as the Goldman or Detsky examples are not useful in the care of an individual who needs the operation. A functional (rather than actuarial) approach to the patient as proposed by Fleisher and Barash seems to be a more sensible and useful way to evaluate patients. This approach assigns specific cardiologic testing to patient groups with particular histories such as recent MI. This approach is further stratified into the age and type of the infarction and magnitude of the surgery. (The reference is given at the end of this chapter.) It must be kept in mind that there is no "correct" approach to the patient at risk for perioperative ischemia or infarction and that the number and invasiveness of tests do not necessarily have a strong positive correlation with patient outcome and do always involve additional discomfort, inconvenience, and expense. Sometimes it is probably adequate to know that the patient has significant but stable coronary artery disease that is well-controlled medically and that a reasonable course is to go ahead with a careful anesthetic without further testing. It takes seasoned and confident clinicians to make this call and buck the current trend of a preoperative workup as expensive as the gross national product of small island nations.

The anesthesiologist often has the role of identifying patients whose risk for carotid surgery justifies cardiologic consultation. These include patients with a recent MI (<6 months, vide infra), unstable angina, undiagnosed chest pain, or simply on the grounds of clinical judgment. The risk of anesthesia and surgery in patients with a recent MI has probably decreased since the initial study from the Mayo Clinic over 20 years ago. Furthermore, it is probably reasonable to stratify these patients on the basis of factors such as Q wave vs. non-Q wave MI and the presence of significant coronary disease in areas not affected by the MI. It is likely that a patient who has had a transmural inferior wall MI 2 months ago with normal or minimally stenosed coronary vessels elsewhere is at less risk than a patient who had a non-Q wave infarction 5 months ago and has significant coronary disease in areas not involved by the infarction. A knowledgeable cardiologic consultant can assist in this stratification with ECG stress tests, evaluation of myocardial perfusion with a thallium scan (exercise, dipyridamole, adenosine, or dobutamine), stress echocardiography, or even coronary arteriography. The new sestamibi scan uses a technetium analog that produces a brighter image but has about the same general utility as thallium (John Dent, M.D., University of Virginia, personal communication). In addition to optimizing medical therapy, options include coronary angioplasty, coronary artery bypass graft (CABG) surgery, or proceeding with intensified monitoring such as a pulmonary artery (PA) catheter or transesophageal echocardiography. The cardiac risk of carotid surgery is not as great as that for aortic or infrainguinal vascular surgery and few patients will require PA catheters or CABG (unless the latter operation was indicated in any case, surgery or not). The timing of CABG vs. endarterectomy is a matter of some controversy; clinical evaluation of signs and symptoms should dictate which operation is done first, whereas combined procedures are indicated for those selected patients who have a great and urgent need for both operations. Some clinicians maintain that endarterectomy under regional anesthesia followed by CABG at a later date is optimal in reducing overall cardiac and neurovascular risk. We would make the strong point that carotid endarterectomy performed in the presence of truly unstable angina is an extremely (perhaps unacceptably) risky undertaking that should only be performed with full awareness of risk on the part of physicians, surgeons, patient, and family.

The patient with no cardiac history, clearly stable angina with reasonable exercise tolerance (i.e., able to climb up eight to 10 steps without stopping), or with a remote (>6 months) MI generally proceeds directly to surgery under general anesthesia in our institution. There is a possibility of false-negative screening test results, such as dipyridamole thallium while caring for these patients. In general, our approach is to care for the patient with the knowledge that undiagnosed, significant CAD may be present and therefore we attempt to avoid undesirable hemodynamic scenarios such as the combination of tachycardia and hypotension. It is important to continue antianginal drugs such as beta-blockers, nitrates, and calcium channel blockers on the day of surgery.

MYOCARDIAL FUNCTION

In this population congestive heart failure is most likely to be a result of hypertensive or ischemic heart disease. Significant valvular disease or right-sided failure from cor pulmonale are less common but must be kept in mind. Importantly, the heart that functions acceptably at rest may become dysfunctional during exercise or ischemia. Although carotid endarterectomy does not involve large fluid shifts or aortic cross-clamping, major hemodynamic changes may occur when the carotid sinus is manipulated, when the blood pressure falls unacceptably (as occurs commonly during the course of an anesthetic), or when a controlled blood pressure increase is indicated while the carotid is clamped. Finally, ischemia is always a possible cause for cardiac dysfunction in this population (unless the patient has a negative coronary catheterization report and even then coronary vasospasm can develop).

The classic signs and symptoms of CHF are well known to clinicians. In this population diastolic dysfunction is probably quite prevalent, primarily as a result of chronic hypertension. Although the optimal anesthetic approach to the patient with diastolic myocardial dysfunction has not yet been defined, it is clear that these patients require adequate filling pressures and do not do well with the combination of inadequate preload in the face of negative inotropic agents. The hypertrophied myocardium may also contribute to the production of ischemia by decreasing effective subendocardial blood flow independently of the reduced flow produced by coronary stenoses. Because it is essential to maintain reasonable systemic blood pressure before a critical carotid stenosis is repaired, the anesthesiologist must have some idea of cardiac pump function as the surgeon preps the neck and the systolic blood pressure drifts down into the 60s.

Most often, the history is sufficiently informative that further testing is not necessary. As with CAD, the ability to walk up eight to 10 steps seems to indicate that the patient is likely to survive the stress of an anesthetic and an operation like endarterectomy. The problem is that there are so many complicating extracardiac factors that compromise the patient's ability to exercise, such as cerebrovascular disease itself, pulmonary, other neurologic, peripheral vascular, and rheumatologic problems. Although nuclear or angiographic evaluation of cardiac function is possible, two-dimensional echocardiogram has become the usual means of assessing the situation. In addition to providing excellent information on ejection fraction, the echocardiogram can give information on valvular and pericardial disease and myocardial wall thickness and motion abnormalities. If there is truly serious doubt about myocardial function and echocardiography is not feasible, a PA catheter can be used to obtain information on stroke volume and filling pressures that can be assessed in tandem to give a reasonable idea of the state of the heart. In fact, preoperative echocardiography and PA catheters are required fairly infrequently in this setting.

HYPERTENSION

Many of these patients have hypertension that may be variably well controlled. The clinician should seek to have the blood pressure under acceptable control before proceeding with all but the most urgent or emergency cases. In fact, endarterectomy is rarely an emergency unless the thrombosis is the result of a clearly defined event such as cerebral arteriography or postendarterectomy itself. It is essential to avoid rapid or severe decreases in systemic blood pressure in a patient whose cerebral autoregulation curve has been shifted to the right by chronic hypertension and who possesses critical cerebrovascular disease. It is probably the common experience of most clinicians that the poorly controlled hypertensive patient often provides a most uncomfortable hemodynamic roller coaster ride marked by soaring heights and frightening dips.

A reasonable goal is a systolic blood pressure of no more than 200 mm Hg and a diastolic pressure of no more than 110 mm Hg. These do not constitute criteria for good pressure control by a practicing internist but generally seem to afford a reasonable compromise between adequate perfusion and overcontrol. If there is time, the details of care can be left to the medical consultant. The particular drugs selected in a patient should generally be continued through the morning of surgery. The ultimate goal is the avoidance of blood pressure changes of magnitude and duration sufficient to result in myocardial or cerebral ischemia, left heart failure, or intracranial hemorrhage. If coronary disease is present or strongly suspected (most patients), beta-blockers and nitrates are probably first choice as antihypertensives.

Cerebrovascular Function

It is a good idea to have a rough baseline of the patient's preoperative neurologic status documented in the preoperative note. Obviously, this does not require the meticulous detail of a neurologist's examination but should include the gross elements of motor and mental function. Patients who are acutely experiencing a stroke (rarely operated on at present), who have had a stroke within 6 weeks, or who have had a more remote stroke with residual neurologic dysfunction appear to be at higher risk for perioperative stroke. Angiographic characteristics such as severe stenosis, high or extensive stenosis, and significant contralateral stenosis also appear to increase neurologic risk. Currently stenosis of >70% of internal diameter with neurologic symptoms consistent with transient ischemic attack(s) is a clear-cut indication for endarterectomy in that outcome is better than with medical therapy alone. Surgery for asymptomatic stenosis of any magnitude has been controversial but a recent unpublished study (Asymptomatic Carotid Atherosclerosis Study) has found that asymptomatic males with severe carotid stenosis have significant benefit from endarterectomy. The issue is especially likely to arise when cardiac or major vascular surgery is contemplated in that the risk of stroke is presumably exacerbated in the perioperative period. The new findings in asymptomatic patients, especially men, will likely alter the belief of some neurosurgeons that surgery is never indicated in the asymptomatic patient. In patients with <70% internal diameter stenosis, the indications for surgery appear to be a matter of clinical judgment. The presence of a large ulcerated plaque may lower the surgical threshold as may particularly ominous or frequent neurologic events.

Chronic Obstructive Pulmonary Disease

Many of these patients have concomitant COPD because it is smoking that has so strongly contributed to their current vasopathic state. The operation does not impair respiration by major fluid shifts (causing left- or right-side heart failure) or an unfortunately placed incision so that pulmonary disease should not contraindicate surgery unless the patient is a virtual pulmonary cripple. Although pulmonary function tests are therefore generally not necessary, a preoperative arterial blood gas (drawn before the administration of depressant premedications) may be useful to determine the normal resting carbon dioxide tension.

Although a complete discussion of perioperative pulmonary management is not to be found here, these patients often have the problems of excessive secretions, bronchospasm, and relative hypoxia. They also may be particularly sensitive to ventilatory depressants. It must be kept in mind that the usual treatments for these disorders (anticholinergics, $beta_2$-agonists and to a less useful degree aminophylline) are likely to produce tachycardia, which is most undesirable in a population so ridden with coronary disease. If possible, inhaled delivery of anticholinergics and beta-agonists is preferable because less tachycardia is produced. Additional prophylactic measures include introducing, or increasing, steroid doses, adequate levels of anesthesia that may include lidocaine and narcotics as well as volatile agents to the extent hemodynamically tolerated, and avoidance of provocative stimuli such as mainstem intubation, carinal-endotracheal tube contact, and rough or rapid head-turning in the lightly anesthetized patient. Nitroglycerin may provide some bronchodilation and be a useful drug when myocardial ischemia is present or threatening. In these patients myocardial ischemia and hypotension may occur at the same time as wheezing, high airway pressures, and hypoxemia. Measures to reduce postoperative complications include incentive spirometry and coughing or deep breathing, but the endarterectomy population is not nearly so prone to postoperative problems as that for aortic surgery, for example. Loss of protective airway reflexes from cranial nerve damage may result in aspiration that would be tolerated in a normal patient but produce bronchospasm or hypoxemia in this population, which has so little respiratory reserve.

Renal System

A mild degree of renal insufficiency caused by chronic hypertension or atherosclerotic renal artery stenosis is not uncommon in this population. Although it is important to avoid large doses of renally excreted drugs (especially the older muscle relaxants), anesthetic management is not usually markedly affected. More severe degrees of renal dysfunction introduce problems of volume status, need for dialysis, coagulation problems because of platelet dysfunction, anemia, and cardiac problems such as arrhythmias and pericarditis. Obviously, the possibility of neurologic problems because of uremia should be eliminated by dialysis before surgery is undertaken.

Diabetes

Another common problem is diabetes, because these patients so often have significant vascular disease. It is essential to avoid glycemic control so poor that ketoacidosis or nonketotic, hyperosmolar coma occurs perioperatively. The stress of surgery can produce these conditions even in patients whose diabetes was controlled preoperatively by diet alone. We prefer not to administer oral hypoglycemics on the day of surgery because resultant severe hypoglycemia intraoperatively or, more likely, postoperatively is such a devastating and avoidable complication. Nearly all of these patients have arterial cannulas so that checking blood sugars intraoperatively on an hourly basis is a reasonable, easy option. In view of recent data that hyperglycemia exacerbates cerebral ischemia, it is probably advisable to attempt to keep blood glucose levels <200 mg/dl. In fact, it may be important to establish normoglycemia an hour or more before cerebral ischemia occurs because cerebral glucose levels may lag behind systemic levels. Other clinicians may choose to attempt tighter control with glucose levels <150 mg/dl, but tighter control increases the likelihood of intraoperative hypoglycemia, which may be difficult to detect in an anesthetized patient. Although the sympathetic manifestations of tachycardia and hypertension can occur even when anesthesia obliterates the neurologic manifestations of hypoglycemia, the patient who is receiving beta-blockers may only manifest excessive sweating in the presence of dangerously low blood glucose levels.

The perioperative administration of insulin will not be covered in detail here but practical possibilities include:

1. Withhold insulin from patients who are not control problems, administer nonglucose containing fluids, and check blood glucose frequently
2. Administer one half the usual morning dose of intermediate- or short-acting insulin along with a glucose-containing maintenance fluid, check blood glucose frequently
3. For those with a taste for infusions, begin an insulin infusion at 1 to 2 units/hour with a glucose-containing fluid, check blood glucose frequently

It should be clear from the above that we believe the method of insulin administration is not critical so long as it is consistent with common sense and blood glucose levels are checked hourly during this relatively short operation.

PREMEDICATION

Sedation

Because it is usually the goal to have the patient awake and extubated immediately after this operation, premedication is kept to a minimum. Most of our patients need and receive no sedative premedication. Other practitioners routinely use a "heavier" premedication, but we have not found this necessary or desirable. A benzodiazepine can be given orally or parentally as indicated.

Administration of Usual Medications

In general, a patient's usual drugs are continued through the morning of surgery and given orally with a sip of water. Exceptions to this include oral hypoglycemics (generally held by us), diuretics, and digoxin (held or administered according to individual clinical judgment regarding volume status and possibility for toxicity).

MONITORING

Cardiovascular Monitors

BLOOD PRESSURE

An arterial cannula is generally inserted to enable blood gas sampling and continuous monitoring of blood pressures. It is most convenient to insert the cannula in the radial artery of the nonoperative side to facilitate access and to avoid the rare but reported possibility of the proximal shunt tip occluding blood flow to the arm on the operative side. However, it is probably just as important to insert the cannula in the nondominant side, again for a rare possibility—the loss of digits or even a hand from the cannula. We insert the cannula before the induction of anesthesia so that the induction period can be closely monitored. With the near universal availability of automated oscillometers and capnometers, it may in fact be excessively conservative to insist on an arterial cannula in all patients undergoing endarterectomy. The inability to insert an arterial cannula should not present a contraindication to proceeding with surgery so long as noninvasive pressures are readily available.

ELECTROCARDIOGRAPHY

It is optimal in these cases to have the capability to monitor lead II and a frontal lead (V_4 or V_5) to have a reasonable chance of detecting myocardial ischemia. In addition, these patients are prone to sudden episodes of bradycardia or occasionally even asystole when the carotid sinus is surgically manipulated. Computerized programs that monitor ST segments are available and appear to be helpful in monitoring for and quantifying ischemia. Because ischemia is more likely to be detected in the frontal than the limb leads, a modified V lead can be assembled from a standard 3 lead ECG by placing the left arm lead in the V_4 or V_5 position and putting the monitor on lead I. Ischemia is usually evidenced by ST segment depression but can also produce ST elevation, conduction abnormalities, and arrhythmias. Minor T wave changes (i.e., flattening) may not represent ischemia, but distinct T wave inversion is worrisome if not diagnostic. Minor T wave changes and minimal (<1 mm) ST segment depression can be produced by drugs, electrolyte and ventilatory changes, stress, or surgery itself, and part of the art of intraoperative medicine is the avoidance of overinterpretation and overtreatment of minor, meaningless monitoring phenomena. On the other hand, myocardial ischemia demands urgent attention and treatment to avoid progression to infarction, significant myocardial dysfunction, and severe arrhythmias.

CENTRAL VENOUS PRESSURE AND PULMONARY ARTERY CATHETERS

Although carotid artery surgery may produce wide swings in hemodynamics, these are not generally the result of major fluid shifts or blood loss. A central venous catheter (CVP) is therefore not usually indicated for this purpose. As noted in Chapter 16, the arterial pulse waveform can be analyzed for volume deficits or overload in any case. If the reason for insertion of a CVP includes planned or likely administration of drugs best given centrally, this may well be a patient who requires a PA catheter. A PA catheter might be inserted in patients with severe compromise of myocardial function or with recent MI or unstable angina. All these instances would presumably constitute situations in which a cardiologic consultation had already been obtained and options explored for improvement of coronary disease or myocardial function before proceeding to surgery. In our experience a PA catheter is very infrequently required for this operation.

The site of placement for either of these catheters represents a problem because the operated side is obviously unavailable and a catheter positioned in the opposite internal or external jugular vein may be prone to kinking when the head is positioned for surgery. The subclavian veins are possible sites but are prone to serious insertion problems, and even a small pneumothorax may expand with mechanical ventilation. The antecubital site is ideal in some ways and is certainly used successfully for CVP placement. Successful PA catheter placement from this site is challenging.

The PA catheter is primarily a monitor of cardiac function and volume status and secondarily a monitor of myocardial ischemia in that filling pressures will rise and function decrease when ischemia occurs. The pulmonary capillary wedge pressure (PCWP) is used to approximate left ventricular end-diastolic pressure, which itself is an approximation of left ventricular end-diastolic volume, which is the true preload of the left side of the heart. As is the usual case in medicine, problems and errors arise in the transformation of preload to PCWP that must be considered in the care of the patient. In fact, echocardiography provides a more accurate depiction of preload, and careful analysis of the arterial pressure pulse waveform may furnish a more accurate picture of overall volume status. However, the absolute PCWP is useful for evaluating the likelihood that the patient is near or in cardiogenic pulmonary edema. Furthermore, when thermodilution cardiac outputs are obtained by the PA catheter, the actual state of myocardial function can be assessed because stroke volume (normally 60 to 80 ml) is compared with the filling pressure (normally 5 to 12 mm Hg). For example, a low stroke volume with low filling pressures most likely represents hypovolemia, whereas the same stroke volume at high pressures represents myocardial dysfunction. A normal stroke volume with normal filling pressures may indicate to the clinician that myocardial function is not as bad as anticipated. This sort of simple analysis can be used repeatedly to provide an analysis of myocardial function in the face of anesthesia and surgery. On the other hand, although myocardial ischemia may produce an increase in filling pressures (possibly with decreased function), the PA catheter is not a particularly good or useful monitor for ischemia.

ECHOCARDIOGRAPHY

Transesophageal echocardiography has become a commonplace monitor for cardiac anesthesia and in some centers a common one during major vascular surgery and procedures where myocardial function or ischemia risk may justify its use. Most of us mere mortal, regular-old-anesthesiologists are not yet expert in its use or do not have this expensive (but still unproved) modality available to use. Not only can global left ventricular function be monitored, segmental wall motion abnormalities may represent a more sensitive monitor for ischemia than the usual two-lead cardiogram. However, changes in cardiac loading conditions may also produce changes that mimic ischemia and provoke unnecessary and possibly even deleterious therapy. It is not known whether having a large tube in the esophagus may affect the likelihood of cranial nerve damage during the operation. The echocardiogram may be particularly useful for endarterectomy in those cases in which a PA catheter seems to be possibly indicated because the echo can be used initially as a substitute or later when a catheter cannot be successfully inserted.

Respiratory Monitors

There is less uniqueness concerning the respiratory monitoring of endarterectomy patients since capnometry has come into routine use. As will be discussed, the clinician is aiming for normocapnia or mild hypocapnia in most instances and the capnometer provides a guide to the arterial carbon dioxide level once an arterial blood gas has been drawn to establish a baseline arterial end-tidal carbon dioxide gradient. In healthy anesthetized patients this gradient is generally <5 mm Hg but may be quite a bit more in the heavy smokers who present for pipe cleaning. The increase in gradient is due to an increase in dead space that often occurs in these patients. The gradient may change during the course of surgery, but this will be due to an event worthy of recognition itself, such as a severe fall in cardiac output, endobronchial intubation, emboli to the pulmonary vasculature, or breathing circuit problems (e.g., leak with low end-tidal carbon dioxide but a hypoventilated patient). In the past, if capnometry was unavailable, the endarterectomy patient was monitored with several blood gases. Today, if capnometry is not available, the question is whether general anesthesia should proceed at all.

Neurologic Monitors
ELECTROPHYSIOLOGIC MONITORS

The details of electroencephalographic (EEG) and evoked potential (EP) monitoring are outlined in the monitoring chapter. In carotid surgery they are intended to monitor for potentially reversible cerebral ischemia. As the normal cerebral blood flow (CBF) of 50 ml/100 g/min falls, there is no (or minimal) change until flow is about half of normal when EEG changes begin to occur. Between about a 50% and 70% decrease in CBF, changes occur that include an overall decrease in the prevalent EEG frequencies and a decrease in amplitudes. At approximately a 70% decrease level, the EEG will become totally flat (isoelectric if there is total electrical silence but suppressed if varying small degrees of activity persist) because the brain enters the so-called ischemic penumbra when there is still sufficient energy for basal metabolism but not for luxury items such as electrical activity. This represents a reversible stage, but at this point the electroencephalographer is flying blind because the EEG cannot distinguish the ischemic penumbra from a flat EEG, which represents a more severe level of ischemia with >80% flow reduction. The latter may in fact represent an irreversible state of ischemia when cell membranes start to leak, calcium enters the cell like a malicious vandal, and the entire enterprise is not for long. Because the EEG changes, including generalized flattening, may represent reversible ischemia or neuronal death (which is especially complicated in the anesthetized patient because anesthesia itself may contribute to these changes), the EEG is likely to register false-positive changes. Because the EEG monitors very superficial neuronal activity, ischemia in deeper cell layers may be missed. Unless a sufficient number of leads are correctly (or fortuitously) placed, the area of ischemia may simply not be included in the monitored field. Baseline EEG changes in the patient who has had prior ischemia may make the tracing difficult to interpret. Finally, the computerized EEG tracings most of us use to monitor compressed or density spectral array (see Chapter 4) may lose some information in the process of converting the complex EEG into its component sine waves and plotting these data as bar graphs, hills and valleys, or dashes of differing densities. Evoked potential monitoring has been reported by the University of Washington group to be as sensitive (valuable?) as the computerized EEG when the EP tracing is evaluated for >50% amplitude reduction in the cortical component of the first negative peak. Other workers (see Kearse et al. in Suggested Readings) have not found this to be the case.

The hope with EEG or EP monitoring is that they will detect reversible deficits caused by a reduction in regional CBF during cross-clamping or during excessive hypotension during the course of the anesthetic, which should then allow for insertion of a surgical shunt that will preserve CBF when the carotid artery is cross-clamped. Other surgeons never insert shunts, place shunts routinely, or insert shunts on the basis of preoperative data such as the cerebral arteriogram. Unfortunately, about 60% of perioperative neurologic deficits are estimated to be caused by embolic phenomena that are not necessarily reversible when blood pressure is raised or the cross-clamp is removed. Of the remaining 40%, perhaps one fourth occur postoperatively as a result of thrombosis or hemorrhage. Therefore about one third of patients who have neurologic deficits present a situation that is theoretically amenable to monitoring for and correction of cerebral ischemia. The perioperative stroke rate may vary greatly among surgeons. Assuming a stroke rate of approximately 1%, which has been the case in our institution for several years, one in 300 patients may potentially benefit from EEG monitoring. This rate does not include false negatives (which our last two strokes were), which generate a false sense of security, or false positives, which may generate a series of maneuvers that can lead to myocardial ischemia (e.g., administration of phenylephrine) or real cerebral ischemia (insertion of a shunt that has a low but genuine incidence of neurologic injury).

The above discussion represents an extreme position in the world of neuroanesthesia. Other authors would maintain that EEG monitoring is absolutely essential and useful in this situation. They could make the case that the ECG or the pulse oximeter may be similarly inessential in the majority of cases, but would you do a case without them? In fact, more EEG leads (16 rather than four often used with density or compressed spectral array) placed and monitored directly (without computer analysis) by experts may yield better numbers than the above. However, the key factor that a neurologist in the operating room cannot replace is surgical skill, which is by far the most important factor in outcome. Skilled and experienced neurovascular or vascular surgeons will have a stroke rate near 1%, which is hard to improve with EEG monitoring. This appears to be independent of whether patients are always shunted, never shunted, or shunted selectively as indicated by EEG monitoring. Patient selection is another critical factor because the patient with a recent stroke, unresolved older stroke, or a particularly awful cerebral vasculature is more likely to have a perioperative deficit. Obviously severe, prolonged hypotension (before repair) and hypertension (after repair) are to be avoided.

OTHER MONITORS

Perhaps the "best" monitor is neurologic examination of the conscious patient who has received a local or regional anesthetic. There is no debate about the significance of EEG or EP findings when the patient becomes hemiplegic. Unfortunately, the deficit may be embolic and not reverse with removal of the carotid clamp.

Stump pressure, which represents the intravascular pressure on the far side of the distal carotid clamp, makes theoretic sense as a good monitor but it has simply not proved to be so in practice. Its performance may represent as much of a surgical ritual as it does a monitor. A few research centers use clearance methods to measure regional CBF, but this is limited in availability. Finally, noninvasive methods such as Doppler flow studies are being applied to this situation, with questionable utility at this time.

INDUCTION AND MAINTENANCE OF ANESTHESIA

Choice of Induction Agents

In addition to the usual goals in anesthetizing patients with CAD and varying degrees of left ventricular dysfunction, it is important to avoid significant sustained hypotension before the critical carotid stenosis is repaired. A variety of agents may be used to block a severe tachycardic response to laryngoscopy and intubation, including narcotic pretreatment, beta-blockers, and vasodilators. Esmolol has become a popular beta-blocker because it is effective and short acting in doses of 0.5 to 1.0 mg/kg as a bolus. Labetalol provides alpha-blockade as well, but it is difficult to select a dose that will prevent adverse induction hemodynamics and yet not persist and result in hypotension while the patient is being prepped, etc. A preinduction dose of about 10 to 20 mg will generally provide some blunting of undesirable hemodynamics without excessive postinduction hypotension. Finally, an intravenous bolus of 50 to 100 μg of nitroglycerin is an effective way to prevent or treat hypotension in the patient with coronary disease. Topical anesthesia of the airway (as described in the airway management chapter in Dr. Ronald Miller's text [see Suggested Readings]) with glossopharyngeal, superior laryngeal, and translaryngeal analgesia represents another approach to the prevention of excessive hypertension and tachycardia. As a general principle, these patients deserve a more careful induction than the general population, and a slow, controlled induction with mask ventilation, nondepolarizing relaxant, and careful titration of intravenous drugs as dictated by the patient's cardiovascular response is recommended. This can generally be accomplished with small doses of thiopental (1 to 4 mg/kg as judgment dictates), narcotic (of choice, in doses that will not result in a requirement for postoperative ventilation), or +/− lidocaine. The aforementioned antihypertensive adjuncts may or may not be required in any individual and only careful monitoring and response to adverse hemodynamics will prevent routine overtreatment.

Drug doses need to be modified for individuals, and as a general rule it is easier to give more drug than to remove what's already there. Etomidate now presents an alternative induction agent in patients even with fairly severe CHF. The occasional patient may "crump" even with this relatively safe agent, so vigilance cannot be abandoned because it is used. Significant hypertension may develop after an etomidate induction, and this hypertension is least desirable in the afterload-sensitive patient with left ventricular dysfunction. We have found that it is essential to have some thiopental in the room to deal quickly with this severe hypertension. Etomidate is especially useful for those patients who will not tolerate a standard thiopental or propofol induction but in whom we wish to avoid large narcotic doses, because it is a relatively short operation after which we would like to quickly evaluate neurologic status.

The patient with significant bronchospasm and coronary disease represents a special challenge because the therapeutic maneuvers for the former may provoke the latter (e.g., glycopyrrolate, theophylline, beta-agonists) and air trapping may reduce venous return to the heart and result in systemic hypotension. Lidocaine, steroids, and narcotics are especially useful adjuncts if this combination of problems is present. However, inhaled beta$_2$-agonists and small doses of intravenous glycopyrrolate can be used as well. Caution should be applied to the use of beta-blockers, but esmolol appears to be the safest of these drugs in regard to bronchospasm. Topical anesthesia is again an option, including intratracheal lidocaine application under direct vision.

If a difficult airway is suspected, the situation should be handled as in any difficult airway situation with strong consideration given to some form of conscious intubation. A slow, careful conscious intubation can produce results equal or superior to anesthetized intubation with regard to provocation of tachycardia, hypertension, or bronchospasm. Our surgeons occasionally request placement of a nasotracheal tube in patients with high carotid lesions so that they have access to a bit more blood vessel because the mouth can then fully close. Placement of a nasotracheal tube may not be a common practice elsewhere but can be approached either with a full anesthetized-paralyzed induction and insertion under direct laryngoscopy with Magill forceps or by a conscious nasal intubation with or without a bronchoscope. Some patients will have severe nosebleeds after anticoagulation, so we have attempted to discourage this practice.

Relaxants

If a rapid-sequence intubation is required for risk of aspiration, succinylcholine can certainly be used in the patient free of neurologic deficits (without other contraindications). Rocuronium has become a commonly used drug when a relatively rapid onset is desired with a nondepolarizing agent. Vecuronium in a large dose (0.25 mg/kg) may produce slightly less tachycardia but is slower in onset. In most cases a slow induction is used to control hemodynamics so that an intubating dose of a nondepolarizing agent is a reasonable choice. Because of the likelihood of underlying coronary disease, pancuronium would not be among our first choices. Because this is a relatively brief operation, the old long-acting relaxants or the combination of metocurine and pancuronium may present problems with complete reversal at the end. In this population it is especially important to check renal function before administering doses of the older nondepolarizing relaxants (curare, metocurine, pancuronium), which might prove to be excessively long acting for the combination of case and patient. Patients receiving phenytoin or carbamazepine will require a double dose of nondepolarizers to achieve an equal pharmacodynamic effect.

It is always important to consider the possibility that succinylcholine is contraindicated, especially in this population. Succinylcholine should be avoided for at least 6 months in patients who have had a neurovascular ischemic deficit that has not resolved. It is not clear to us when it becomes safe to resume the use of succinylcholine so that it is probably prudent to continue to avoid its use if a deficit judged to be significant remains after 6 months. In patients who have had a stroke that has completely or nearly completely resolved in the last 6 months, the use of succinylcholine becomes a matter of judgment between benefits (rapid onset and offset) and hazards (severe hyperkalemia leading to cardiac arrest). The treatment of succinylcholine-induced hyperkalemia depends most importantly on recognition because it may be misinterpreted to be ischemia-related ventricular tachycardia. Expert cardiopulmonary resuscitation is critical if cardiac arrest has occurred so that the heart and brain can continue to be perfused while the potassium is redistributed back intracellularly. Calcium, bicarbonate for alkalinization, and glucose +/− insulin to accelerate intracellular movement constitute the standard pharmacologic treatment. In addition, epinephrine provides cardiovascular support and $beta_2$-agonism to drive potassium into cells. Magnesium may also be considered to counteract the electrophysiologic effects of hyperkalemia on the heart.

If there is doubt about the use of succinylcholine and the airway does not appear to present difficulties, it may be best to simply use a nondepolarizer for intubation. Note that a pretreatment dose of nondepolarizer does not prevent hyperkalemia from succinylcholine. If the airway appears problematic, consider a careful conscious intubation that preserves hemodynamics and the airway.

Note that in stroke patients the paralyzed side is relatively "resistant" to the effects of relaxants so that the twitch monitor will continue to display an inadequate block while an overdose of relaxant is administered. This is due to the same postsynaptic spread of receptors that contributes to succinylcholine-related hyperkalemia. The monitor should be placed on an unaffected limb and the administration of relaxants limited to a clinically reasonable dose in any case as muscle relaxation is not essential to the surgery itself.

Maintenance of Anesthesia

In general, the goal of anesthesia is to avoid significant decreases in cerebral perfusion before the endarterectomy is performed and to avoid severe increases in blood pressure during closure and emergence that might contribute to cerebral or cervical hematomas. Although somewhat controversial in the past, it is generally agreed currently that normocarbia is a reasonable goal so that unpredictable changes in focal CBF produced by hypocarbia or hypercarbia are avoided. However, if electrophysiologic monitors appear to indicate that ischemia is present during cross-clamping and controlled hypertension is not helpful, a reduction in carbon dioxide may be reasonable in an attempt to divert blood flow away from well-perfused to ischemic areas of brain.

Because many of these patients are elderly and fragile and have some degree of CHF or hypovolemia from diuretics, it is often a challenge to keep the blood pressure (and presumably cerebral perfusion) at adequate levels in the ventilated, anesthetized patient, especially before the incision is made. Even when surgical stimulation is present, blood pressure may fall to less than acceptable levels. The neurosurgeons at our institution are particularly concerned about postoperative hypertension and sometimes give these patients a preoperative dose of clonidine or captopril, which, however, makes the maintenance of blood pressure difficult during the operation and is not recommended by us. We find that acceptable hemodynamics are least difficult to achieve with a nitrous oxide and narcotic (usually fentanyl) technique supplemented as necessary, with low doses of isoflurane. The narcotic dose should be kept to a level consistent with the resumption of adequate postoperative ventilation. Some clinicians prefer to avoid nitrous oxide on the theoretic basis that it may have a negative impact on brain protection. Although this may be so, it is more certain that severe and prolonged hypotension has a negative impact on brain protection. Isoflurane is an effective way to keep the blood pressure down to the lower range of acceptable limits, which we would define as the patient's usual level minus about 20% to 30%. The occasional patient in whom tachycardia develops can be carefully treated with small doses of esmolol after adequate anesthesia and intravascular volume levels are affirmed. If hypertension is a problem in addition to tachycardia, labetalol in very small doses (start at 1.25 to 2.5 mg) is also reasonable.

We use isoflurane commonly but not in the hope that it provides a significant degree of brain protection. In spite of very encouraging early reports from the Mayo Clinic, more recent work indicates that the cerebral protective effect of isoflurane is probably minimal. However, we prefer not to use halothane in this age group (because of hepatitis) and generally avoid enflurane because of possible epileptogenicity (with high levels and hypocarbia) and because we generally find it harder to maintain blood pressure with enflurane than with isoflurane at an equi–minimum allowable concentration level. The volatile agents remain useful drugs because, unlike intravenous agents, their elimination can be rapidly accelerated. Coronary steal from isoflurane was a "hot" topic several years ago but appears to have fallen to the wayside in spite of the impassioned editorials of those times. We have not found it to be a problem but, given the correct steal-prone coronary anatomy, significant hypotension, tachycardia, and an adequate level of isoflurane, it may be a possibility and should be considered whenever myocardial ischemia occurs during isoflurane anesthesia.

Regional Anesthesia

Regional or local anesthesia represents an alternative approach to the anesthetic care of the endarterectomy patient. Issues of concern include technical administration of the anesthetic, concomitant sedation, management of complications in the conscious patient, and possible differences in outcome. It is critically important that the operation proceed with efficient dispatch in these patients, and it may be a poor choice if the surgeon is slow, the patient is anxious (or otherwise not well disposed), or if trainees are performing the operation.

The simplest approach is infiltration of local anesthetic by the surgeon, which, however, may not provide optimal pain relief and is probably best used when the regional block has worn off but the operation is not yet completed. Cervical epidural anesthesia is an excellent way to provide pain relief but is not in the armamentarium of most neuroanesthetists. Complete analgesia is produced by the combination of superficial and deep cervical plexus blocks to block the cervical nerves (C2, C3, and C4) on the operative side. We suggest the use of 1.5% mepivacaine for these blocks because it provides the rapid onset of lidocaine with a longer duration ($\cong$ 3 hours) than lidocaine. However, any local anesthetic may be used with the usual considerations to patient allergy and total dose.

The superficial cervical plexus (SCP) innervates the skin and superficial structures from the lower border of the mandible to just below the clavicle. To perform the block, the patient is positioned with the head slightly elevated, extended, and rotated to the opposite side. The SCP is blocked by infiltrating 10 to 15 ml of anesthetic solution at the midpoint of the posterior border of the sternocleidomastoid muscle, usually where it is crossed by the external jugular vein, with care taken to inject the drug under the vein (Fig. 17-1). The drug is injected superiorly, medially, and inferiorly behind the posterior border of the sternocleidomastoid with care to stay in a superficial tissue plane.

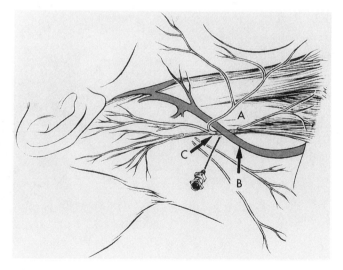

FIG 17-1.
Superficial cervical plexus block *(C)* is accomplished at lateral border of sternocleidomastoid muscle *(A)* at level where external jugular vein *(B)* crosses muscle. (From Carron H, Korbon GA, Rowlingson JC: *Regional anesthesia,* Orlando, Fla, 1984, Grune & Stratton.)

The deep cervical plexus (DCP) can be blocked with three separate injections or a single injection at C4 as described by Winnie. The DCP block is also accomplished by maintaining the head of the patient rotated away and the neck extended (Fig. 17-2). The lower tip of the mastoid process is identified and marked. A line is then drawn from the mastoid process to the supersternal notch. In adults the larynx overlies the cervical vertebrae of C4 to C6 with the upper border of the larynx at the level of C4 and the lower border of the larynx at C6 (the level of the cricoid cartilage). A line drawn from the cricoid cartilage perpendicular to the previous line should overlie the C6 process. The C4 process is likewise markable: a point 1.5 cm below the mastoid process marked along the original line indicates the position of the C2 process. The C3 process is then identified as the midpoint between the two previously noted points at C2 and C4.

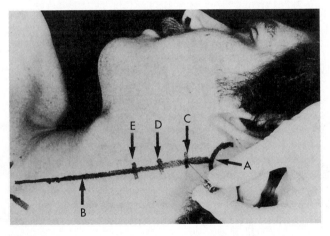

FIG 17-2.
Deep cervical plexus block. A line *(BA)* is drawn from tip of mastoid process *(A)* to suprasternal notch. Injection at C4 process (at *E*) is obtained by drawing line perpendicular to previous line at level of top of larynx. C2 process (at *C*) is on original line 1.5 cm below mastoid process. C3 process *(D)* lies halfway between *C* and *E*. (From Carron H, Korbon GA, Rowlingson JC: *Regional anesthesia,* Orlando, Fla, 1984, Grune & Stratton.)

To perform a DCP block, a 1.5-inch, 22-gauge needle is inserted perpendicular to the skin and slightly caudad to a depth of approximately 2 cm. Contact with the C2 and C4 processes is accomplished in sequential penetrations. Parasthesias may or may not be obtained. The needle is withdrawn approximately 1 to 3 mm after bony contact and 5 ml of local anesthetic is injected at each of these sites after aspiration for blood or spinal fluid. Anesthesia onset is rapid and evident within 5 minutes. Some clinicians advocate the injection of the C3 process also, as previously described, with 5 ml of drug, whereas others advocate the use of 10 ml of drug at C2 and C4, which allows the drug to migrate and cover the C3 process. Still others believe that injection of the total dose in only one of these processes is needed to produce a deep cervical plexus block with the drug (see reference by Winnie). By use of any of these anesthetic techniques deeper structures are well anesthetized. As an alternate technique, an interscalene block is carried out by the technique of Winnie with 30 ml of local anesthetic injected in the interscalene groove.

Several complications are possible as a result of SCP and DCP block. For the SCP block, the major potential problem is intravascular injection. Therefore the usual precautions to identify intravenous injection are essential. The most common complication of the DCP block is the paralysis of the recurrent laryngeal nerve and the production of a stellate ganglion block, which can be symptomatic. Respiratory distress may infrequently occur in patients with severe COPD because this technique can produce hemidiaphragmatic elevation. If bilateral blocks are attempted, bilateral stellate ganglion block may also occur and result in profound bradycardia from the loss of the cardioaccelerator fibers. In addition, the nerve root sleeve can be entered and the local anesthetic will produce a subarachnoid block. Injection into the vertebral artery is also possible, and such injection, even with very small quantities of local anesthetic, will result in convulsions or apnea.

Sedation for the procedure may range from no additional medication to a propofol infusion to maintain a light sleep. In the fragile elderly patient, diphenhydramine (12.5 to 25 mg) may provide adequate sedation. Alternatives include midazolam, fentanyl, droperidol, or the clinician's personal favorite. It is essential to avoid oversedation in the patient with an uncontrolled airway and an exposed carotid artery, much as one would do in the eye room. Oxygen should generally be administered.

In addition to the aforementioned complications of the blocks themselves, difficulties may arise in that the patient may not be able to further tolerate the procedure under regional anesthesia or that the patient may have lost consciousness because of oversedation or neurologic mishap. In all cases the clinician must be prepared to take control of the airway and administer general anesthesia, which is difficult in this situation and may represent the most important reason for the reluctance of many anesthetists and surgeons to perform the procedure under regional anesthesia. In addition to conventional endotracheal intubation, alternative approaches to control of the airway include the laryngeal mask airway and the Combitube.

The major impetus for the use of regional anesthesia has been the obvious ability to monitor the awake patient for severe ischemia during carotid cross-clamping. However, the majority of ischemic events are not a result of simple reduction in blood flow from cross-clamping. Furthermore, ischemia that apparently results from cross-clamping may actually be embolic and not reverse when the clamp is removed. Improved cardiovascular stability and less myocardial ischemia or infarction are possible advantages for surgery under regional anesthesia but do not appear to be significant. The major advantage may be that patients appear to have a quicker postoperative recovery and leave the hospital, on average, a day sooner than patients receiving general anesthesia. In these days of cost cutting this result may turn out to be an important consideration, which may simply be because surgeons tend to handle tissue more carefully and gently in the awake patient. In any case, regional anesthesia for carotid endarterectomy requires a willing surgeon, anesthetist, and patient before it is undertaken and should probably not be performed if one of the above three characters is not suitable for the role.

Special Considerations During Surgery

As previously noted, it is important to keep blood pressure at or not far below baseline levels in the period before cross-clamping, although it appears that systemic hypotension is not a major contributor to perioperative stroke. Surgery and mechanical stimulation in the area of the carotid sinus may result in bradycardia or hypotension, although not a common problem in our practice. Administration of an anticholinergic, cessation of and resumption of gentler surgical stimulation, and injection of local anesthetic may provide the solution to this problem.

When the carotid artery is actually cross-clamped, it is reasonable to avoid hypotension; we generally provide a blood pressure that is slightly above baseline (10% to 30% increased) to provide for improved perfusion by the available collaterals to the distal circulation. We provide this pressure with phenylephrine in small boluses (25 to 100 μg), but if repeated boluses are required it may be simpler and more efficacious (in the sense of a more constant pressure) to start an infusion beginning at 20 μg/min and titrate upward to maintain the desired pressure. Any vasopressor can be used with the knowledge that myocardial ischemia may be produced by increasing afterload and even direct coronary vasoconstriction. In the patient with known severe coronary disease, it may be reasonable to administer nitroglycerin by skin patch or infusion concomitantly to reduce the direct coronary effect of the vasoconstrictor.

Currently we do not provide any particular pharmacologic agent in an attempt to improve brain protection. In general, isoflurane is used as the volatile anesthetic agent but not in any hope that this will provide anything more than minimal brain protection. The patient's temperature may drift down to 35° C simply from general anesthesia, but no further hypothermia is intended so that the patient can be quickly reawakened after this relatively short operation. Clinicians at some centers may administer a bolus of thiopental or etomidate before cross-clamping, but the results of this practice are unknown. Certainly it is important to avoid thiopental-related hypotension during cross-clamping.

If the EEG is monitored and changes interpreted as ischemia are produced by cross-clamping, some surgeons choose to insert a shunt to bypass the occluded segment. Ischemic changes may be subtle but it appears to be major changes such as a 50% decrease in amplitude (or greater, including EEG flattening) that are "significant." Unfortunately, the insertion of the shunt itself appears to contribute to the occurrence of stroke in some small ($\cong 1\%$) number of cases. Other surgeons, including the neurosurgery staff at our institution, choose never to shunt in that they prefer not to replace an unknown injury with a known one. Some surgeons decide to shunt on the basis of preoperative factors such as the arteriogram or they decide to place a shunt in virtually all patients. The differences between these practices are difficult to know but are probably dependent on the technical skills of the surgeon. Recent work by Riles and Imperato at New York University indicates that surgical technical failure may have even a greater role in perioperative stroke than previously thought.

In any case, the insertion of a shunt is a surgical decision. If the EEG is not monitored, it is reasonable to keep blood pressures at slightly supernormal levels and the arterial partial pressure of carbon dioxide at normal levels. If significant EEG changes are detected, our options basically are limited to increasing the blood pressure and perhaps hyperventilating the patient to divert blood from normal to ischemic areas. It is essential to use reasonable judgment and not hurt the heart in overzealous but perhaps futile or even misguided attempts to salvage a brain that is beyond our help or not even injured.

Emergence

One of the goals of anesthesia for carotid endarterectomy is rapid emergence so that a rough neurologic examination can be performed as soon as possible. In addition to the usual airway concerns, special problems include the possibility of cervical hematomas and bilateral hypoglossal nerve damage (after carotid endarterectomies performed in the presence of an existing contralateral hypoglossal nerve injury). It is important to maintain reasonable hemodynamics at this time to avoid myocardial ischemia and intracranial hemorrhage. Patients who suddenly have resumption of flow to a previously poststenotic area may have difficulty with autoregulation and be prone to hemorrhage with excessive hypertension postoperatively. Labetalol is a good choice at this time if tachycardia is part of the picture; it can be given in 5, 10, 20, etc., mg doses at approximately 5-minute intervals. Less frequently, bradycardia or hypotension are so significant that treatment is required. These problems are dealt with in more detail in Chapter 19.

Extracranial-Intracranial Bypass

Extracranial-intracranial bypass is virtually no longer performed for purposes of treating cerebral vascular disease per se. Rather, it may be performed prophylactically before extensive craniobasal surgery to preserve a distal blood supply. For this reason, there is a brief discussion of this procedure in Chapter 14.

Suggested Readings

Blume WT et al: Significance of EEG changes at carotid endarterectomy, *Stroke* 17:891, 1986.

Breslow MJ et al: Changes in T-wave morphology following anesthesia and surgery: a common recovery room phenomenon, *Anesthesiology* 64:398, 1986.

Ferguson GG: Intraoperative monitoring and internal shunts: are they necessary in carotid endarterectomy? *Stroke* 13:287, 1982.

Fleisher LA, Barash PG: Preoperative cardiac evaluation for noncardiac surgery, *Analg Anesth* 74:586, 1992.

Fleisher LA et al: Failure of negative dipyridamole thallium scans to predict perioperative myocardial ischemia and infarction, *Can J Anaesth* 39:179, 1992.

Gelabert HA, Moore WS: Occlusive cerebrovascular disease: medical and surgical considerations. In Cottrell JE, Smith DS, editors: *Anesthesia and neurosurgery,* ed 3, St Louis, 1994, Mosby.

Goldstein LB et al: Multicenter review of preoperative risk factors for carotid endarterectomy in patients with ipsilateral symptoms, *Stroke* 25:1116, 1994.

Herrick IA, Gelb AW: Occlusive cerebrovascular disease: anesthetic considerations. In Cottrell JE, Smith DS, editors: *Anesthesia and neurosurgery,* ed 3, St Louis, 1994, Mosby.

Kearse LA et al: Somatosensory evoked potentials sensitivity relative to electroencephalography for cerebral ischemia during carotid endarterectomy, *Stroke* 23:498, 1992.

Lam AM et al: Monitoring electrophysiologic function during carotid endarterectomy: a comparison of somatosensory evoked potentials and conventional electroencephalogram, *Anesthesiology* 75:15, 1991.

Miller RD, editor: *Anesthesia,* ed 4, New York, 1994, Churchill Livingstone.

North American Symptomatic Carotid Endarterectomy Trial Collaborators: Beneficial effect of carotid endarterectomy in symptomatic patients with high-grade carotid stenosis, *N Engl J Med* 325:445, 1991.

Riles TS et al: The cause of perioperative stroke after carotid endarterectomy, *J Vasc Surg* 19:206, 1994.

Silbert BS et al: The processed electroencephalogram may not detect neurologic ischemia during carotid endarterectomy, *Anesthesiology* 70:356, 1989.

Winnie AP et al: Interscalene cervical plexus block: a single injection technique, *Anesth Analg* 54:370, 1975.

ANESTHESIA FOR HEAD TRAUMA

18

Marcel E. Durieux

Head injury and its treatment comprise an area of considerable importance to the neuroanesthesiologist. As with other forms of major trauma, the anesthesiologist will often be involved in patient care before the patient's appearance in the operating room. Also, head injury is one of the few true emergencies in neurosurgical practice, necessitating a plan of action well thought out in advance and executed flawlessly and rapidly if the patient is to survive without major deficit. Because these patients often have other major injuries that may compete for attention, both cooperation and communication with the various surgical subspecialties are essential for optimal results.

In this chapter I will, after reviewing the pertinent demographics and pathophysiologic features, discuss the initial assessment, diagnosis, and management of the patient with head injury, followed by a detailed description of anesthetic care. Outcome will be addressed briefly in the final section.

INCIDENCE OF INJURY

Defining the incidence of head injury is not straightforward. First, a continuum of severity exists, ranging from the many thousands of injuries that are never seen in the hospital because of their insignificance to those injuries that never reach the emergency department because the patient died at the scene of injury or in transit. Second, the exact definition of head injury used determines the incidence reported: are facial or skull injuries included; is computed tomographic (CT) evidence of injury required to classify a patient as having head trauma, or is a clinical constellation of symptoms sufficient? Because criteria vary, numbers will always reflect the specific population included in the study design. Third, the geographic locale will influence the reported results significantly because injury patterns differ. Despite these variables, most studies find a head injury incidence of approximately 200 per 100,000 residents per year. The estimated annual frequency of brain injury for 1990 was as follows: 1,975,000 medically attended head injuries were sustained, of which 366,000 patients were hospitalized and 75,000 patients died. Thus the vast majority of head injuries seen at hospitals are minor, but of those patients admitted a significant percentage (>20%) dies. A similar number of patients with head injury die before hospital admission. Overall, one third of trauma deaths in the United States are due to head injury.

When stratified by age, the incidence of brain injury is invariably found to be highest in young people, peaking between the ages of 15 and 25 years. Two secondary peaks include infants and children on one side and the elderly on the other. Most studies have shown a preponderance of male over female victims of at least 2:1. In contrast to these universal findings, stratification as to cause depends on several variables. In most studies motor vehicle accidents are the most common cause of head injury (approximately 50% of cases), but in urban areas violence (assaults and firearms) takes the primary place. Falls are the second most common cause, particularly in elderly patients. There is conclusive evidence that restraint of automobile passengers, and persuasive evidence that helmet use by cyclists and motorcyclists, decreases the number of head injuries significantly. On the other hand, alcohol use has been shown to increase the number of automobile accidents and resultant head trauma. Intoxication also makes neurologic assessment more difficult. Approximately 50% of patients with head injury show detectable blood alcohol levels. Most head injuries are seen in the emergency department between 4 PM and midnight, and the peak incidence is between Friday and Sunday.

PATHOPHYSIOLOGY

Brain damage as a result of head injury can be divided into primary and secondary injury. *Primary injury* is the injury occurring during the traumatic event itself. Direct impact of the head, although a common occurrence, is not essential for bringing about the pathologic findings of primary injury; it has now been shown that virtually all forms of primary injury—macroscopic disruption of blood vessels as well as microscopic shearing damage to axons and dendrites—can be replicated in experimental systems by subjecting the head to rapid rotation and deceleration forces. One exception is epidural hematoma, which most times results from damage to the skull rather than from direct damage to the brain. Primary injury has already occurred by the time the patient is first seen by medical or paramedical personnel and therefore cannot be minimized, except through preventive measures. The only therapeutic goal that can be attained is to provide the best environment possible for recovery. *Secondary injury,* on the other hand, is the injury occurring after the traumatic event, as a result of hypoxia, hypercapnia, and ischemia induced by hypotension, vasospasm or increased intracranial pressure (ICP). The importance of secondary injury to outcome is most clearly demonstrated by those patients who, at some point after injury, are conscious and talk, only to subsequently deteriorate and die. In these patients death can be attributed in its entirety to secondary injury. Because secondary injury may still be developing during the patient's treatment in the hospital, it offers opportunities for active intervention. The most important contributors to secondary injury are *hypoxemia* and *hypovolemia with hypotension,* which should be actively searched for and corrected as rapidly as possible.

Much recent research has addressed the issue of *diffuse axonal injury* (i.e., the microscopic disruption of neurons and neuronal connections). In almost half of patients with severe head injury diffuse axonal injury is the main finding; the patients show no demonstrable intracranial mass lesion but remain in prolonged coma and have a high mortality. Unfortunately, it has been shown that diffuse axonal injury occurs at the moment of injury (i.e., it is a primary injury and as such not amenable to therapeutic intervention). However, better understanding of the exact mode of damage might allow the development of more effective regimens to enhance neuronal regeneration.

Increased ICP is a final common pathway of many pathophysiologic processes and a frequent precursor to death. It results from edema or swelling. *Edema* can have multiple causes: (1) vasogenic edema results from impairment of the blood-brain barrier; (2) hydrostatic edema occurs after disruption of autoregulation, most often after rapid decompression of a mass lesion; (3) cytotoxic edema results from ischemia and inability to sustain cellular metabolism; and (4) osmotic edema results from a decrease in serum osmolality, usually associated with hyponatremia. *Swelling* is a consequence of obstruction to outflow of blood or cerebrospinal fluid (CSF). Because these different causes of increased ICP require different treatments, it is of obvious importance to determine the cause of increased ICP in each patient before therapy is instituted. The pathophysiologic processes and treatment of increased ICP are detailed in Chapter 2.

In summary, mechanical injury, hemorrhage, edema, and ischemia are the most important causes of brain damage in patients with head injury. Particularly the last two are forms of secondary injury that are of concern to the anesthesiologist.

TYPES OF INJURY

Skull and Scalp Injury

Several types of nonpenetrating injury are of importance to the anesthesiologist. *Open skull fractures* (and depressed skull fractures) should not be disturbed until in the operating room because the bone or a foreign body may be causing tamponade of a disrupted blood vessel. Therefore particular care should be taken when patients with these injuries are intubated. Patients with documented or expected *basilar skull fractures* should, if possible, not be intubated nasally because of the risk of introducing bacteria into the CSF or the tracheal tube into the cranial vault. The presence of hemotympanum, otorrhea, mastoid ecchymosis (Battle's sign), and ecchymoses around the eyes without extension beyond the orbit (raccoon's eyes) should be warning signs. Whether nasally draining fluid is CSF can be confirmed by the "double ring" sign on blotter paper. A glucose test will give a false-positive reaction in 75% of patients without CSF leak, but if negative, it rules out the presence of CSF. If oral intubation is deemed impossible (e.g., because of facial injuries), a cricothyroidotomy or tracheostomy should be considered. *Scalp lacerations,* although they can bleed profusely, are not usually the cause for systemic hypotension (except in small children), and internal injury should be strongly suspected in such cases.

Traumatic Intracranial Mass Lesions

Although classic descriptions of the symptoms of various types of penetrating injury are widely known, recent studies have shown that there is in fact little correlation between the type of lesion and clinical symptoms. As an example, approximately 20% of patients with an intracerebral hematoma will have a lucid interval, a number higher than that reported for patients with an epidural hematoma, for which it was classically described. Most forms of traumatic intracranial mass lesion will cause some degree of decreased level of consciousness and increased ICP, with or without localizing symptoms. Thus correct diagnosis and treatment is largely dependent on radiologic procedures, primarily CT. Neurosurgical consensus prescribes evacuation of virtually all clinically significant lesions (i.e., those associated with symptoms or with a midline shift ≥ 5 mm).

Epidural Hematoma

Epidural hematoma (EDH) occurs as a result of injury to the skull, not injury to the brain. It is fairly uncommon, occurring in approximately 3% of hospitalized head trauma patients. Bending or fracture of the skull results in tearing of meningeal vessels, causing a hematoma with lentiform appearance on CT. Because the bleeding is often arterial, neurologic deterioration can be rapid and preclude

CT scanning. Exploratory burr holes may need to be drilled immediately if the patient is to survive. In such cases the anesthesiologist will most likely already be in attendance to provide airway management, and transfer to the operating suite for evacuation of the hematoma should be accomplished in a very short time. Outcome from EDH is dependent on the rapidity with which symptoms develop; mortality decreases from up to 60% in those patients in whom symptoms develop rapidly to <10% in those with slowly expanding lesions. Acute EDH is a true neurosurgical emergency.

SUBDURAL HEMATOMA

In contrast to EDH subdural hematoma (SDH) results from acceleration-deceleration injury to the brain, resulting in stretching of and damage to parasagittal bridging veins. SDH is divided in acute and chronic forms. Although operative treatment is generally indicated for both forms, their presentation is quite different. An intermediate form, *subacute SDH,* is seen between 3 and 15 days after injury, with symptoms primarily related to increased ICP. *Acute SDH* manifests within 72 hours after injury and is seen on CT as a diffuse lesion over the cerebral convexity. It is found in up to 13% of head-injury victims and in approximately 30% of those in coma. Although symptoms usually develop slower than with EDH, mortality is higher because of underlying brain injury. In fact, mortality of acute SDH is higher than that of any other mass lesion after head injury and is generally reported as ≥50%. The association with brain injury makes it unclear how much of this mortality is due to the expanding hematoma and how much to primary brain injury. Thus there is no consistent relationship between hematoma size and outcome. *Chronic SDH* is seen more than 20 days after injury, often in alcoholics, epileptics, or the elderly, after relatively minimal trauma. In fact, 25% to 50% of patients have no history of head injury at all. The symptoms can be variable, but headache and other symptoms of increased ICP, slowly developing focal neurologic lesions, dementia, inappropriate behavior, amnesia, and gait disturbances are commonly seen.

INTRACEREBRAL HEMORRHAGE

The incidence of intracerebral hemorrhage (IH) is largely dependent on the effort expended to find small lesions, but if only clinically significant hemorrhages are taken into account it occurs less frequently than SDH or EDH. A most important feature of IH is its propensity to develop later in the course of hospitalization, although 80% of these hemorrhages will become apparent within 48 hours after admission. Thus patients with head injury must be monitored closely for neurologic deterioration, and there should be a low threshold for repeat CT scanning if delayed hemorrhage is suspected. This is particularly so because it often will be impossible to distinguish clinically between IH and mass effect from other causes, such as the development of edema around a preexisting hemorrhage.

Vascular Lesions

Although the hematomas described above are caused by rupture of small blood vessels, injury to the major vessels of the brain may also be caused by head trauma. The *carotid* or *vertebral arteries* may be damaged by penetrating or nonpenetrating trauma to the neck. Intimal dissection or hemorrhage in the media may occur, resulting in thrombosis. Thrombosis of the vertebral artery may involve the anterior spinal artery with resulting ischemia or infarction of the cervical spinal cord. *Venous sinus* disruption can lead to massive blood loss and carries a high risk of air embolism during surgery. Many of these lesions can be repaired, and they provide challenging cases for the anesthesiologist. *Fistulas,* particularly between the carotid artery and cavernous sinus, and *aneurysms* can also result from head trauma. Close communication with the surgical team is essential for proper management of these complex cases.

Associated Injuries

Up to 50% of head trauma victims will have significant, often life-threatening, associated injuries. Even if emergency surgical evacuation of an intracranial mass lesion has to take precedence over treatment of other injuries, the anesthesiologist should be fully aware of these other issues because their presence may have a significant impact on anesthetic management. In addition, the possibility should be kept in mind that potentially life-threatening but undiagnosed injuries may exist and could reveal themselves during surgery or postoperatively. Examples of relevant associated injuries are the following, chosen with particular emphasis on the head-injured patient who has been involved in a motor vehicle accident. *Cervical spine injury* is present in 10% of head trauma victims and should always be suspected in any patient with an injury above the clavicle. It can result from the head hitting the windshield or dash-board. *Aortic disruption* and *cardiac tamponade* can develop after impact on the steering column. *Pulmonary contusions, cardiac contusions, pneumothorax,* and *hemothorax* can occur by the same mechanism. *Lumbar spine injury, splenic injury,* and *retroperitoneal bleeding* may result from seatbelt impaction. *Hypovolemia* from profuse hemorrhage should always be kept in mind. *Aspiration* of blood and vomitus is also common. Some of these problems are discussed in greater detail in Chapters 19 and 20.

INITIAL ASSESSMENT

There has been major emphasis in recent years on standardizing initial assessment and treatment of the trauma victim, including the head-trauma victim. This trend follows from findings indicating the existence of a trimodal distribution of trauma deaths. A first peak occurs within seconds or minutes of injury (in head injury patients this corresponds to primary injury). A second peak occurs within a few minutes to hours of injury (representing secondary injury). This period has been referred to as the *golden hour.* The third peak, days to weeks after injury, results from sepsis or organ failure. As primary injury cannot be addressed by medical management, and the third mortality peak appears related to the efficacy of earlier treatment, any major impact on trauma mortality will have to come from more effective treatment in the first hours after injury. This is best accomplished by efficient teamwork, which requires the use of standardized treatment protocols. The most dramatic of such attempts to standardize care has been the development of the Advanced Trauma Life Support Course by the American College of Surgeons. This course includes a special section on management of the patient with head injury. Because most trauma centers now follow the protocols outlined in this course, I will use them as a base for describing the approach to treatment of these challenging patients, focusing particularly on items of specific interest to the anesthesiologist. The overall goal is to allow optimal integration of the effort of the anesthesiology team with that of the trauma team as a whole.

History

The essential issues in the patient's history are as follows. The *mechanism of injury* is helpful in determining prognosis and directing a search for other injuries. For example, a patient injured in a fall has a four times higher chance of having an intracerebral hematoma than one involved in a motor vehicle accident. The patient's *immediate postinjury status* serves as a baseline for repeated assessments; particularly the level of consciousness provides critical information. The *preinjury status,* if known, is similarly helpful. Any *prehospital treatment* the patient has received, such as airway management, the use of paralyzing agents and sedatives, and the adequacy of fluid resuscitation, should be known. Other items in the history that are of importance to the anesthesiologist are summarized by the acronym AMPLE: *A*llergies, *M*edications currently taken, *P*ast illnesses, *L*ast meal, and *E*vents related to the injury. Symptoms of intracranial hypertension should be sought: nausea, vomiting, tinnitus, headache, and visual symptoms.

Physical Examination

Vital signs should be assessed immediately and reassessed frequently. Hypotension almost invariably points to associated systemic injuries. Hypertension, particularly when associated with bradycardia, suggests increased ICP resulting from a mass lesion (the classic Cushing's triad), which may necessitate immediate surgical exploration. A rapid *neurologic examination* will provide the baseline for repeated assessments. It should consist of a measure of the patient's level of consciousness, such as the Glasgow Coma Scale (GCS, Table 18-1) or even the simple AVPU method (*A*lert, responsive to *V*ocal stimuli, responsive to *P*ainful stimuli, or *U*nresponsive), assessment of pupils for equality and response to light, and a check for lateralized extremity weakness. Papilledema is distinctly unusual in the head trauma population, even in the presence of increased ICP, and pupillary abnormalities may be unreliable in patients with severe hypotension. A quick *head examination* will reveal any obvious injuries to the scalp and palpable depressed skull fractures. The possibility of a basilar skull fracture, with its implications for intubation, should be considered when compatible signs are observed. Gross damage to the face, mouth or neck, which could interfere with airway management, should be noted.

EARLY MANAGEMENT AND STABILIZATION

The goals of early management of the patient with head trauma are twofold. First, prevention of secondary injury must be attempted aggressively. Second, a rapid decision needs to be made as to whether emergency surgical exploration is required. At the same

TABLE 18-1. Glasgow Coma Scale

Eye Opening (E)	
Spontaneous	4
To speech	3
To pain	2
None	1

Best Verbal Response (V)	
Oriented	5
Confused conversation	4
Inappropriate words	3
Incomprehensible sounds	2
None	1

Best Motor Response (M)	
Obeys	6
Localizes	5
Withdraws	4
Abnormal flexion	3
Extensor response	2
No movement	1

NOTE: Best motor response for any extremity is used for scoring. Eye opening scoring is not valid if eyes are swollen shut, and verbal scoring is invalid if speech is impossible (e.g., in presence of tracheal tube). Maximal GCS is 15; minimal score is 3. All patients with GCS <8 and most with GCS = 8 are in coma (i.e., no eye opening [M = 1], no ability to follow commands [M = 1 to 5], and no word verbalizations [V = 1 to 2]. GCS ≤8 is classified as severe head injury, GCS between 9 and 12 as moderate head injury, and GCS between 13 and 15 as minor head injury.

time other, potentially life-threatening injuries should be sought and addressed, and essential laboratory data (hemoglobin or hematocrit, platelets, blood chemistry, arterial blood gas, coagulation parameters, toxicology screen, and blood type and cross-match for transfusion) collected. Electrocardiographic (ECG) and blood pressure monitoring and pulse oximetry should be applied as early as possible.

Prevention of Secondary Injury

Although our understanding of the factors involved in the development of secondary injury is incomplete, the two most important variables thus far identified are the inability of the circulation to maintain cerebral metabolic needs and the development of intracranial hypertension.

MAINTENANCE OF CEREBRAL METABOLIC NEEDS

The primary factors resulting in insufficient cerebral metabolism are hypoxia and cerebral ischemia. The presence of either hypoxia or ischemia, but particularly both in combination, affects outcome adversely. A single episode of hypotension occurring between injury and resuscitation has been shown to be associated with an increase in mortality of almost 50%. Although this is an association only and not a proven cause-effect relationship, similar data have been generated in controlled animal studies. Hypoxia and hypotension occur remarkably commonly, and either or both are present in at least 50% of head trauma victims. Clearly anesthesiologists should play a major role in the attempt to decrease the incidence of these detrimental factors.

Hypotension should be treated by the administration of crystalloid solution or, in the case of extensive injuries, blood. Administration of free water should be avoided because it can lead to hyponatremia and hypoosmolarity, with subsequent cerebral edema. As a temporizing measure, MAST (*m*ilitary *a*ntishock *t*rousers) can be applied to increase venous return, and they have been shown to be effective. The head-down position, on the other hand, is contraindicated because it raises ICP significantly and leads to cerebral edema. In addition, cerebral perfusion is not necessarily improved by this maneuver because arterial and venous pressures generally are increased by the same amount. It should be realized that blood pressure, although easily measured, may not be an adequate indicator of blood flow and volume. Pulse pressure, strength of the pulse, and the waveform of an arterial catheter tracing provide qualitative information on these aspects. Because increased glucose concentrations have been associated with poor outcome after cardiac arrest and other instances of decreased cerebral perfusion, supplemental glucose generally should not be given, unless documented hypoglycemia is present. Hypertension can be as detrimental for the head-injured patient as hypotension because it increases edema formation and ICP. Excessive increases in blood pressure should be treated once a compensatory blood pressure response to high ICP has been ruled out. As discussed in the section on cardiovascular complications, adrenergic blocking agents are the therapy of choice because they have minimal cerebral effect and address the underlying pathophysiologic processes.

Hypoxia, often clinically apparent as restlessness, should be treated by supplying supplemental oxygen. In the head trauma patient this often will be combined with tracheal intubation to allow full ventilatory control. Early intubation is encouraged because a large study showed that intubation within the first hour after injury rather than after the first hour decreased mortality from 38% to 22%. Although intubation will temporarily raise ICP, this effect is minimal in comparison to the changes resulting from hypoventilation and hypoxia. Nonetheless, the decision when, and how, to intubate can be difficult. Intubation is often necessary for (1) relief of airway obstruction, (2) protection from aspiration, (3) prevention of hypoventilation, (4) administration of hyperventilation to control ICP, and (5) for allowing paralysis of the combative patient for diagnostic procedures. Some clinicians recommend that all patients with a GCS <8 be intubated. Irregular respirations and tachypnea can herald impending respiratory failure and should also be considered indications for intubation because prevention of hypoxia is far better than correction.

Intubation of the head trauma patient can be a significant challenge. To a large extent the technique selected will depend on the urgency with which ventilatory control is required. Because previous hypoventilation and existing hypoxia can lead to rapid hemoglobin desaturation during the intubation attempt, optimal denitrogenation is required. Any airway obstruction, usually from the tongue falling back, but occasionally from blood or oropharyngeal trauma, should be relieved. Jaw thrust, placement of an oropharyngeal airway, or removal of vomitus and debris will often provide a patent airway. At times mouth opening will be difficult because of either muscle spasm resulting from trauma or temporomandibular joint damage. The former will disappear with neuromuscular blockade, but if the temporomandibular joint is involved, awake intubation is required. The observation that *succinylcholine* modestly increases ICP has made some experts argue against its use and recommend awake intubations. However, the intracranial hypertension induced by a struggling, gagging, partially conscious patient during awake intubation will most likely increase ICP much more than succinylcholine will. In addition, the potentially difficult airway and full stomach of the head trauma patient warrant rapid and optimal intubating conditions, which should be balanced against the perceived likelihood of inability to ventilate or intubate after the patient is paralyzed. Although each patient should be assessed individually, succinylcholine (1 mg/kg) is often a useful adjunct in airway management. This issue is discussed further in the section on anesthetic management.

Cervical spine fracture is present in 10% of head trauma patients and in up to 20% of severely injured patients and should therefore always be suspected. Techniques minimizing neck movement must be used, as detailed in Chapter 8, but concern about a cervical fracture should never take precedence over relieving hypoxemia. It is of critical importance that the anesthesiologist ensure that appropriate monitoring and suction are present because these adjuncts, always immediately available in the operating room, might not be present or in working order in the crowded, busy trauma room in the emergency department. In addition, the presence of a skilled assistant can be extremely important under these circumstances, and particularly trainees should assure themselves of available backup. If the situation warrants, surgeons should be prepared to perform a rapid cricothyroidotomy if intubation attempts fail.

TREATMENT OF INTRACRANIAL HYPERTENSION

The second variable responsible for secondary injury is intracranial hypertension. There are many causes of increased ICP, as discussed in the section on pathophysiologic mechanisms, and different treatment modalities are advocated for different causes. However, during the initial assessment and stabilization of the head-trauma victim, it may not be possible to determine the exact etiology. Indeed, the presence of increased ICP may have to be judged by limited clinical signs only. Therefore treatment involves those measures that will be efficacious for most causes. In patients with a GCS <7, ICP monitoring should be strongly considered because physical examination may not reflect the actual level of ICP in the comatose patient. ICP levels up to 20 mm Hg are generally considered acceptable, although some will advocate more aggressive treatment and use a maximally acceptable level of 15 mm Hg. ICP values should not be overly depended on because the implications of a certain ICP level vary with the site of the intracranial lesion. For example, patients with frontal lobe hematomas tolerate high levels of ICP, whereas those with temporal lobe masses are prone to brainstem compression at much more moderate ICP values.

Hypocapnia induced by hyperventilation is a standard mode of treatment. By constricting cerebral blood vessels it decreases intracranial blood volume and thus ICP. Although difficult to determine in the emergency department, optimal levels of hypocapnia are probably between 25 and 30 mm Hg. Below 25 mm Hg the possibility of cerebral ischemia exists, at least in theory. Induced hypocapnia is an extremely rapid way to decrease ICP. The effects are transient, however, and CSF pH generally returns to normal within 24 hours.

Diuretics form the second mainstay of ICP treatment, with mannitol and furosemide the drugs used most frequently. *Mannitol* is a six-carbon sugar that is too large in size to pass through the intact blood-brain barrier or cell membrane, does not undergo metabolism, and is eliminated by renal filtration without reabsorption. It increases plasma osmolality and induces osmotic diuresis. In turn, fluid is drawn from intracellular to extracellular spaces, resulting in decreased brain swelling. In addition, mannitol is thought to improve the rheologic properties of blood by decreasing viscosity and erythrocyte rigidity and to act as a free-radical scavenger. Dosage is 0.25 to 1 g/kg given over 10 to 20 minutes, repeated as necessary every 3 to 6 hours. Higher doses do not decrease ICP any further but have a longer duration of action. Some rebound effect may be seen. There is concern that disruption of the blood-brain barrier would allow mannitol to enter brain tissue, resulting in localized edema and increased ICP, but unfortunately this effect is difficult to evaluate in the individual patient. In children with increased ICP resulting from head trauma, mannitol may not be indicated because in these patients intracranial hypertension is caused primarily by hyperemia, not brain edema. *Furosemide* is a loop diuretic acting on the distal tubule where it inhibits sodium reabsorption. It also inhibits carbonic anhydrase, thereby reducing the rate of CSF production. A total of 0.5 to 1 mg/kg may be given before mannitol to prevent a rebound in ICP and cerebral blood volume (CBV). The drug should be titrated to raise osmolality by approximately 30 mOsm. Potassium levels should be monitored because excessive diuresis can lead to hypokalemia.

Use of the head-up position in an attempt to decrease ICP may be counterproductive because mean arterial blood pressure tends to drop more than ICP when the head is raised, thereby decreasing cerebral perfusion pressure (CPP). However, modest head elevation (10% to 20%) appears to be beneficial.

Adjuvant Therapy

After intubation and control of ventilation, it is appropriate to use small doses of *fentanyl* (50 to 100 μg) or a benzodiazepine such as *midazolam* (0.01 to 0.05 mg/kg) to relieve some of the pain-induced hypercatecholaminergic state and also to sedate the patient.

Seizures are common after head injury, particularly after missile injury, when the incidence can reach 40% to 60%. Posttraumatic seizures do not necessarily develop into epilepsy. Because seizures are associated with increases in cerebral metabolism and ICP, thus further compromising already precarious brain tissue, prophylactic *phenytoin* is given routinely. A total of 10 to 15 mg/kg is injected slowly (50 mg/min) as a loading dose; further dosing is based on blood levels. Phenytoin has the added advantage of modestly reducing CBV and cerebral metabolic rate (CMR). Should seizures develop despite prophylaxis, acute treatment may consist of a rapidly acting benzodiazepine (midazolam, 0.01 to 0.05 mg/kg) or barbiturate (thiopental, 1 to 3 mg/kg). Succinylcholine (1 mg/kg) will block the muscle activity of seizures and allow adequate ventilation, but it should be realized that cerebral hyperactivity is not affected.

The evidence for the effectiveness of *steroids* in the head trauma patient is weak, and most centers, including ours, have stopped using them for this indication. In other places selected patients (adults with GCS <8, children with GCS <6) receive 1 to 1.5 mg/kg dexamethasone, which is then tapered rapidly.

Use of *barbiturates* in the management of increased ICP is discussed in Chapter 3. Although these drugs are able to control otherwise unmanageable increases in ICP in about 25% of patients, this therapy has not resulted in improved outcome, and consequently they are used rarely for this purpose.

Surgical Triage

Although not the responsibility of the anesthesiologist, it is important to be aware as early as possible in the course of resuscitation which patients will need an emergency or urgent neurosurgical operation. This will allow the anesthesiologist to be adequately prepared for rapid transfer to the operating room and conversion of the early management described thus far to surgical anesthesia.

Patients with massive depressed or open skull fractures and those with large focal mass lesions will need emergency surgery. Mass lesions are not easily assessed clinically, yet often there will be no time for radiologic diagnosis. Therefore a *triage scheme* has been developed that allows determination of the need for surgery on the basis of the patient's level of consciousness and the existence of a lateralized motor deficit. Knowing whether the trauma was vehicular or nonvehicular is important because victims of nonvehicular trauma are much more likely to sustain focal mass lesions than are patients involved in vehicular trauma, who more often have diffuse brain injury. If a patient is comatose (GCS <8) and has either unequal pupils or a lateralized motor deficit, a focal lesion requiring surgery must be presumed present (80% of nonvehicular and 30% of vehicular trauma victims will require surgery). Thus these patients should be intubated and hyperventilated, receive mannitol, if at all possible undergo a rapid CT scan, and then be operated on. In contrast, comatose patients without lateralizing signs most likely have diffuse axonal injury, although a CT scan is still required to rule out a mass lesion. They will need aggressive ICP management, but generally no surgical intervention is required. Noncomatose patients with lateralizing signs must be suspected of having a small focal lesion, and urgent CT scanning is required. In contrast, the absence of lateralizing signs allows a more expectant approach.

DIAGNOSTIC PROCEDURES

Although at times the decision to operate will have to be made on clinical grounds alone, it is highly preferable to obtain a radiologic diagnosis first. Usually this will be done by performing a *CT scan* of the head. In addition to localizing intracranial mass lesions, CT scanning provides important prognostic information by determining the degree of midline shift and basal cistern compression. *Skull x-ray films* are useful for localizing bullet fragments or other penetrating objects. They do not show intracranial mass lesions. Although linear fractures may help indicate the site of an epidural hematoma, the presence or absence of skull fractures has not been shown to correlate sufficiently with intracranial events to make them a practical diagnostic tool. Much more useful is a lateral *cervical spine film,* although it should not be overly relied on because 20% of cervical fractures will still be missed. For the film to be useful, all vertebrae from C1 through T1 should be visible. Further radiologic evaluation of the cervical spine will be performed after initial stabilization. To rule out the presence of a hemothorax or pneumothorax and assess trauma to thoracic organs, a *chest x-ray film* should be obtained as early as possible. *Magnetic resonance imaging* can provide anatomic information supplemental to that obtained with the CT scan. It is particularly sensitive in differentiating white and gray matter and in the diagnosis of contusions and shearing injuries. However, this added sensitivity has not translated into better diagnosis during the acute stage of head trauma management. The longer scanning times, relative inaccessibility of the patient during the scan, and the technical difficulties related to the powerful magnetic field have made the technique less popular for this patient population. *Cerebral angiography* may be performed when vascular damage is suspected or in the occasional event that a CT scanner is not available.

Radiologic diagnostic procedures undertaken on severely injured patients can create a significant challenge for the anesthesiologist. Most of these patients should be intubated and paralyzed before undergoing CT scanning. Adequate monitoring is essential but can be difficult to accomplish because the anesthesiologist cannot be in the room during actual scanning. Resuscitation may have to be continued while diagnostic studies are in progress. In the less severely injured patient, when the presence of an anesthesiologist is not required during the study, it is important that care of the patient is assigned and responsibility shifted appropriately, so that the patient is not left in the radiology department without proper attention. Detailed information on anesthetic management of patients undergoing neuroradiologic procedures is provided in Chapter 15.

ANESTHETIC MANAGEMENT

Premedication

Generally the patient with head injury who breathes spontaneously should not receive sedative premedication because the decrease in ventilation and resultant hypercapnia will increase ICP. In addition, neurologic assessment would become more difficult. The patient who is intubated and paralyzed can be treated more liberally with a benzodiazepine such as *midazolam* (0.01 to 0.05 mg/kg) or a narcotic such as *fentanyl* (100 to 200 μg).

Glycopyrrolate (0.2 to 1 mg) is useful to dry airway secretions. It causes less tachycardia and has a longer duration of action than atropine.

A major concern with any patient undergoing emergency surgery is the possibility of a full stomach, with the potential for aspiration. *Metoclopramide* (10 mg) can be given to increase gastrointestinal motility and thereby decrease gastric volume. If the patient is able to take oral medication, a nonparticular antacid such as *Bicitra* will help increase gastric pH. In addition, it may decrease gastric volume. If surgery is delayed because of diagnostic testing, *ranitidine* (50 mg by infusion) may be useful. However, because H_2 histamine antagonists do not affect preexisting stomach contents, at least 1 hour is required for its action on gastric pH to be noticeable.

Monitoring

Standard monitors used include an *ECG, pulse oximeter, esophageal or precordial stethoscope, temperature monitor, urinary catheter, capnograph,* and *blood pressure cuff*. In virtually all cases *invasive arterial blood pressure* monitoring will be useful, particularly because it also allows sampling of arterial blood for pH and blood gas analysis (including determination of the capnograph offset) and electrolyte and osmolarity determinations during diuretic therapy. The arterial catheter should be placed before induction, to monitor the sometimes profound hemodynamic changes during this period. The transducer should be placed at ear level to track cerebral perfusion pressure. If the patient's cardiovascular status is in doubt, or the requirement for large volume shifts is anticipated, placement of a *central venous pressure* (CVP) or *pulmonary artery catheter* should be considered. A long-arm CVP catheter can usually be placed rapidly, although exact positioning can be difficult. A basilic vein approach avoids both the risk of pneumothorax associated with the subclavian approach and the potential disruption of carotid blood flow or obstruction of venous return associated with the internal jugular approach. The head-down position to facilitate catheter placement is absolutely contraindicated in the head trauma victim. If there is a significant risk of development of air embolism (e.g., disruption of a venous sinus or operation in the sitting position), a multiorifice CVP catheter for air aspiration may be placed. Under those circumstances a *precordial Doppler probe* and measurement of *end-tidal nitrogen* are additional useful diagnostic modalities. At times, *ICP monitoring* can be helpful, particularly during anesthetic induction.

Induction of Anesthesia

The goal of anesthetic induction in the patient with head trauma is to make the transition from wakefulness to surgical anesthesia without major swings in blood pressure or increases in ICP. At the same time a potentially difficult airway in a patient with a presumed full stomach must be managed. This requires meticulous planning, including consideration of contingencies, and careful selection of drugs and techniques. The cerebral effects of anesthetic drugs and neuromuscular blockers are described in Chapter 3. I will assume in this discussion that a cervical spine injury has been ruled out. If not, then the precautions mentioned in Chapter 8 should be followed. Of course, if the patient arrives in the operating room intubated, the task is remarkably simplified.

To minimize increases in ICP, painful maneuvers (such as tracheal tube suctioning and manipulation of traumatized areas) should be avoided as much as possible. Coughing, bucking, and straining are similarly detrimental and can increase the risk of cerebral herniation. Placing the head in a neutral position and avoiding flexion and rotation of the neck, which would limit venous return, will help prevent decreases in CPP.

After all monitors have been applied, the patient is denitrogenated and, if able, directed to hyperventilate. *Lidocaine* (1 to 1.5 mg/kg) may be given at this point to blunt changes in blood pressure and ICP during laryngoscopy. *Thiopental* is the induction drug of choice because it rapidly reduces CBV and ICP. In addition, it acts as a free-radical scavenger. However, in the hypovolemic patient the drug can cause severe hypotension, which may result in decreased CPP. Because the circulating blood volume may be difficult to assess before induction and a hyperdynamic state may mask hypovolemia, a reduced dose (2 to 4 mg/kg) is recommended, and small repeated doses might be safer than a single bolus. The imidazole *etomidate* (0.2 to 0.4 mg/kg) is a suitable alternative in the hypovolemic or cardiovascularly compromised patient. It also decreases cerebral blood flow (CBF), CMR, and ICP yet maintains systemic blood pressure and thus CPP. Ketamine is relatively contraindicated because of its tendency to increase CBF and ICP.

Narcotics will help maintain cardiovascular stability because they blunt the hemodynamic response to laryngoscopy and allow the use of smaller doses of induction agents. *Fentanyl* (1 to 4 μg/kg), given 3 to 4 minutes before laryngoscopy, will serve this purpose. Morphine, sufentanil, and alfentanil may cause cerebral vasodilation and therefore are less desirable.

Choosing a muscle relaxant for intubation can be a difficult decision. *Succinylcholine* (1 mg/kg) would appear the obvious choice in a patient at risk for aspiration. However, fasciculations induced by the drug lead to increases in muscle spindle activity and cerebral afferent input, translating into increases in CBF, ICP, and carbon dioxide tension. This effect can be prevented by defasciculation with metocurine (0.03 mg/kg) but apparently not by pancuronium. Defasciculation might to some extent defeat the purpose of succinylcholine use: to have an unprotected airway for the shortest period of time. Hyperkalemia in the head trauma patient after administration of succinylcholine has been reported occasionally, even within the classically accepted 24 hours after injury, and the drug certainly should not be used after this time. If the use of succinylcholine is considered inadvisable, *rocuronium* (0.6 to 1 mg/kg) may be the relaxant of choice. This drug allows intubation within 60 to 90 seconds after administration. When used immediately after thiopental in rapid sequence, adequate flushing of the intravenous line must be ensured to prevent precipitation and obstruction of venous access. Rocuronium has a modest vagolytic action but does not release histamine. If the vagolytic action, with possible associated hypertension, is not considered acceptable, *vecuronium* (0.1 mg/kg) can be used. Atracurium can, when given in large doses, result in histamine release and in addition is metabolized to laudanosine, which, in high doses, causes seizures in animals. Although the clinical relevance of these issues is debatable, better drugs are available.

Whatever the relaxant chosen, the airway should be secured as rapidly as possible while cricoid pressure is maintained. Before intubation it may be appropriate to ventilate by mask with low peak pressures until muscle relaxation is complete, to prevent increases in carbon dioxide tension. Intubation should be as atraumatic as feasible. Only when correct placement of the tube has been confirmed by auscultation, capnography, and presence of vapor in the tube should cricoid pressure be released. Additional small doses of thiopental can be given to blunt excessive blood pressure responses to intubation.

Maintenance

Much of anesthetic management during surgery in the patient with head trauma will be directed toward maintaining cardiovascular stability because hypertension and hypotension may have detrimental effects on areas of the brain with disrupted autoregulatory mechanisms. This cardiovascular stability should, if possible, be maintained with drugs that themselves have little effect on cerebral hemodynamics and that decrease ICP and CMR. Intravenous drugs often serve this purpose best, especially in patients with severe head trauma. Missile injury, for example, will temporarily increase ICP to 2000 to 3000 mm Hg, and patients with such trauma require continuous maintenance of cerebral vasoconstriction. A combination of *narcotics, barbiturates,* and *benzodiazepines* will lower CBF, CMR, and ICP. These drugs can be given as small boluses or continuous infusions. For example, fentanyl delivered at 1 to 4 μg/kg/hr significantly decreases the need for a volatile agent. Residual narcotic effects will smooth emergence and ease postoperative hyperventilation. Thiopental (1 to 6 mg/min) and lidocaine (1 to 4 mg/min) are similarly useful.

In less severely damaged patients volatile agents can be used. *Isoflurane* is presumably the most appropriate of these. Although it is a direct cerebral vasodilator, inhibition of cerebral metabolism with resultant vasoconstriction is so pronounced that the net effect is virtually unchanged CBF, particularly at lower concentrations of the drug. The existence of a clinically relevant cerebral protective effect of isoflurane is still debated. Because it maintains cerebral responsiveness to carbon dioxide, hyperventilation-induced vasoconstriction in normal brain tissue might divert blood to traumatized areas where reactivity is lost. If the injury is ischemic, the resultant increase in flow may be beneficial. However, it may also lead to increased edema formation in these areas, thereby worsening ICP. In the individual patient the balance of these effects cannot be determined in advance, which may explain why isoflurane has not consistently affected outcome. Nonetheless, on theoretic grounds it is the most appropriate volatile anesthetic for use in the head trauma patient. Although its primary side effect is hypotension resulting from peripheral vasodilation, the other volatile drugs currently in use have more pronounced detrimental effects. Halothane is a potent cerebral vasodilator and has undesirable arrhythmogenic side effects in patients with high catecholamine levels. Enflurane is similarly a vasodilator and has the disadvantage of inducing seizure-like activity, particularly in hypocapnic patients. Experience with desflurane and sevoflurane is still limited, but they do not appear to show benefits over isoflurane.

The use of *nitrous oxide* (N_2O) remains controversial. When used in isolation, it has cerebrovascular dilating effects, but these are usually blunted by the concomitant use of hyperventilation and intravenous anesthetics. Therefore increases in ICP are rarely seen. Nonetheless, use of the drug has little benefit in these patients, and concern about ICP effects and potential tension pneumocephalus has led some centers to avoid use of N_2O.

During anesthesia *fluid balance* should be monitored with attention, using the clinical signs of pulse rate, blood pressure, pulse pressure, and particularly the respiratory variation of the systolic arterial blood pressure waveform, which is a more sensitive indicator of hypovolemia than central venous pressure is. Diuretics most times make urinary output an undependable monitor. Preferred crystalloid solutions are lactated Ringer's solution, normal saline solution, Plasmalyte, or Normosol-R. Administration of free water should be minimized to prevent the development of cerebral edema. Overhydration in a patient with a disrupted blood-brain barrier will have a similar effect. Solutions containing glucose should be avoided as well because high blood glucose levels (>150 mg/ml) have been associated with poor outcome in patients with cerebral ischemia caused by stroke, cardiac arrest, and head trauma. This result is thought to be due to increased lactate production through anaerobic pathways in the presence of glucose but absence of oxygen. The resulting acidosis may increase neuronal damage. Even in the absence of glucose administration these patients may be hyperglycemic because of high circulating catecholamine levels. Hypokalemia is often seen. If it results from high catecholamine levels and hypocapnic alkalosis, no treatment is needed, but diuretic-induced urinary potassium losses may need to be replaced. In the patient with head trauma, circulating volume may change dramatically during surgery. Initially the patient will often be hypovolemic because of blood loss, which should be corrected rapidly. Administration of mannitol will lead to a rapid, transient increase in circulating volume, followed by a decrease once diuresis is initiated. The use of furosemide will enhance this effect. After decompression of an intracranial mass lesion, sympathetic outflow may decrease suddenly and hypovolemia may become unmasked. Serum electrolyte levels and osmolality may change as well and should be monitored. Glucose levels should be determined at regular intervals for the reasons mentioned above. A urinary catheter should always be present, and in selected patients a central venous catheter or pulmonary artery catheter may be indicated to guide fluid management, as discussed above. If excessive urine output cannot be explained by diuretics, the possibility of diabetes insipidus should be considered. If confirmed by an increased serum sodium and osmolality values and decreased urine osmolality, administration of DDAVP (desmopressin acetate) is indicated, as described in Chapter 12.

Blood loss during surgery should be replaced as soon as it occurs to prevent anemia and ischemia. A hematocrit of approximately 30% is thought to result in optimal oxygen delivery to brain tissue, balancing the rheologic properties of blood with its oxygen carrying capacity. Significant decreases in hematocrit will lead to increases in ICP. For example, in head-injured animals replacement of one half the blood volume with normal saline solution or 5% dextrose solution will elevate ICP by 90% and 150%, respectively. Thus, although initial blood loss can be replaced by crystalloid or colloid solutions, hematocrit should be checked frequently. There is no definite evidence that any particular nonblood solution is preferred over any other. Colloids are more practical than crystalloids when blood loss is rapid, because smaller volumes have to be infused, and they have the theoretical advantage of remaining outside an intact blood-brain barrier. On the other hand, loss of blood-brain barrier function in damaged areas could lead to movement of the fluid into brain tissue with subsequent edema formation. In addition, the cost of colloids is remarkably higher than that of crystalloids. This issue is discussed in more detail in Chapter 5. Hypertonic saline solution (3% to 5%) shows promise as an effective resuscitation fluid in trauma patients. If the hematocrit decreases below 30, blood should be administered. Preferably, typed and cross-matched packed red blood cells should be used. However, if a cross-match is not available, type-specific blood can be given, and if there has been no opportunity for typing, O-type blood is used, rhesus negative for women and rhesus positive for men. Platelets and fresh-frozen plasma preferably should be given only when indicated specifically (i.e., when laboratory tests show a clear coagulation abnormality). Unfortunately, the emergent nature of head trauma may make empirical treatment necessary.

Ventilation should be controlled to maintain arterial carbon dioxide tension between 25 and 30, and arterial blood gases should be checked at regular intervals. Positive end-expiratory pressure may increase ICP, but this is rarely a problem if levels <10 cm H_2O are used, and it should not be withheld if necessary to maintain adequate oxygenation. *Temperature* should be measured continuously and maintained as close to normal as possible. Hyperthermia should be prevented aggressively because it increases CMR and carbon dioxide production. As discussed in Chapter 2, a modest reduction in temperature (2° to 3° C) may be of benefit.

Emergence

Generally, if the patient was awake and breathing spontaneously at the beginning of the operation, he or she should be in the same condition postoperatively. To allow neurologic examination as soon as possible after surgery, reversal of neuromuscular blockade and tracheal extubation should be accomplished as soon as it is considered safe. Close communication between the anesthesiologist and neurosurgeon is necessary to determine the optimal moment of extubation. Many patients can be extubated safely in the operating room. Arguments against early extubation include associated chest injury, facial fractures, cervical spine injury, anticipated brainstem or cranial nerve damage, postoperative brain swelling, and hypothermia. These should always be balanced against the realization that continued hyperventilation and sedation may obscure early signs of rebleeding and other serious postoperative complications.

Although removal of a mass lesion will decrease the preoperative high ICP, excessive increases in blood pressure as well as coughing and bucking should be avoided. Lidocaine (1 to 1.5 mg/kg) will help smooth emergence, as will small doses of a short-acting narcotic and thiopental. The patient should be transported to the postoperative care unit or intensive care unit with the appropriate monitors applied and supplemental oxygen administered.

COMPLICATIONS

A number of complications can detrimentally affect the patient's intraoperative or postoperative course and adversely affect outcome. The most important of these are cardiovascular complications, neurogenic pulmonary edema, and venous air embolism. Complications most commonly seen in the intensive care setting are discussed in Chapter 20.

Cardiovascular Complications

The most common cardiovascular response to head injury consists of *sympathetic hyperactivity*. It results in elevated systolic and diastolic blood pressure and heart rate and increases in cardiac output, oxygen consumption, intrapulmonary shunt, and $\dot{V}/\dot{Q}$ mismatch, as well as a variety of arrhythmias. Systemic vascular resistance often decreases.

The central hyperadrenergic state can lead to a large variety of *cardiac arrhythmias* and ECG changes. Most common are increased P wave amplitude and prolonged QT intervals. Widened QRS complexes, elevated ST segments, inverted T waves, and U waves are also seen frequently. Such changes are associated with diffuse subendocardial hemorrhagic necrosis and increased mortality and should not be considered innocuous epiphenomena. Treatment consists of adequate oxygenation and careful adrenergic blockade. If ventricular arrhythmias are troublesome, a loading dose of lidocaine (1 to 1.5 mg/kg) followed by a lidocaine infusion (1 to 4 mg/min) may be beneficial. Halothane should be avoided. It is important that a cardiac contusion be ruled out.

Hypertension resulting from adrenergic drive can have a number of detrimental consequences, including increased cerebral edema and hemorrhage. Therefore control of blood pressure to somewhat above normal levels (i.e., a systolic pressure of approximately 150 mm Hg in the previously normotensive patient) is important, both during surgery and postoperatively. The combined alpha-beta blocker labetalol (5 to 20 mg) is preferred because it has little cerebral effect. Beta-blockers such as esmolol or propranolol are similarly useful. Direct vasodilators such as hydralazine or nitroprusside induce cerebral and systemic vasodilation, which makes them undesirable for the patient with head trauma.

Neurogenic Pulmonary Edema

The syndrome of neurogenic pulmonary edema consists of increases in pulmonary venous pressure and increased pulmonary capillary permeability, and, like the cardiovascular changes described above, is apparently caused by massive sympathetic outflow after head injury, although other causes are still being debated. The pathophysiologic changes result in the rapid development of interstitial edema and subsequent increased pulmonary shunt, decreased compliance, and loss of lung volume. Symptoms and signs include dyspnea; cyanosis; pallor; sweating; a weak, rapid pulse; and the production of pink, frothy sputum.

Development of neurogenic pulmonary edema can be remarkably rapid and is usually associated with a significant and abrupt increase in ICP. Primary treatment therefore consists of ICP normalization by *surgical decompression* or removal of the offending mass lesion, combined with aggressive *pharmacologic management of ICP.* Patient positioning with the head elevated 10% to 20% may be beneficial in decreasing ICP. Because the syndrome is associated with a hyperadrenergic state, administration of *adrenergic-blocking drugs* may be beneficial. Appropriate *ventilator management* is essential. This includes increasing the inspired oxygen concentration as necessary to maintain an arterial oxygen partial pressure (PaO_2) of 70 to 80 mm Hg and controlling arterial carbon dioxide partial pressure between 25 and 30 mm Hg. PEEP should be adjusted to provide maximal increases in oxygenation with minimal effects on ICP and cardiac output.

The possibility of *fat embolism* should also be entertained in the differential diagnosis of pulmonary complications in the patient with head trauma. Because one of its major signs is decreased consciousness, it can be a difficult diagnosis to make in the head trauma victim. Fracture of the long bones of the extremities or pelvis leads to the release of lipid-rich bone marrow into the circulation. The circulating fat globules become lodged in the pulmonary circulation where free fatty acids are released, causing increased pulmonary capillary leakage. Fluffy infiltrates are seen on chest x-ray films, and hypoxemia and pulmonary edema occur clinically. Cerebral edema and disseminated intravascular coagulation may follow, usually at least 12 to 24 hours after the initial injury. Treatment is supportive. Steroids may be of some benefit, although morbidity and mortality remain high.

Air Embolism

Venous air embolism has been shown to be a common occurrence when venous sinuses or bony sinusoids are opened and exposed to air. The risk is increased when the operative site is above heart level. Although embolism is common, clinically significant episodes are rare. Nonetheless, because unexpected massive air entrainment can occur during surgery in head-trauma victims and can lead to rapid cardiovascular collapse, the anesthesiologist should monitor for air embolism and be prepared to treat it if necessary. Paradoxical arterial embolization has been shown to occur even in the absence of a patent foramen ovale, presumably by air movement through pulmonary capillaries, so all patients should be considered at risk for this potentially disastrous event.

Precordial or transesophageal Doppler probes provide the earliest warning signs, followed by the characteristic changes in end-tidal nitrogen and carbon dioxide levels, increases in pulmonary artery and CVPs, and finally decreases in mean arterial pressure and PaO_2. The classically described "mill-wheel" murmur will be heard only in cases of massive entrainment. Treatment includes the following steps, which should be executed in rapid succession:

1. The anesthesiologist should notify the surgeon of the problem.
2. The surgeon should flood the operative field with saline solution and search for an entrainment site.
3. If possible without contaminating the surgical field, the patient's head should be lowered below heart level.
4. Compression of the jugular veins may prevent further air entrainment.
5. N_2O, if used at all, should be discontinued.
6. Oxygen (100%) should be administered.
7. Aspiration of entrained air through a multiorifice central line placed at the junction between superior vena cava and right atrium may be tried.
8. Although not proved to be effective, the patient may be turned left side down to keep air from moving into the pulmonary outflow tract.
9. If cardiovascular collapse occurs, symptomatic treatment with vasopressors, inotropes and, if necessary, cardiopulmonary resuscitation, should be started immediately.

The syndrome is described in more detail in Chapter 11.

OUTCOME

Data on outcome after head injury are at least as difficult to interpret as those on incidence. Part of the reason is that a large variety of factors apart from the injury determine the final outcome, and the presence of these is variable (Fig. 18-1). The other factor making interpretation difficult is that, apart from death and complete recovery, the various degrees of disability after head injury cannot easily be categorized. Finally, it is essential that the time after injury when outcome assessment takes place be taken into account because recovery occurs gradually over time.

Several *premorbid factors* affect outcome. Age has a major impact, leading to an increased incidence of poor outcome in elderly

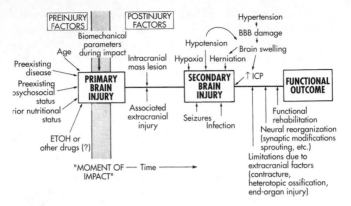

FIG 18-1.
Schematic representation of factors and events that influence outcome after head injury. *ETOH,* Alcohol; *BBB,* blood-brain barrier. (From Vollmer DG, Dacey TG: Prediction and assessment of outcome following closed head injury. In Pitts LH, Wagner FC Jr, editors: *Craniospinal trauma,* New York, 1990, Thieme Medical Publishers, pp 120-140.)

patients and improved prognosis in pediatric victims. It is as yet unclear whether high age is a risk factor per se or whether risk is increased because of coexisting disease. Pre-accident functioning is also important. Patients with higher levels of education, higher income, or professional occupation show a higher rate of return to work. The *level of consciousness after injury,* as determined by the GCS, is the most important factor in determining outcome. Death rates in patients with GCS scores of ≥11 are virtually nil, but with lower scores mortality increases linearly to approximately 80% with a GCS score of 3. Attempts are being made to provide more sophisticated prognostic indicators by including such items as the duration of unconsciousness and the duration of posttraumatic amnesia. Other factors, such as *associated injuries* or the presence of *hypoxemia* and *hypotension* also affect outcome detrimentally. As a result of these variables, the mortality rate in hospitalized head trauma patients has been reported as ranging from 4% to 25%.

However, many more patients are left with permanent deficits by head injury than are killed by it, and these patients should be included in outcome determinations. The Glasgow Outcome Scale attempts to do this by dividing patients with head injury into five classes (Box 18-1). Of those disabled by head injury, a high proportion sustain neuropsychologic rather than neurologic deficits. These disorders of memory, attention, reaction time, language function, perception, and intellectual ability require neuropsychologic testing for proper quantification and follow-up. Generally, such deficits are considered by patients to be more disabling and to interfere more with functioning than neurologic deficits do. The incidence is high. If fatal cases are excluded, cognitive deficits are found in at least 60% of those patients with head injury admitted to the hospital when they are tested 2 years after injury. The GCS has some predictive value; severe cognitive deficits are unlikely to persist for more than 2 years in patients with GCS ≥8 at 24 hours after injury.

Many attempts have been made to develop comprehensive prognostic models based on clinical, radiologic, and laboratory data available at admission. Thus far, however, none has sufficient specificity to be able to predict outcome in the individual patient with any degree of accuracy. This fact should serve as a reminder that every head injury patient should receive optimal care as rapidly as possible, both in and out of the operating room. Only in this way can secondary injury be prevented and outcome improved. Of the anesthesiologist this requires a thorough understanding of the principles and practice of anesthetic management of the head injury victim, and a willingness and ability to function as an effective team member.

BOX 18-1.
Glasgow Outcome Scale

Dead (D)
Persistent vegetative state (PVS)
　　Wakefulness without awareness
Severe disability (SD)
　　Conscious but dependent
Moderate disability (MD)
　　Independent but disabled
Good recovery (GR)
　　Reintegrated (may have nondisabling sequelae)

Suggested Readings

Adams RW, Cucchiara RF, Gronert GA, et al: Isoflurane and cerebrospinal fluid pressure in neurosurgical patients, *Anesthesiology* 54:97, 1981.

Alexander RH et al: *Advanced trauma life support program,* ed 5, Chicago, 1993, American College of Surgeons.

Bedford RF, Persing JA, Pobereshin L, et al: Lidocaine or thiopental for rapid control of intracranial hypertension? *Anesth Analg* 59:435, 1980.

Borel C, Hanley D, Diringer MN, et al: Intensive management of severe head injury, *Chest* 98:180, 1990.

Cooper PR: *Head injury,* ed 3, Baltimore, 1993, Williams & Wilkins.

Cottrell JE, Hartung J, Giffin JP, et al: Intracranial and hemodynamic changes after succinylcholine anesthesia in rats, *Anesth Analg* 62:1006, 1983.

Demann D, Leisman G, et al: Biomechanics of head injury, *Intern J Neurosci* 54:101, 1990.

Donegan MF, Bedford RF, et al: Intravenously administered lidocaine prevents intracranial hypertension during endotracheal suctioning, *Anesthesiology* 52:516, 1980.

Faden AI, Salzman S, et al: Pharmacological strategies in CNS trauma, *Trends Pharmacol Sci* 13:29, 1992.

Murdoch J, Hall R, et al: Brain protection: physiological and pharmacological considerations. I. The physiology of brain injury, *Can J Anaesth* 37:663, 1990.

Rose J, Valtonen S, Jennett B, et al: Avoidable factors contributing to death after head injury, *BMJ* 2:615, 1977.

Sutin KM, Ruskin KJ, Kaufman BS, et al: Intravenous fluid therapy in neurologic injury, *Crit Care Clin* 8:367, 1992.

Vernon DD, Woodward GA, Shjonsberg AK, et al: Management of the patient with head injury during transport, *Crit Care Clin* 8:619, 1992.

THE POSTANESTHESIA CARE UNIT

19

George S. Leisure
Burkhard F. Spiekermann

Excellent anesthetic care of the neurosurgical patient must continue in the postanesthesia care unit (PACU) to ensure optimal outcome. Although the general principles of management are the same as for other postoperative patients, there are concerns unique to the neurosurgical patient. This chapter will address the initial evaluation of the postoperative neurosurgical patient and then focus on concerns related to the airway, pulmonary system, and cardiovascular system and on problems associated with specific neurosurgical procedures.

TRANSFER TO POSTANESTHESIA CARE UNIT

Ideally patients should be extubated in the operating room, which allows for the immediate assessment of neurologic function, and if reintubation becomes necessary it can be performed in the safest possible setting. However, many patients cannot be extubated in the operating room, including patients with inadequate blood gas values, elevated intracranial pressure (ICP), hemodynamic instability, hypothermia, a preexisting medical condition, or surgical complications. If there is any question as to whether the patient will tolerate extubation, he/she should remain intubated.

Unless otherwise contraindicated, neurosurgical patients should be transferred to the PACU in a 30-degree head-up position. This position facilitates cerebral venous drainage, thereby decreasing ICP, and improves oxygenation by increasing the functional residual capacity of the lungs. Supplemental oxygen should be administered, and vital signs should be continuously monitored.

In the PACU a full report is made to the staff assuming care of the patient. This report should include a pertinent past medical history with special reference to the patient's preoperative neurologic status, a summary of all preoperative and intraoperative medications, a history of allergies, and a description of the patient's intraoperative course, including blood loss, fluid administration, and urine output.

The initial evaluation in the PACU should include a basic neurologic assessment. The examination should focus on determining the patient's level of consciousness, the degree of motor activity, and the pupillary light response. A more comprehensive examination may be limited by residual anesthetic effects. Focal motor weakness may be the earliest sign of a developing supratentorial lesion. Unequal pupils are an ominous sign and must be evaluated promptly. Regional increases in ICP can cause transtentorial herniation of the uncus and may be heralded by dilation of the ipsilateral pupil. Pathologic processes involving the midbrain may cause pupillary constriction. It is important, however, not to be led astray by benign causes of anisocoria. Phenylephrine (Neo-Synephrine) nose drops, commonly used to provide mucosal vasoconstriction before nasal intubation can cause mydriasis if inadvertently placed into the eyes. Anisocoria may have been present preoperatively and should be documented in the preoperative record. Systemically administered atropine, epinephrine, and trimethaphan may cause bilateral pupillary dilation, whereas narcotics may cause bilateral, naloxone-reversible pupillary constriction.

The examination of blood chemistry data, hemoglobin level, and arterial blood gases are helpful to rule out metabolic causes of postoperative neurologic dysfunction. In any case, the clinician must remain with the patient until his/her condition is stable and patient care responsibilities are transferred to the appropriate PACU personnel.

UPPER AIRWAY COMPLICATIONS

Airway obstruction in the immediate postextubation period is usually due to a problem that falls into one of three categories: (1) pathologic processes involving the respiratory control pathways in the brain, (2) damage to cranial nerves responsible for the maintenance of airway reflexes, or (3) mechanical obstruction.

The control of respiration involves pathways within the reticular formation of the medulla and the ventrolateral portions of the spinothalamic tract of the cervical cord, as well as two pontine areas, the apneustic and pneumotactic centers. Any surgical procedure that causes interruption or compression of these structures can lead to postoperative apnea or highly irregular respiratory patterns. Patients with a history of sleep apnea may show disturbances of central control of respiration and close observation in the immediate postoperative period is imperative. Residual anesthetic agents and neuromuscular blockers can impair proper return of protective airway reflexes.

Damage to cranial nerves or their nuclei can lead to difficulty maintaining the airway postoperatively. Procedures involving the posterior fossa, tumor resections along the base of the skull, and carotid endarterectomies can lead to cranial nerve damage. The fifth (trigeminal), seventh (facial), ninth (glossopharyngeal), tenth (vagus), and twelfth (hypoglossal) cranial nerves are important in maintaining airway integrity. Damage to the ninth and tenth cranial nerves can cause difficulty with swallowing, and damage to the twelfth cranial nerve can cause poor control of the tongue, all of which may predispose to aspiration. Damage to the vagus nerve can cause bilateral vocal cord paralysis, possibly precipitating postobstructive pulmonary edema. If postoperative cranial nerve damage is suspected, the endotracheal tube should be left in place until swallowing and vocal cord function can be assessed. This may be especially important in the obese patient or the patient with a difficult airway. After cervical spine surgery, the patient must not be extubated until fully awake because reintubation may be difficult because neck extension is contraindicated.

Airway obstruction can also be due to mechanical causes. A common problem is postoperative swelling of the tongue. This condition may result from venous outflow obstruction, particularly in patients operated on while in the prone position for protracted periods or in those positioned with extreme neck flexion. The oral airway, if left in place for the duration of the operation, may also interfere with venous drainage of the tongue. Upper airway obstruction can also occur in patients with a history of obstructive sleep apnea because of enlarged anatomic structures. If not contraindicated, as with a cervical spine injury, neck extension and jaw thrust may relieve the obstruction. Positioning the patient on the side or the insertion of a nasal or oral airway are other potentially beneficial maneuvers. Remnants of surgical throat packing must always be considered as a possible cause of airway obstruction, especially after transsphenoidal surgery.

PULMONARY COMPLICATIONS

Pulmonary problems in the immediate postoperative period resulting in hypoxemia and hypercarbia are generally caused by (1) bronchospasm or clinical entities that may mimic it, (2) hypoventilation, and (3) intrinsic lung dysfunction. Other causes of hypoxemia include pulmonary thromboembolism, markedly depressed cardiac output, diffusion hypoxia, and the use of a low inspired oxygen concentration.

Bronchospasm

Bronchospasm as a result of airway hyperreactivity can present in the PACU with wheezing, although not all wheezing is a result of bronchospasm. Upper airway obstruction may present with inspiratory wheezing. Wheezing can also occur with pulmonary edema either from cardiogenic (high pulmonary venous pressures) or noncardiogenic (increased capillary permeability) causes. Cardiogenic causes are unlikely in the absence of underlying cardiac disease. Causes of noncardiogenic pulmonary edema unique to the neurosurgical patient include edema resulting from venous air embolism and neurogenic pulmonary edema. Neurogenic pulmonary edema is associated with insults to the medulla or hypothalamus. Its etiology is not entirely clear, but studies suggest that heightened sympathetic tone from the central nervous system (CNS) injury may increase pulmonary capillary permeability. Other causes of noncardiogenic pulmonary edema include pulmonary aspiration, allergic reactions to drugs or transfusion components, sepsis, and postobstructive pulmonary edema. Clinically, pulmonary edema can mimic bronchospasm because the small airways are mechanically compressed by peribronchial edema, resulting in obstruction of expiratory airflow and wheezing. Wheezing can occur from obstruction of the endotracheal tube by mucus, a clot, a foreign body, a kinked endotracheal tube, an overinflated cuff, or by clenched teeth. Pneumothorax and endobronchial intubation must also be considered in the differential diagnosis of wheezing.

Once bronchospasm has been identified and other causes of wheezing have been ruled out, humidified 100% oxygen and appropriate pharmacologic therapy should be instituted:

1. Inhaled beta$_2$-agonists: nebulized metaproterenol (0.2 to 0.3 ml in 2 ml of normal saline solution) or isoetharine (0.5 ml in 2 ml of normal saline solution). Aerosolized beta-mimetic agents are generally considered the first line of therapy for airway hyperreactivity.

2. Anticholinergics: glycopyrrolate 0.4 to 1 mg intravenously (IV) or nebulized glycopyrrolate 0.4 to 1 mg in 2 ml of normal saline solution. In addition to blocking vagal afferents, the anticholinergics decrease airway secretions without increasing their viscosity.

3. Corticosteroids: hydrocortisone 2 to 3 mg/kg IV or an equivalent dose of another preparation. These agents are not useful for acute bronchospasm because they may require 4 to 6 hours to show a clinical effect.

4. In the intubated patient, lidocaine 1 to 1.5 mg/kg IV or fentanyl 1 to 2 μg/kg may decrease reactivity to the endotracheal tube.

5. Parenteral beta$_2$-agonists: terbutaline 0.25 mg subcutaneously.

6. IV beta$_2$-agonists: isoproterenol or epinephrine. Infusions should start at 0.5 μg/min and be titrated. As with parenteral beta$_2$- agonists, tachyarrhythmias, and myocardial

ischemia are possible and careful hemodynamic monitoring is important.

7. Aminophylline: loading dose of 5 mg/kg over 20 minutes followed by an infusion of 0.5 mg/kg. The dose may need to be adjusted in those previously on aminophylline and in patients with liver or heart failure and the elderly. Tachyarrhythmias and nausea are common side effects.

Hypoventilation

Any neurosurgical procedure that leads to injury of the central respiratory centers may lead to hypoventilation with subsequent hypoxemia and hypercarbia. In addition, residual anesthetic effects may contribute to hypoventilation. In fact, the neurosurgical patient, because of preexisting CNS disease, may be particularly prone to the respiratory depressant effects of the potent inhalational agents, narcotics, benzodiazepines, and barbiturates. Naloxone in doses of 20 to 40 μg IV can be carefully administered to reverse narcotic-induced respiratory depression. However, because of naloxone's short half-life, renarcotization must be closely watched for. Severe hypertension, arrhythmias, and pulmonary edema are other complications reported with naloxone administration. Flumazenil, a specific benzodiazepine antagonist, may be useful if these agents are thought to be contributing significantly to hypoventilation. Postoperative hypoventilation can also occur from residual neuromuscular blockade. This may be from incomplete pharmacologic reversal of the neuromuscular blocking agents or extreme drug sensitivity. In either case the trachea should remain intubated until the patient demonstrates adequate muscle strength. Myasthenia gravis, the Eaton-Lambert syndrome, and many other neuromuscular diseases may cause exceptional sensitivity to muscle relaxants. The possibility of a pseudocholinesterase deficiency should be considered after a prolonged neuromuscular blockade with succinylcholine. Other causes of muscle weakness include preexisting myopathies, and metabolic causes such as hypermagnesemia and hypomagnesemia, hypocalcemia and hypercalcemia, or hypercarbia.

Intrinsic Lung Dysfunction

Surgical patients with underlying pulmonary dysfunction such as chronic bronchitis and emphysema may be particularly susceptible to postoperative hypoxemia. Even in normal patients undergoing surgical procedures not involving the abdomen or thorax, lung volumes may be reduced by half for up to 4 hours after general anesthesia. As a result $\dot{V}/\dot{Q}$ mismatching may be exacerbated. The magnitude of this problem is further compounded in patients with already diminished pulmonary reserves. In this group of patients resting hypercarbia (arterial partial pressure of carbon dioxide >45 mm Hg) noted on a preoperative arterial blood gas test is a sensitive indicator for the development of postoperative pulmonary problems.

As the etiology of hypoxemia is being evaluated, the fraction of inspired oxygen should be increased with nasal prongs, face mask, or endotracheal intubation, as clinically indicated. Positive end-expiratory airway pressure (PEEP) may be used in the mechanically ventilated patient, or continuous positive airway pressure (CPAP) may be used in the spontaneously breathing patient to improve oxygenation. (CPAP can be applied by mask in the unintubated patient.) The lowest level of PEEP needed to achieve adequate oxygenation should be applied because higher levels (>10 to 15 cm H_2O) may cause an increase in ICP. Any airway maneuvers, including suctioning through the endotracheal tube, may exacerbate intracranial hypertension and must be performed with caution. Spikes in ICP can be attenuated with the administration of lidocaine, 1 to 1.5 mg/kg IV, 60 to 90 seconds before stimulation of the airway.

CARDIOVASCULAR COMPLICATIONS

Postoperative cardiovascular instability is a common occurrence in the neurosurgical patient. The most frequent problems include hypertension, hypotension, cardiac arrhythmias, and myocardial ischemia. Myocardial ischemia will be discussed in the section on carotid endarterectomy, where it is a particularly common postoperative complication.

Hypertension

Hypertension is a common and serious occurrence in the neurosurgical patient; as many as 80% of patients undergoing elective craniotomy require prompt evaluation and treatment postoperatively. Hypertension can precipitate cerebral hemorrhage and myocardial ischemia or it may result from cerebral hemorrhage. In patients with increased ICP hypertension must be treated adequately to lower ICP without decreasing cerebral perfusion pressure (CPP) and causing further cerebral ischemia. Before pharmacologic treatment is instituted, other causes of hypertension such as pain, shivering, bladder distension, hypothermia, hypercapnia, hypoxia, or residual vasopressor effects should be ruled out. A serious cause of hypertension in the neurosurgical patient is the Cushing reflex, which involves extreme blood pressure elevations along with reflex bradycardia caused by an increased ICP. This reflex may signal brainstem herniation and demands immediate surgical attention. Treating Cushing reflex–associated hypertension pharmacologically may actually be detrimental because it may decrease CPP and increase cerebral ischemia. Invasive blood pressure measurements with the transducer placed below the level of the left atrium will make blood pressure determinations inaccurate.

Alpha- and beta-blockers can be used to lower blood pressure with minimal effects on cerebral blood flow (CBF). Propranolol in 0.5 mg increments or metoprolol in 5 mg increments can be administered and titrated intravenously. Labetolol, a combined alpha- and beta-blocker, may be the best choice in neurosurgical patients because of its rapid onset of action (usually <5 minutes) and because it does not increase ICP even in the face of reduced intracranial compliance. Labetolol reduces blood pressure by decreasing cardiac output and systemic vascular resistance. Its $beta_1$ effect allows for preservation and possibly reduction of myocardial oxygen consumption by preventing any reflex tachycardia and its $alpha_1$ effect causes a reduction in afterload, thus diminishing myocardial wall tension. These drugs are limited in their usefulness, however, by their relatively long half-lives and by their potential for causing bronchoconstriction and myocardial depression. Esmolol, an IV short-acting cardioselective beta-blocker may be a desirable agent in cases where a short half-life is necessary. It has a rapid onset and is quickly metabolized and eliminated by red blood cell esterases independently of the patient's renal or hepatic function. It is administered by continuous IV infusion at a dose of 50 to 300 μg/kg/min. It is important to note that beta-blockers can blunt the normal hemodynamic response to acute postoperative blood loss.

Direct acting vasodilators, such as sodium nitroprusside (SNP) are often used postoperatively to control hypertension. SNP is very potent, acts rapidly, and has a very short elimination half-life. Dosage is in the range of 0.5 μg/kg/min to 5 μg/kg/min IV. Its mechanism of action is primarily arteriolar dilation mediated by nitric oxide. Because of its potency, SNP should only be used when an arterial line is in place and reliable and accurate blood pressure readings are available. Elderly and hypovolemic patients can be sensitive to the hypotensive effects of this drug. SNP has several features that may not make it the ideal agent for blood pressure control in the neurosurgical patient. SNP should be used with extreme caution in patients at risk for intracranial hypertension; although SNP decreases CBF by decreasing mean arterial pressure (MAP), it may increase cerebral blood volume and ICP by dilating cerebral capacitance vessels.

Other problems associated with SNP are impaired hypoxic pulmonary vasoconstriction, decreased platelet function, reflex tachycardia, and rebound hypertension after therapy is discontinued. Rebound hypertension is due to increased renin excretion with the increased production of angiotensin II. This rebound effect can be limited by slowly tapering the SNP infusion and by adding a beta-blocker or angiotensin-converting enzyme inhibitor.

SNP can cause cyanide toxicity (cyanide inhibits cytochrome oxidase, thereby interfering with tissue oxygen use) at doses >8 μg/kg/min. Signs of cyanide toxicity include tachyphylaxis, metabolic acidosis, hypotension, and increased mixed venous oxygen saturation. Treatment of SNP toxicity includes discontinuation of the drug, hemodynamic support, and IV administration of sodium nitrite, 5 mg/kg, followed by IV sodium thiosulfate, 150 mg/kg, in cases of severe toxicity.

Nitroglycerin (0.25 to 10 μg/kg/min IV) can also be used to treat hypertension. It has a short plasma half-life (2 minutes) and a more favorable effect on distribution of coronary blood flow in patients with coronary artery disease than SNP. It acts by dilating capacitance vessels rather than resistance vessels, thus decreasing venous return, stroke volume, and cardiac output. Nitroglycerin, however, has a less potent and less predictable antihypertensive effect than SNP and may not achieve the desired blood pressure reduction, especially in younger patients. The drug may increase ICP by the same mechanism as SNP but produces no toxic metabolites or rebound hypertension.

Trimethaphan, a ganglionic blocker with a plasma half-life of 1 to 2 minutes, started at 1 mg/min IV, causes relaxation of both capacitance and resistance vessels. It is rapidly inactivated by plasma cholinesterase and renally excreted. Unlike nitroglycerin and SNP, trimethaphan rarely raises ICP. Side effects include histamine release, bronchospasm, tachyphylaxis, and fixed, dilated pupils.

Hydralazine (5 to 20 mg IV) and nifedipine (10 to 20 mg sublingually) can be used to treat postoperative hypertension. However, they may be more difficult to titrate and can increase ICP. Enalaprilate (1.25 to 2.5 mg IV) is also very effective in decreasing blood pressure and does not increase ICP. Its time to onset is between 10 and 15 minutes.

Hypotension

Causes of hypotension include the persistent effects of anesthetic or antihypertensive drugs, peripheral vasodilation from rewarming, cardiac tamponade, tension pneumothorax related to central venous catheter insertion, myocardial ischemia, arrhythmias, sepsis, anaphylaxis, hypoxia, hypocalcemia, and adrenal and thyroid failure. By far the most common cause of postoperative hypotension is hypovolemia.

The diagnosis of hypovolemia begins with a review of the patient's preoperative history and intraoperative course with special emphasis on medications and fluids received and blood lost. Artifactually low blood pressure readings caused by measurement errors should be ruled out. Oliguria, supine hypotension, tachycardia, and marked variation in pulse pressure with positive pressure ventilation all support the diagnosis of hypovolemia. However, patients with autonomic dysfunction, such as those with long-standing diabetes mellitus or patients on antihypertensive therapy, may not exhibit these expected cardiovascular responses to hypovolemia. The presence of lactic acidosis may indicate severe hypovolemia with systemic hypoperfusion. A central venous or pulmonary artery catheter may aid in the diagnosis (and therapy) of hypovolemia. Other diagnostic tools include transthoracic or transesophageal echocardiography.

Treatment of hypotension is directed at correcting the underlying cause. In the case of hypovolemia, a fluid challenge with an isotonic crystalloid or colloid solution (or blood in cases of severe anemia) is the first therapeutic step. The legs may be raised in the acute setting to provide autotransfusion of volume into the central circulation. The Trendelenburg position is contraindicated in the patient at risk for increased ICP. In addition, this position has not been shown to be effective in raising the central circulating blood volume. A vasopressor such as ephedrine (5 to 10 mg IV) or phenylephrine (25 to 50 μg IV) may be judiciously used as a temporizing measure to increase blood pressure, but it should not replace adequate volume resuscitation.

Arrhythmias

Arrhythmias are a common postoperative occurrence and may be a result of hypoxemia, hypercarbia, acid-base disturbances, electrolyte abnormalities, administration of anticholinesterases, digitalis toxicity, preexisting organic heart disease, myocardial ischemia, pain, stress, cranial nerve injuries, or hypothermia. Because the spectrum of arrhythmias ranges from benign to lethal it is extremely important to (1) identify the type of arrhythmia correctly, (2) determine its underlying cause, and (3) treat promptly if necessary. Arrhythmias refractory to initial treatment may warrant a cardiology consultation.

PREMATURE ATRIAL CONTRACTIONS

Premature atrial contractions are not usually a serious rhythm disturbance and rarely necessitate treatment.

PREMATURE VENTRICULAR CONTRACTIONS

Premature ventricular contractions (PVCs) may be benign but may also be an early sign of myocardial ischemia, especially when polymorphic and multifocal. If a central venous catheter is in place, its position should be confirmed because PVCs may result from the catheter irritating the endocardium. Frequent PVCs that cause hemodynamic compromise should be treated. Correction of underlying abnormalities and the administration of lidocaine, 1.5 mg/kg bolus IV, followed by an infusion of 1 to 4 mg/min, are done. Lidocaine may cause significant sedation.

SINUS BRADYCARDIA

Benign causes of sinus bradycardia include beta blockade, narcotics, and cholinesterase inhibitors. Underlying sinus node dysfunction (especially in the elderly population) and bradycardia associated with Cushing's triad should be ruled out.

SUPRAVENTRICULAR TACHYARRHYTHMIAS

Supraventricular tachyarrhythmias may require immediate treatment. Therapy includes beta blockers such as esmolol (0.5 to 1 mg/kg bolus IV, followed by an infusion of 50 to 300 μg/kg/min), adenosine (3 to 6 mg bolus IV), verapamil (5 to 10 mg IV), digoxin (0.125 to 0.25 mg IV every 15 minutes to a total dose of 1 mg), carotid sinus massage, and cardioversion.

ATRIAL FIBRILLATION

Atrial fibrillation is characterized by fragmented and disorganized atrial electrical activity and is often due to disease processes that cause stretching of the atria or a high catecholamine state. The hemodynamically unstable patient should be cardioverted (starting at 50 joules). Drug therapy includes digoxin, verapamil, or beta-adrenergic blockade.

OTHER POSTOPERATIVE COMPLICATIONS

Hyperthermia

Hyperthermia is relatively uncommon in the recovery room, although it may be seen in patients, especially small children, who have been in a warm operating room and were covered with drapes for a long period of time. A preoperative fever, aspiration pneumonitis, infections, atelectasis, thyroid storm, and pheochromocytoma are other causes of postoperative hyperthermia. Malignant hyperthermia, although rare, must be ruled out. An arterial blood gas usually shows a mixed respiratory and metabolic acidosis. The administration of phenothiazines (chlorpromazine) or butyrophenones (droperidol and haloperidol) can cause the malignant neuroleptic syndrome. Anticholinergics, especially the tertiary amines such as atropine can cross into the CNS and cause toxicity manifested by fever, flushing, delerium, and anhydrosis. Treatment consists of the administration of physostigmine, 1 to 4 mg IV. Meperidine in combination with monoamine oxidase inhibitors may cause hyperpyrexia with seizures and death. Neurogenic hyperthermia may be a result of brainstem or hypothalamic damage or intraventricular or subarachnoid blood accumulation.

Fever should be treated to improve patient comfort and to avoid an increase in carbon dioxide production, an associated increase in cerebral metabolic rate of oxygen consumption ($CMRO_2$) and CBF with a potential increase in ICP. Fever may also cloud the patient's mental status and interfere with the neurologic examination. Acetaminophen can be administered orally or rectally at a dose of 650 to

1000 mg. In children a dose of 10 to 15 mg/kg is suggested. Uncovering the patient and the use of cooling blankets may also be helpful.

Hypothermia

Hypothermia is a common postoperative finding because of heat loss from convection, conduction, and radiation, and from the infusion of cold IV solutions. In addition, compensatory thermoregulatory mechanisms initiated by the hypothalamus are suppressed during general anesthesia. Moderate hypothermia may occasionally be used intentionally intraoperatively to protect the brain from ischemic injury. Even mild hypothermia can prolong emergence from general anesthesia. Shivering will increase oxygen consumption by as much as 400%, will raise $CMRo_2$ and possibly ICP, and will place the patient with coronary artery disease at increased risk for myocardial ischemia. The hypothermic patient can be warmed with warming lights, a warming blanket, head covers, and warmed IV fluids. If deliberate hypothermia is used intraoperatively and rewarming of the patient cannot be established, it is our preference to transport the patient directly to the intensive care unit and keep him/her intubated and sedated until normothermia has been secured.

Oliguria

Postoperative oliguria is most frequently caused by hypovolemia. Obstructive causes like a kinked Foley catheter or urinary retention must be ruled out. A fluid challenge is given to optimize the patient's intravascular volume and to prevent acute tubular necrosis. The use of diuretics to increase urine output in the face of hypovolemia is dangerous and may actually precipitate renal damage. If the etiology of oliguria is unclear, a pulmonary artery catheter may help determine the cause. Appropriate laboratory studies should be performed (urine sodium, urine creatinine, urine osmolarity, urine specific gravity, serum sodium, and serum creatinine) to determine which therapy should be instituted.

Nausea and Vomiting

Nausea and vomiting should be treated promptly in the neurosurgical patient because it may cause an increase in systemic blood pressure and ICP. However, it should also be kept in mind that refractory nausea and vomiting may be caused by intracranial pathologic processes and high ICP. Commonly used drugs to treat nausea and vomiting include droperidol (Inapsine), 0.625 mg to 2.5 mg IV, promethazine (Phenergan), 12.5 mg to 25 mg IV or intramuscularly (IM), prochlorperazine (Compazine), 5 to 10 mg IV or IM, and metoclopramide (Reglan), 10 mg IV. All of these agents are dopamine antagonists and may cause dystonic reactions or an exacerbation of Parkinson's disease. Dystonic reactions may be treated with diphenhydramine (Benadryl), 25 to 100 mg IV or IM, or benztropine (Cogentin), 1 to 2 mg IV. The serotonin antagonist ondansetron has also been used successfully to treat nausea and vomiting in the neurosurgical patient in doses of 4 mg IV in adults or 0.15 mg/kg IV in children. It seems to be more effective in preventing and treating nausea and vomiting than both droperidol and metoclopramide.

SPECIAL CONCERNS RELATED TO SPECIFIC NEUROSURGICAL PROCEDURES

Carotid Endarterectomy

The most frequent serious complications after carotid endarterectomy (CEA) are stroke, cranial nerve damage, myocardial ischemia, hypertension, hypotension, and hemorrhage. The incidence of neurologic and cardiovascular complications after CEA is similar whether patients received general or regional anesthesia.

The incidence of perioperative stroke ranges from 2% to 10% and represents the major source of operative morbidity in patients undergoing this procedure. Cerebral ischemia is more frequent in patients with preexisting neurologic risk factors such as transient ischemic episodes, multiple previous cerebral infarctions, a progressing neurologic deficit, or a new deficit of <24 hours' duration. New postoperative deficits most often occur as a result of cerebral ischemia caused by emboli resulting from intraoperative manipulation of the diseased blood vessel. Other causes of stroke include intraoperative or postoperative hypotension, carotid cross-clamping, carotid thrombosis, or intracerebral hemorrhage caused by hyperperfusion of an area that has been previously supplied by a stenotic vessel (i.e., sudden restoration of a high perfusion pressure to a vascular bed that has been chronically perfused at a low pressure). During the immediate postoperative period a regular assessment for the development of new neurologic deficits should be performed. The presence of a new deficit should prompt immediate diagnostic evaluation with either Doppler ultrasound or angiography and the surgeon must be notified.

Hypoglossal (twelfth cranial) nerve palsies are the most common cranial nerve injury after CEA. Treatment is supportive because this complication usually resolves spontaneously. If bilateral CEA is performed and the ninth and tenth cranial nerves are damaged, difficulty with swallowing, vocalization and airway protection may occur. In addition, bilateral CEA may lead to damage to both carotid bodies, resulting in a diminished or absent hypoxic respiratory drive. Hemidiaphragmatic paresis has also been reported in 60% of patients undergoing CEA under cervical plexus blockade.

Myocardial ischemia is a common problem in CEA patients because they frequently have concomitant coronary artery disease. Operative mortality associated with CEA is about 1% to 2%, and it is most often due to perioperative myocardial infarction (MI). The risk of a perioperative MI is highest in patients with a history of unstable angina, congestive heart failure, or a recent (<6 months) MI. Combined coronary artery bypass grafting and CEA is reserved for patients with severe carotid stenosis and medically untreatable coronary artery disease because this procedure carries a higher mortality.

Myocardial ischemia is often first diagnosed in the PACU by changes in the patient's baseline electrocardiogram (ECG) (i.e., S-T segment changes, T-wave inversion, new Q waves, or certain arrhythmias). However, T-wave changes after CEA are nonspecific and may not reflect myocardial ischemia. Surgery in close proximity to the stellate ganglia may alter their autonomic output, which may cause ECG changes without ischemia. Stress, surgery, drugs, temperature, raised ICP, and electrolyte shifts may all nonspecifically alter the ECG. If ischemia is suspected from the ECG monitor display, a 12-lead ECG must be obtained and compared with the preoperative study. Substernal chest pain associated with dyspnea in the awake patient and a rise in pulmonary artery diastolic blood pressure (if a pulmonary artery catheter is in place) may also be suggestive of ischemia. Transesophageal (in the anesthetized patient) or transthoracic echocardiography may be used as a more sensitive tool to confirm the diagnosis of myocardial ischemia. As with the ECG, comparison to a preoperative study is helpful.

Treatment of ischemia involves adjusting the delicate balance between myocardial oxygen demand and supply. Supply can be improved by administering supplemental oxygen, maintaining an adequate circulating blood volume, and treating tachycardia and hypotension. IV nitroglycerin may provide coronary artery vasodilation.

Demand is decreased by reducing preload, afterload, and heart rate. Nitroglycerin may be helpful in reducing preload. SNP, hydralazine, enalaprilate, and nifedipine (10 mg sublingually) can effectively reduce afterload. The heart rate can be slowed with beta blockade. However, beta blockade may profoundly depress cardiac output, and beta blockers must be used carefully. The consultation of a cardiologist to aid in the postoperative care of a patient with suspected or active myocardial ischemia is suggested.

Preexisting hypertension is present in 60% to 80% of patients undergoing CEA. Postoperative hypertension is more common in those with inadequately treated preoperative hypertension. It has been suggested that new neurologic deficits after CEA are more common in patients who have postoperative hypertension. Others have found no association between perioperative hypertension and stroke, and it remains controversial as to whether preoperative blood pressure control changes postoperative morbidity. Acute hypertension after CEAs may be due to denervation of the carotid sinus with resultant loss of tonic baroreceptor activity. Blood pressures >200 mm Hg were reported in one series in 33% of patients after CEA. Pain, bladder distension, hypercarbia, and hypoxemia are other causes of hypertension.

Postoperative hypotension occurs in 15% to 20 % of patients after a CEA. Sudden exposure of the carotid sinus to true arterial pressures after removal of the plaque may result in a vagally mediated reflex vasodilation and bradycardia. Cardiac output is usually normal or elevated and fluid administration is the initial therapy. Vasopressors (ephedrine or phenylephrine) may be used if fluid administration is unsuccessful in restoring a normal blood pressure. In most cases the hypotension resolves spontaneously within 12 to 24 hours.

Hemorrhage at the surgical site can be life threatening, and the surgeon must be immediately notified. Reintubation should be considered very early because the expanding hematoma can quickly distort airway anatomy, making intubation difficult or impossible. In a life-threatening situation the skin sutures should be removed to decompress the hematoma and relieve airway obstruction to facilitate reintubation.

Craniotomy

One of the goals of neuroanesthesia is to deliver anesthetic care that allows for prompt awakening, extubation, and early neurologic evaluation. If awakening after a craniotomy is unexpectedly delayed or a new focal neurologic deficit is detected after awakening, the differential diagnosis includes the effects of residual anesthetic drugs, metabolic derangements, and structural causes that may require immediate surgical attention. Severe hypotension and hypoxemia are obvious causes for delayed awakening, and the initial evaluation should focus on cardiorespiratory function.

Metabolic abnormalities are more likely to cause global neurologic dysfunction rather than focal findings. However, the combination of a vascular stenosis and a metabolic derangement such as hypoglycemia, hypercarbia, or hyponatremia can result in a focal deficit. An arterial blood gas and serum glucose and sodium concentrations will assist with the diagnosis.

Structural problems that may cause delayed awakening or neurologic deficits include bleeding, cerebral edema, hydrocephalus, tension pneumocephalus (TPC), and cranial nerve damage. Seizures and the postictal state are other causes of postoperative neurologic dysfunction.

Although postoperative bleeding is uncommon, the most consistent manifestation is a decreased level of consciousness. A large percentage of intracranial hematomas present within the first 6 hours after a craniotomy. The bleeding can be epidural, subdural, intraparenchymal, or intraventricular. Risk factors associated with bleeding after surgery for brain tumor resection include perioperative hypertension and an existing coagulopathy. Patient position during the operation has no influence on the incidence of postoperative bleeding. Most postoperative hematomas occur at the operative site. If monitored, ICP may not always rise with the development of intracranial bleeding despite clinical deterioration of the patient. The clinical examination remains the most important tool in evaluating the patient. The definitive diagnosis and the decision to reoperate is made by computed tomographic (CT) scan. Postoperative hypertension should be treated to minimize the occurrence of postoperative bleeding.

Brain edema is common within the first 24 to 72 hours after elective intracranial surgery and reaches its peak approximately 16 hours postoperatively. Risk factors for postoperative brain edema and ICP elevation include protracted surgery longer than 6 hours and repeat surgery. The ICP measured in the supratentorial compartment may not accurately reflect the pressures in the infratentorial compartment because of the lower compliance of the latter. In one study the monitored pressure in the posterior fossa was up to 50% greater than that of the supratentorial space during the first 12 hours postoperatively. Diagnosis of cerebral edema is made by CT scan. Treatment of increased ICP includes hyperventilation, the administration of mannitol, positioning the patient with the head up, steroid therapy and, if refractory, a continuous IV infusion of lidocaine, propofol, or sodium pentothal, as outlined in a previous chapter. Endotracheal tube suctioning should be avoided.

Acute hydrocephalus can occur after a craniotomy because of obstruction of flow of cerebrospinal fluid resulting from edema or blood clots. It is diagnosed by CT scan and may need to be treated surgically with a ventriculostomy or ventricular shunt.

New-onset seizures occur postoperatively in approximately 13% of patients undergoing intracranial surgery. The seizure occurs within the first 24 hours in 50% of these patients. Patients with a preexisting seizure history have a 35% incidence of seizures in the immediate postoperative period. Seizures are more likely to occur if surgery involved the sensory or motor cortex. Prevention of seizures is critical because they may precipitate serious complications such as aspiration, hypoxemia, increased ICP, and intracranial bleeding. Maintaining a patent airway and oxygenation are essential. Incremental doses of sodium pentothal (25 to 100 mg IV), diazepam (2 to 20 mg IV), or midazolam (1 to 5 mg IV) can be used to arrest the seizure, and phenytoin should be administered to prevent recurrence (the loading dose is 10 to 15 mg/kg). Neuromuscular blockers will successfully stop motor activity and may be required for airway management and intubation, but they will not halt seizure activity and seizure associated increases in $CMRo_2$ and CBF.

Special Concerns with Infratentorial Craniotomies

Bleeding and edema may also occur with posterior fossa surgery, which may lead to brainstem compression or ischemia. Irregular respiratory patterns, hypotension or hypertension and arrhythmias are often the first signs. Immediate surgical decompression may be indicated.

Tension pneumocephalus (TPC) occurs when an excessive amount of air accumulates in the subdural space and is trapped during dural closure. TPC is more common after operations performed with the patient in the seated position and is exacerbated by aggressive intraoperative cerebrospinal fluid drainage, diuretic administration, and other attempts to collapse the brain to improve surgical exposure. As the brain swells postoperatively, the pressure increases within the cranium because of the fixed amount of space available. Patients may have either focal or global neurologic dysfunction. The diagnosis can be made with skull films or CT, and treatment involves placement of a burr hole under local anesthesia to vent the air and relieve the pressure. Nitrous oxide (N_2O) has been implicated in the development of TPC, although TPC can occur in the absence of N_2O. If N_2O has been used throughout the operation and the partial pressure of N_2O is high in the trapped gas under the dura, then no further N_2O will enter the subdural space after dural closure. However, if N_2O is only used during closure, it will equilibrate with the subdural space, possibly worsening the TPC. Consequently, if N_2O has not been used from the beginning of the case, it should not be used during or after dural closure.

Cranial nerve damage during posterior fossa surgery may involve the fourth through twelfth cranial nerves. If airway integrity is a concern because of cranial nerve dysfunction, extubation may not be possible or safe.

Patients who have undergone craniotomy in the sitting position are at risk for several other complications. Intraoperative venous air embolism may precipitate noncardiogenic pulmonary edema and right ventricular failure as a result of pulmonary hypertension. Paradoxical emboli may present with cerebral, myocardial, and other tissue infarction. Peripheral tissue ischemia can occur at position related pressure points. Sciatic, brachial plexus, and peroneal nerve injury have been described with the sitting position. Spinal cord ischemia resulting in quadriplegia has been reported and is thought to be related to decreased blood flow from a lower MAP in combination with extreme neck flexion. Head and tongue swelling from position-related venous obstruction has also been reported and may make immediate extubation impossible.

Intracranial Vascular Surgery

At our institution mild hypothermia is commonly used during neurosurgical procedures for aneurysm clipping and resections of arteriovenous malformations. Persistent postoperative hypothermia of the patient prevents fast emergence, and these patients are routinely brought directly to the neurosurgical intensive care unit. Their care and specific postoperative concerns are discussed in detail in Chapter 16.

Pituitary Surgery

The pituitary gland is approached surgically either by a frontal craniotomy or, more commonly, by the transsphenoidal approach. Special PACU considerations arise with this group of patients because of the nature of their disease and the surgery.

A major concern in posttranssphenoidal surgery patients is that they will be unable to breathe through the nose after extubation because of the presence of nasal packs. This places the patient at increased risk for hypoxemia, postobstructive pulmonary edema, and pulmonary aspiration. Extubation should only be performed in the fully awake patient. Acromegalic patients may be difficult to reintubate should the need arise because of tongue enlargement, mandibular overgrowth, and glottic narrowing.

After transsphenoidal resection of a pituitary tumor, the remaining intrasellar cavity is often packed with exogenous fat or muscle to prevent a cerebrospinal fluid leak or prolapse of the optic chiasm into an empty sella. As a result, chiasmal compression can occur and surgical decompression may be required. It is therefore important to monitor the patient for the development of visual field deficits.

A cerebrospinal fluid leak (with an increased risk of meningitis) and the development of sinusitis are known complications after pituitary surgery. Damage to the third, fourth, fifth, and sixth cranial nerves as a result of tumor removal near the lateral wall of the cavernous sinus or from direct surgical trauma can occur. The cavernous portion of the carotid artery may be injured during transsphenoidal surgery. The development of a carotid-cavernous fistula or a false aneurysm of the cavernous carotid artery have been reported, as well as complications related to intraoperative venous air embolism. Severe central neurogenic hyperthermia is a rare complication after pituitary surgery.

Endocrine abnormalities after pituitary surgery may manifest themselves as adrenal insufficiency (presenting with hypotension, fever, hyperkalemia, hyponatremia, and nausea), and perioperative replacement therapy with hydrocortisone (100 mg IV every 6 to 8 hours) is standard at our institution for all patients who undergo pituitary surgery. Patients with Cushing's disease may exhibit hyperglycemia, hypokalemia, and hypertension and obesity-related anesthetic complications. Hypothyroidism is rarely a problem in the immediate postoperative period. For a more detailed discussion on endocrine abnormalities, including the diagnosis and treatment of diabetes insipidus and the syndrome of inappropriate antidiuretic hormone secretion, refer to Chapters 5 and 12.

Spinal Surgery

Special problems associated with the postoperative care of spinal surgery patients are primarily related to airway management after cervical spine surgery, hemodynamic instability of the quadriplegic patient, postoperative respiratory care of the scoliosis patient, and the evaluation of new neurologic deficits resulting from hematomas or direct nerve trauma. The special postoperative concerns related to positioning of the patient and other specific management problems are discussed in Chapter 8.

Pediatric Patient

Most postoperative concerns after craniotomies in the pediatric age group are similar to those in the adult patient. If surgery was extensive and prolonged or the child was intubated in the intensive care unit before surgery, we generally leave the child sedated and intubated and transport her/him directly to the pediatric or neonatal intensive care unit.

Children are more likely to have postoperative airway edema and postintubation croup, characterized by inspiratory stridor and respiratory distress. Treatment consists of the administration of humidified 100% oxygen, nebulized racemic epinephrine (0.25 to 0.5 ml in 2 ml of normal saline solution every 20 to 30 minutes) and IV dexamethasone (0.5 mg/kg). If severe, reintubation may be necessary.

Laryngospasm after extubation is also more common in the pediatric age group. Initially, gentle mask CPAP with 100% oxygen and jaw extension should be tried. A small dose of succinylcholine (0.5 to 1 mg/kg, maximally 10 mg) and reintubation may be required if the initial interventions fail.

Children who have undergone myelomenigocele repair should receive careful attention as to their respiratory status. About 80% have an associated Arnold-Chiari malformation (causing brainstem and cranial nerve compromise) predisposing them to airway obstruction and respiratory arrest.

A ventriculoatrial shunt procedure, especially in small infants, can precipitate congestive heart failure if a large amount of cerebrospinal fluid is shunted into the central circulation. Tachycardia is often the first sign of fluid overload, and the shunt mechanism may have to be disconnected.

Other issues related to the postoperative care of the pediatric patient are discussed in Chapter 13.

Suggested Readings

Ahuja A, Guterman LR, Hopkins LN: Carotid cavernous fistula and false aneurysm of the cavernous carotid artery: complications of transsphenoidal surgery, *Neurosurgery* 31:774, 1992.

Alon E, Himmelseher S: Ondansetron in the treatment of postoperative vomiting: a randomized, double-blind comparison with droperidol and metoclopramide, *Anesth Analg* 75:561, 1992.

Asiddao CB, Donegan JH, Whitesell RC et al:Factors associated with perioperative complications during carotid endarterectomy, *Anesth Analg* 61:631,1982.

Bedford RF: Perioperative air embolism, *Semin Anesth* 6:163, 1987.

Castresana MR, Masters RD, Castresana EJ et al: Incidence and clinical significance of hemidiaphragmatic paresis in patients undergoing carotid endarterectomy during cervical plexus block anesthesia, *J Neurosurg Anesth* 6:21, 1994.

Colice GL: Neurogenic pulmonary edema, *Clin Chest Med* 6:473, 1985.

Craig DB: Postoperative recovery of pulmonary function, *Anesth Analg* 60:46, 1981.

Donegan MF, Bedford RF: Intravenously administered lidocaine prevents intracranial hypertension during endotracheal suctioning, *Anesthesiology* 52:516, 1980.

Malik AB: Mechanisms of neurogenic pulmonary edema, *Circ Res* 57:1, 1985.

Matthew E, Sherwin AL, Weiner K et al: Seizures following intracranial surgery: incidence in the first postperative week, *Can J Neurol Sci* 7:285, 1980.

Stone DJ: Recovery room care. In Sperry RJ, Stirt JA, Stone DJ, editors, *Manual of neuroanesthesia,* Philadelphia, 1989, BC Decker.

Towne JB, Weiss DG, Hobson RW: First phase report of Cooperative Veterans Administration Asymptomatic Carotid Stenosis Study: operative morbidity and mortality, *J Vasc Surg* 11:252, 1990.

NEUROSCIENCE INTENSIVE CARE

Cherylee W.J. Chang
Thomas P. Bleck

The neuroscience intensive care unit (ICU) deals primarily with postoperative neurosurgical patients, although many centers triage neurologically ill patients to these units rather than to medical ICUs. The rationale for this choice involves the specialized training required for ICU nurses to understand the neurologic examination, which often remains the most sensitive method for evaluating neurologically and neurosurgically critically ill patients. This chapter focuses on problems most frequently encountered in a neurosurgical ICU.

TRANSPORT AND INITIAL ADMISSION ASSESSMENT

During transport careful attention to the patient's vital signs and clinical examination is essential. Sudden hypertension, with or without bradycardia, may be an early sign of postoperative hemorrhage or increased intracranial pressure (ICP). Although the patient may be under the influence of neuromuscular blockading agents, pupillary reflexes remain unaltered and should be evaluated for changes.

Once the patient is admitted to the unit, admission blood samples, an electrocardiogram (ECG), and a baseline neurologic examination should be performed. The Glasgow Coma Scale (Table 20-1), initially developed as a prognostic indicator in head-injured patients, is most commonly used for this evaluation; however, extraocular movements, corneal reflexes, pupillary size and response, and extremity strength testing are also important components to recognize, localize, and follow-up neurologic deficits.

NEUROLOGIC CONSIDERATIONS

Intracranial Hypertension
PHYSIOLOGY

ICP changes are described by the Monro-Kellie hypothesis that the skull is a semiclosed compartment that contains brain and interstitial fluid (80%), cerebrospinal fluid (CSF) (10%), and blood (10%). Under pathologic conditions, where one or more of these components is increased (e.g., hemorrhage or edema after trauma or stroke, or hydrocephalus with CSF outflow obstruction), compensatory mechanisms cause reductions in CSF production or cerebral blood flow (CBF). Once these compensatory mechanisms are overwhelmed, an increase in the volume of the cranial contents results in increased ICP. The compliance in the skull (volume-pressure relationship; see Fig. 20-1) determines the extent that an increase in one component will change ICP. For example, patients with smaller brains (i.e., atrophy) will be on the lower slope of the

TABLE 20-1. Glasgow Coma Scale

Eye Opening (E)	
Spontaneous	4
To verbal stimuli	3
To painful stimuli	2
None	1
Best Verbal Response (V)	
Oriented	5
Confused conversation	4
Inappropriate words	3
Incomprehensible sounds	2
None	1
Best Motor Response (M)	
Obeys commands	6
Localizes pain	5
Withdraws to pain	4
Abnormal flexion	3
Extensor response	2
None	1

NOTE: Best motor response for any extremity is used for scoring. Eye opening scoring is not valid if eyes are swollen shut, and verbal scoring is invalid if speech is impossible (e.g., in presence of tracheal tube). Maximal GCS is 15; minimal score is 3. All patients with GCS <8 and most with GCS = 8 are in coma (i.e., no eye opening [M = 1], no ability to follow commands [M = 1 to 5], and no word verbalizations [V = 1 to 2]. GCS ≤8 is classified as severe head injury, GCS between 9 and 12 as moderate head injury, and GCS between 13 and 15 as minor head injury.

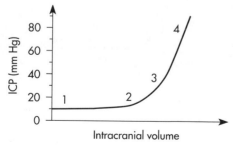

FIG 20-1.
Intracranial volume-pressure relationship is described by compliance curve. Changes in ICP that occur with increases in volume depend on compensatory ability of brain. (Modified from Shapiro HM: Intracranial hypertension, *Anesthesiology* 43:445, 1975.)

compliance curve and may tolerate greater amounts of edema or space-occupying masses without changes in ICP.

Cerebral perfusion pressure (CPP) is determined by the difference between mean arterial pressure (MAP) and the pressure impeding blood flow to the brain (i.e., ICP). When central venous pressure (CVP) exceeds ICP, the intracranial jugular venous and sagittal sinus pressures will rise to equal the CVP. As a result, the ICP increases to the level of CVP. Elevation in ICP is significant when it compromises CPP, causing cerebral ischemia, or when high ICP (>18 to 20 mm Hg) contributes to pressure gradients within the skull, resulting in tissue displacement (i.e., herniation).

A normal CPP ranges between 70 to 100 mm Hg. However, a CPP of 50 to 60 mm Hg is considered adequate for tissue perfusion. A CPP below 30 to 40 mm Hg results in cerebral ischemia.

Autoregulation of the cerebral vasculature follows from the concept that blood flow is directly proportional to pressure and inversely proportional to resistance. In the normal individual the brain is able to maintain a constant CBF by vasomotor control of arteriolar resistance despite changes in mean arterial blood flow (see Fig. 20-2). When MAP and CPP increase, cerebral vasoconstriction oc-

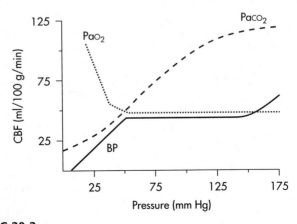

FIG 20-2.
CBF changes caused by alterations in PaO_2, $PaCO_2$, and blood pressure (BP). (Modified from Shapiro HM: Intracranial hypertension, *Anesthesiology* 43:445, 1975.)

curs to maintain a constant CBF with decreased cerebral blood volume (CBV). Similarly, when hypotension occurs, vasodilation occurs, which maintains CBF with increased CBV. Changes in arterial oxygenation (PO_2) and carbon dioxide (PCO_2) will also effect changes in CBF by autoregulative mechanisms. The ability to regulate CBF by these mechanisms is used in the management of intracranial hypertension (see below).

Autoregulation breaks down below an MAP of about 40 or 50 mm Hg and beyond an MAP of 150 mm Hg in normal individuals; in chronically hypertensive patients this entire curve is shifted to the right. An MAP above the level of autoregulative control can result in an increase in intracranial volume as capacitance vessels dilate; depending on intracranial compliance, this may result in an increase of ICP. When the blood brain barrier (BBB) is disrupted, edema may occur at an MAP as low as 100 mm Hg.

MONITORING INTRACRANIAL PRESSURE

ICP monitoring devices differ by the location that they are placed in the cranium and their ability to allow CSF drainage.

The intraventricular catheter, or ventriculostomy, is the most accurate and reliable method for measuring ICP. It is placed blindly into a frontal horn of a lateral ventricle by an acknowledged safe trajectory and is usually placed in patients who have enlarged ventricles. Besides its accuracy, the major advantage of the ventriculostomy is its ability to drain CSF when elevations in ICP occur. Infection is the most common risk involved (see under Infectious Complications). Early removal is essential to decreasing infection. Hemorrhage can also occur, typically during insertion. Correction of coagulation parameters is the rule before placement of any monitoring device. Occasional clogging of the catheter can occur.

Subdural bolts or subarachnoid screws are another fluid-coupled method of monitoring ICP. Typically, they are placed in the frontal area. Their risks for infection are low and they have fewer bleeding complications than ventriculostomy; however, CSF drainage is not feasible. The drawbacks of these devices are inaccurate measurements by obstruction of the device with blood or debris, loss of integrity of fluid coupling by small leaks, and herniation of the brain into the bolt.

Fluid-coupled epidural catheters are rarely used because they provide unreliable information. Their only advantage lies in the rarity of bleeding complications; therefore they have been advocated for patients with coagulopathy.

We most commonly use fiberoptic subdural and intraparenchymal monitoring with a fiberoptic catheter. Zeroed before insertion, it tends to be highly accurate and easy to maintain, with few infectious complications. Drawbacks include expense and the inability to drain fluid. Although placement in the subdural or subarachnoid space is ideal, often these catheters are placed intraparenchymally. Despite this, bleeding complications are infrequent.

Changes in ICP may be compartmentalized because the falx and tentorium provide a semirigid membrane through which increases in ICP may not be transmitted. Occasionally, an ICP monitor placed in one hemisphere may not fully reflect elevated pressures that occur in the opposite hemisphere. Similarly, elevated pressures in the posterior fossa separated from the ICP monitor by the tentorium may not be transmitted to the pressure monitor. Although rare, patients have herniated with normal ICP monitor readings that have good waveforms and appear to be functioning well. Thus the clinical examination continues to remain essential to assessing neurologic status despite placement of monitoring devices.

TREATMENT OF ELEVATED INTRACRANIAL PRESSURE

Normal ICP is <10 mm Hg. Sustained elevations of ICP above 15 mm Hg are abnormal. An acutely elevated ICP of 18 to 20 mm Hg necessitates intervention. The ICP waveform emulates the systolic and diastolic waveforms of arterial tracings, including the dicrotic notch. With progressing intracranial hypertension the waveform deteriorates. Initially the diastolic peak rises above the systolic peak, then the entire waveform elevates, and finally the waveform loses its dicrotic notch and becomes rounded.

In addition, there are three types of ICP waves that vary from baseline: Lundberg A, B, and C waves. Lundberg C waves are rapid, four to eight per minute, rhythmic, and are small in amplitude and change with blood pressure. These are not clinically significant. B waves are sharp, rhythmic elevations to levels of 50 mm Hg that occur at 0.5 to 2 minute intervals and last for only several seconds. These waves herald decreasing cerebral compliance. Finally, Lundberg A waves (also known as plateau waves) require immediate intervention. The baseline ICP when an A wave occurs is typically >15 mm Hg, and the A wave is characterized by pressures over 60 mm Hg that last for 5 to 15 minutes. The A waves occur at varying intervals and may arise spontaneously or be precipitated by noxious stimuli (e.g., suctioning of an endotracheal tube, turning, or painful stimulation). They appear to be associated with a mostly intact cerebral autoregulative mechanism responding to increased ICP and decreased CPP with vasodilation and increased CBV. Neurologic deterioration occurs; these waves often indicate impending herniation.

When the characteristics of the ICP waveform changes or ICP remains elevated above 18 to 20 mm Hg, various maneuvers may be used to decrease pressure. The mainstays of therapy are based on the Monro-Kellie hypothesis (i.e., to decrease either blood, CSF, or brain volume in the cranial vault).

HYPERVENTILATION

Hyperventilation remains one of the fastest therapeutic maneuvers to decrease CBV. Its effect is usually seen within several minutes. Hyperventilation lowers arterial Pco_2, causing a cerebral alkalotic state that results in cerebral vasoconstriction and subsequently a fairly rapid decrease in CBV. The optimal Pco_2 appears to be between 25 and 30 mm Hg. Pco_2 levels <20 mm Hg can result in cerebral ischemia from excessive vasoconstriction. There is some debate as to the duration of effect of hyperventilation. Within 24 hours the kidney will begin to compensate for the respiratory alkalosis, and serum and CSF pH will begin to return to normal. However, rapid normalization of Pco_2 results in rebound vasodilation and intracranial hypertension, so it is reasonable to normalize arterial Pco_2 over 24 to 48 hours.

In patients for whom hyperventilation may be required for several days allowing the Pco_2 to slowly rise from 25 to 30 mm Hg may continue to have some effect in lowering ICP, but give an additional margin for hyperventilation if ICP abruptly rises. In addition, the use of tromethamine (THAM, tris[hydroxymethyl]aminomethane) 1 mg/kg/hr, a weak base and proton buffer, can prolong the effect of hyperventilation on ICP control.

During hyperventilation other ventilatory parameters must be monitored. Because the means to increase minute ventilation requires either higher tidal volumes or higher respiratory rates, excessive hyperventilation may also elevate ICP by raising intrathoracic pressure and impeding venous return. To access this, the CVP should be monitored for increases while hyperventilation is being initiated and maintained.

OSMOTIC AGENTS

Mannitol, long a mainstay for ICP therapy, begins to act within 10 to 20 minutes. One of its actions is to create an osmotic gradient between blood and brain, drawing fluid from the interstitial space and reducing cerebral edema. Mannitol also has a systemic action by acting as an osmotic agent to draw fluid from extracellular compartments throughout the body into the intravascular compartment. This causes elevation in CVP and cardiac preload, which results in increased cardiac output and MAP. This subsequently increases CPP in patients with elevated ICP. Mannitol also has an effect on the rheology of red blood cells and appears to improve viscosity, which results in pial vasoconstriction. In this manner CBV is diminished. This drug is also a free radical scavenger. Finally, CSF production may be decreased by osmotic agents. Which of these mechanisms, if any, explains the reduction of ICP at usual doses remains unknown.

Mannitol is given in 0.25 to 1.0 g/kg boluses through a filtered needle to remove crystals in the solution. It may then be given in 0.25 to 0.5 g/kg every 3 to 6 hours. Although it is rapidly cleared through the urine (84%), there is evidence that mannitol accumulates in cerebral tissue after repeated dosing, especially in areas of BBB disruption. Therefore multiple doses should be avoided, if possible, to reduce exacerbation of vasogenic cerebral edema.

During osmotic therapy serum osmolality should be monitored, and further mannitol should not usually be administered once osmolality reaches 320 mOsm/L; otherwise, renal failure and further cerebral damage may occur. Because an osmotic diuresis results from mannitol therapy, careful attention must be given to fluid status to avoid dehydration and hypotension.

Other osmotic agents have been used. Hypertonic glucose (50%) is rarely used because it is metabolized quickly and because it is possible that excessive glucose may exacerbate cerebral ischemia that occurs with head trauma and stroke; this will be discussed later. Urea is also rarely used because it has a short duration of action, greater brain absorption, and vessel irritant properties. Side effects also include nausea, vomiting, diarrhea, abnormal bleeding, weakness, and seizures.

HEAD POSITION

Simple maneuvers such as ensuring midline position of the head can dramatically decrease ICP because occluding the neck veins may impede venous drainage. Loosening overly tight cervical collars can also decrease ICP in the same manner; at the same time head immobilization in the midline position must be maintained in patients with cervical precautions.

Use of gravity to improve jugular venous return by elevating the head and trunk at the waist can also decrease ICP significantly. Neck flexion should be avoided. It is of tantamount importance, however, to remember the principle that CPP is dependent on MAP. In a patient with hypotension raising the head of the bed may further compromise MAP and decrease CPP. Furthermore, in some circumstances (e.g., fulminant hepatic failure), raising the head may actually elevate ICP.

SEDATION

Agitation and pain can increase ICP. Adequate sedation may attenuate this response; however, hypotension must be avoided. In patients who are not intubated, respiratory drive must be closely monitored because rising PCO_2 will result in vasodilation and increased CBF. Short-acting intravenous agents that can be reversed (e.g., narcotics such as fentanyl) are probably the best agents in this situation. Benzodiazepines and propofol can decrease ICP; however, both can cause significant hypotension and must be used judiciously. Acute reversal of benzodiazepines with flumazenil have been studied in animals and humans with increased ICP; severe and highly significant elevations of CBF and ICP resulted after flumazenil administration. In addition, seizures may be precipitated by abrupt reversal of benzodiazepines.

Inhalational anesthetic agents that should be avoided because of cerebral vascular dilation and increase in blood flow are halothane and nitrous oxide. Isoflurane produces the greatest decrease in cerebral metabolic rate ($CMRo_2$) and has the least increase in CBF.

DIURETICS

Acetazolamide and loop diuretics both decrease CSF production. As with mannitol, diuretics may cause a serum-brain water gradient that reduces brain water.

PARALYTIC AGENTS

In ventilated patients coughing or "bucking" the ventilator can increase intrathoracic pressure and CVP. Neuromuscular blocking agents decrease ICP in these patients and may also improve chest wall compliance, further lowering the CVP.

Depolarizing neuromuscular blocking agents such as succinyl-choline should be avoided because they may increase ICP. Rocuronium is a nondepolarizing neuromuscular blocking agent with fast onset and moderate duration; it may become an alternative to succinylcholine during rapid induction for intubation. The sequelae of neuromuscular blocking agents will be discussed later in this chapter in the section on neuromuscular complications.

OXYGENATION

Poor oxygenation increases CBF and CBV by autoregulative mechanisms. Therefore adequate oxygen delivery is essential in these patients. In mechanically ventilated patients with borderline oxygenation, raising positive end-expiratory pressure (PEEP) may not significantly raise ICP and may be preferable to raising the fraction of inspired oxygen (FiO_2) into a "toxic" range. The degree that PEEP affects ICP depends on pulmonary and cerebral compliance. In patients with reasonable compliance in the intracranial vault, small increases in CVP with diminished cerebral venous outflow may not affect ICP. Conversely, in patients with noncompliant lungs (i.e., adult respiratory distress syndrome or pulmonary edema), PEEP may not be significantly transmitted to the ventral veins and hence may not affect ICP.

TEMPERATURE CONTROL

Each $1°$ C increase in body temperature raises the $CMRO_2$ by 6% to 7%. For this reason fever should be treated aggressively in patients with increased ICP. A fever workup and antimicrobial therapy should be started as clinically indicated; however, acetaminophen should be given to control temperature. If this is inadequate, a cooling blanket may become necessary; however, shivering can also increase ICP. In this setting paralytic agents may become necessary to block the shivering response. Neuroleptic agents may also help to control shivering but also decrease the seizure threshold.

SEIZURE CONTROL

Seizures increase the metabolic demands of the brain and subsequently increase CBF even in paralyzed patients, although clearly the motor manifestations of a tonic-clonic seizure will also raise

ICP by decreasing chest wall compliance and increasing intrathoracic pressures. For these reasons seizure control should be rapidly instituted and maintained. A benzodiazepine can quickly, although transiently, control seizures. Phenytoin has a longer duration of action than the benzodiazepines and has little sedating properties; thus it remains the first-line prophylactic anticonvulsant medication. It must be given through an intravenous line containing normal saline solution. A loading dose of 18 to 20 mg/kg should be administered, best given by direct injection from a syringe into an intravenous line because it can precipitate when diluted into larger volumes of saline solution. In patients with repeated seizures, a barbiturate will not only control seizure activity, but when dosed to electroencephalographic (EEG) isoelectricity, can decrease cerebral metabolic requirements by 50% to 60%, thereby decreasing CBF. Because hypotension is a common side effect of these drugs, vigilance to maintain an adequate MAP is essential. In cases where seizure control requires hypotensive-inducing anticonvulsant drug loading, concomitant pressor administration may be necessary to maintain CPP.

BARBITURATES

In patients with intracranial hypertension barbiturates have a twofold effect by controlling seizure activity and decreasing cerebral metabolic requirements. Thiopental (1 to 5 mg/kg) is usually considered a short-acting barbiturate, but it accumulates in tissues with continuous administration. Pentobarbital is longer acting and can be loaded with 10 to 15 mg/kg with an infusion of 1 to 3 mg/kg/hr. Hypotension from vasodilation and myocardial depression is the most common side effect, but long-term infusions have been associated with poikilothermia, ileus, and increased risk for infection.

CEREBROSPINAL FLUID DRAINAGE

In cases where increased CSF volume (e.g., obstructive hydrocephalus) contributes to increased ICP, a ventriculostomy not only allows monitoring of ICP but provides a means of draining CSF and lowering ICP.

HEMICRANIECTOMY

Decompression of posterior fossa hemorrhages, infarcts, and tumors should be performed quickly in cases where swelling compromises the brainstem. However, in medically intractable intracranial hypertension from massive cerebral hemispheric damage from trauma, ischemia, or hemorrhagic stroke, small case studies and anecdotal reports support the utility of reducing ICP by removing the skull and sometimes nonviable tissue. This technique has been reserved for patients with nondominant hemispheric lesions without underlying severe irreversible medical conditions. Bifrontal craniectomy is sometimes used to manage life-threatening ICP elevations from global cerebral swelling (e.g., head trauma).

CORTICOSTEROIDS

Steroids in cerebral injury remain a debated topic. Three types of cerebral edema exist. Classically, cytotoxic and vasogenic edema have been associated with cerebral injury. Vasogenic edema is formed when the integrity of the BBB is compromised (for example, in the area of neoplasm or abscess). This edema usually is responsive to glucocorticoid administration. It is not clear how steroids act, although they may stabilize the BBB. Cytotoxic edema forms when the integrity of the neuronal or glial cell membrane is disrupted and homeostatic mechanisms are perturbed, as in ischemia. Typically, this edema is not responsive to steroid use. Interstitial edema is not usually associated with acute cerebral injury. This form of edema is seen in patients with increased interstitial cerebral fluid, such as in patients with acute hydrocephalus where obstruction of CSF flow within the ventricular system forces CSF out into the surrounding brain.

Thus steroid use in patients with increased ICP from tumor or abscess may be effective. Studies have shown that steroids worsen outcome in patients with intracerebral hemorrhage. In patients with subarachnoid hemorrhage (SAH), hypoxia, or ischemic strokes, large doses of steroids may affect outcome by mechanisms other than their glucocorticoid effects (i.e., free radical scavenging effect).

Head Injury

Head trauma is responsible for 66% of deaths of people aged 15 to 34 years. Fifteen percent of these die before reaching the hospital. Approximately 50% of head injuries are a result of motor vehicle crashes, whereas 28% are due to falls.

During the patient's initial presentation, in addition to basic and advanced trauma life support, the neurologic evaluation begins with measurement of the Glascow Coma Scale (GCS). A GCS score of 8 or less is defined as severe head injury and implies coma. These patients require intubation before further investigation or management. A GCS between 9 and 12 represents moderate head injury, and a GCS of 13 and above indicates mild head injury. As mentioned previously, the GCS correlates with outcome. In one prospective study of 1311 head-injured patients by Klauber, a GCS of 3 was associated with an 83% mortality, and a GCS of 8 and above was associated with a 0.3% mortality. Other studies have shown similar results. Others have found that further examination, such as presence of reactive pupils or oculocephalic responses can add prognostic information. For example, a patient with a GCS ≤8 with unreactive pupils has a 91% chance of dying, but the presence of reactive pupils decreases this to 39%.

Skull fractures occur approximately three times more commonly in the vault than the base of the skull. Basilar skull fractures may be associated with a CSF leak; 80% of such leaks close spontaneously. Bacterial meningitis complicates a CSF leak in approximately 11% to 25% of cases; some studies show otorrhea to present a slightly higher risk than rhinorrhea, whereas others show the converse. No studies have shown convincing evidence regarding the efficacy of routine antibiotic prophylaxis for skull fractures. At this time it is reasonable to withhold antibiotics for this reason, but constant surveillance for evidence of early meningitis is essential.

Cerebral injury after head trauma can be classified as focal and diffuse injury. Focal lesions include epidural, subdural, intraparenchymal hematomas, and contusions. Diffuse injury involves diffuse axonal injury (DAI) classically attributed to tearing of nerve fibers because white and gray matter decelerate at different velocities within the skull. More recent data by Povlishock suggest that DAI is a dynamic cell biologic process that begins soon after trauma and may not be complete for 24 hours. Two theories include posttraumatic increases in intracellular calcium, which activates proteases causing neurofilament degradation, or a focal accumulation of neurofilaments after trauma, which become disordered and cause neuronal disconnection. The observation that DAI may need hours to fully develop suggests that intervention in this process may be useful. The radiologic diagnosis of DAI reflects capillary bleeding at the sites prone to this sort of injury, rather than the injury itself. The most common sites of DAI include the corpus callosum, the dorsolateral quadrant of the brainstem, the subcortical white matter, the gray-white junction of the frontal, occipital, and parietal lobes, the basal ganglia, and the parahippocampal gyri. This type of injury differs from the focal contusions that occur as the brain hits the skull at the site of impact (coup injury) and then the opposite side during deceleration (contracoup injury). Outcome in head trauma is worse with patients with intracranial mass lesions than those with diffuse brain injury. However, DAI may presage residual neuropsychologic problems.

In the Traumatic Coma Data Bank subdural hematomas (SDHs) accounted for the majority of focal injuries after head trauma. Typically, they are easily seen on noncontrast head computed tomography scans; however, in patients with severe anemia (hematocrit <20% and hemoglobin 6.7 g/dl), an SDH may be isointense. Mortality from SDH appears to decrease if prompt evacuation is performed. In a study by Seelig, surgery within 4 hours of injury decreased mortality from 90% to 30%. Ninety percent of epidural hematomas are associated with skull fractures. They typically arise from laceration of meningeal arteries or venous sinuses that course within the skull. Frank intraparenchymal hematomas and hemorrhagic contusions can present with findings immediately but more often are responsible for delayed neurologic deterioration. Any patient with neurologic decline should be evaluated with a repeat head CT scan.

Hypotension, hypoxemia, and intracranial hypertension are complicating factors that increase mortality after head injury. Review of several studies show that 11% to 13% of patients have significant hypotension, defined as systolic blood pressures <90 mm Hg. In a study by Gentleman the presence of hypotension increased mortality from 34% to 75%. In another study by Kohi, bad outcome (defined as a severely disabled, dead, or vegetative state) increased from 24% to 88% when hypotension was found. Hypoxemia is recorded in 23% to 36% of severely head injured patients and nearly doubled mortality from 34% to 59%. Kohi also showed that hypoxemia increased the chance for poor outcome from 28% to 71%. Increased ICP (>20 mm Hg) is well known to increase mortality. Miller has reported a 92% to 100% mortality in patients whose ICP could not be controlled below this level. Previously, because it is well known that maximal brain swelling occurs 24 to 72 hours after injury, the conventional wisdom had been to gear management toward prophylactic therapy of cerebral edema and intracranial hy-

pertension. There is considerable evidence to show that routine, prophylactic barbiturate coma, hyperventilation, head elevation, and
glucocorticoids do not improve outcome after head injury. However,
barbiturates and hyperventilation, when administered specifically
for known intracranial hypertension, are beneficial. Head elevation
for increased ICP, as stated above, is effective, so long as this maneuver does not lower MAP.

Seizures
PROPHYLAXIS

Seizures are seen in approximately 10% to 26% of patients after
SAH. Because the risk of potential neurologic deterioration after
seizures is high in this group of patients, prophylactic anticonvulsant
medications are used routinely.

After head injury it is widely recognized that early seizures,
which occur within 7 days after injury, represent a different entity
than late seizures that occur weeks, months, or years later. Early
posttraumatic epilepsy (PTE) is less common than late PTE. After
closed head injury early PTE occurs in approximately 3% to 6% of
patients; however, penetrating trauma results in an 8% to 10% incidence of early seizure. Late PTE in the military population varies
between 30% and 50%. In the civilian population the incidence has
been reported between 2% and 30%; differences in the length of
follow-up may be responsible for such disparate numbers. Up to
17% of patients may not have PTE until 5 years after injury. Factors
that appear to play a role in the development of both early and late
PTE are penetrating injury, intracerebral hematoma, or focal damage seen on head CT scan. Twenty-five percent of patients with late
seizures also had early seizures.

There is good evidence to support the prophylactic treatment of
seizures within the first week after head injury. In a randomized,
double-blind study phenytoin reduced the risk of seizure by 73% in
the first week. Between 8 days and 2 years, when follow-up ended,
there was no evidence that phenytoin prevented late seizures.

The incidence of postoperative epilepsy is difficult to study because supratentorial procedures themselves have been widely recognized to increase the risk of seizures; thus prophylactic therapy is
routine. A retrospective study with a follow-up period of 5 years in
1102 patients in the United Kingdom showed that in patients operated on for vascular lesions the risk of seizure was 50% for arterio-

venous malformations (AVMs), 38% for middle cerebral aneurysms, 21% for anterior cerebral vessel aneurysm, and 20% for spontaneous hematomas. No patients with aneurysm surgery had seizures after 2 years. Of tumors, meningiomas carried a 41% preoperative and 36% postoperative risk. Gliomas and brain metastases had similar preoperative (28%) and postoperative risks (20%). Brain abscesses had the greatest incidence of seizures: 92% of 13 patients. Supratentorial neurosurgical procedure patients are routinely given anticonvulsant therapy during the acute postoperative period; the duration of therapy after this remains in debate. Infratentorial procedures carry little risk for seizure because the posterior fossa is anatomically discrete from the cerebral hemispheres (where seizures propagate); thus prophylactic anticonvulsants are not necessary after these procedures.

STATUS EPILEPTICUS

Status epilepticus (SE) is defined as a "condition characterized by an epileptic seizure that is sufficiently prolonged or repeated so as to produce a fixed and lasting epileptic condition." Clinically, this should be interpreted as any patient who either has convulsive activity for >30 minutes or who has a 30-minute period of repetitive seizures without rousing to full awareness and clear mental status. The 30-minute interval has come from recent animal and human studies that show significant neuronal damage occurring after this time. Nonconvulsive SE is an entity to be considered in any patient who has no obvious explanation for an obtunded mental status. Nonconvulsive SE can be considered "electromechanical dissociation" of the central nervous system (CNS), where electrographic seizures have no overt clinical manifestation except a diminished mental status. Occasionally slight rhythmic twitching of an eyelid or lip may provide a clue that rhythmic electrical cerebral discharges are occurring; however, this movement is often the exception. Continuous EEG monitoring is mandatory in these patients, because this provides the only means to detect seizure activity.

SE is most often seen with drug withdrawal (including antiepileptic medication and alcohol), drug intoxication, metabolic disarray, and structural lesions from stroke, tumor, abscess, and trauma. Generalized SE should be considered a medical emergency. It should be noted that focal repetitive seizures *without impairment of mental status,* for example, repetitive localized hand or arm jerking, also known as epilepsia partialis continua, does not in itself constitute an emergency.

Initial treatment of SE starts with basic life support: establishing an airway and determining a pulse and blood pressure. In a patient who is actively seizing, a lateral position may help prevent aspiration. Mouth sticks to ostensibly prevent tongue biting should be considered a historic curiosity and should never be used. Establishing venous access will facilitate diagnostic workup and a mode for therapy. Laboratory tests including a complete blood cell count, blood chemistries (specifically, sodium, glucose, blood urea nitrogen, creatinine, calcium, phosphorus, and magnesium), a toxicology screen, and anticonvulsant levels in a patient known to be taking antiepileptic medication can be helpful. The choice of intravenous fluids should include normal saline solution if phenytoin will be used because phenytoin will precipitate in glucose-containing solutions.

The fastest medications known to terminate seizures are the benzodiazepines. Diazepam has the fastest onset (1 to 3 minutes) and historically was the treatment of choice. However, because of its lipophilicity, diazepam has a very short duration in the CNS (10 to 20 minutes). For this reason, lorazepam has replaced diazepam as the drug of choice. Its onset is only slightly slower (2 to 3 minutes), but its anticonvulsant action typically lasts for more than 4 hours. After 8 mg of lorazepam, if seizures have not been aborted, use of another anticonvulsant medication is indicated. If benzodiazepines are effective in seizure control, further seizures need to be prevented with a long-acting anticonvulsant. In both situations phenytoin remains the agent of choice.

A loading dose of phenytoin is 18 to 20 mg/kg. Even at the recommended rate of administration (50 mg/min), hypotension is the most common side effect and mandates decreasing the infusion rate. Cardiac arrhythmias may also be seen, and continuous cardiac monitoring is routine during the loading dose. Fosphenytoin, a phenytoin precursor, is very water soluble and should be available soon. Because of its water solubility, it can be delivered intramuscularly and is more stable in the intravenous form. It can also precipitate hypotension if administered too rapidly.

If seizures persist despite adequate phenytoin loading, the treatment algorithm varies with the institution. Traditionally, a 20 mg/kg loading dose of phenobarbital has been recommended. Very slow administration is a necessity because of significant hypotension.

Typically this was to be divided into two 10 mg/kg loading doses because 10 mg/kg is occasionally effective. However, interim data from the Veterans' Administration Cooperative Study of SE indicates that, although a first-line medication has a 60% chance of stopping SE, a second-line medication has only a 9% chance, and a third agent only 3%. Because neuronal damage is a certainty after prolonged SE, on the basis of this information, many epileptologists now recommend definitive termination of SE within 60 minutes. One common regimen uses pentobarbital to produce burst-suppression on EEG. Loading doses of 12 mg/kg are given, with an infusion rate starting at 1.0 to 2.0 mg/kg/hr, and titrated as needed. Although many patients will have been intubated for airway protection, by this point all patients should be intubated. Also, continuous EEG monitoring is essential to titrate medications to burst suppression.

There is increasing evidence that continuous intravenous midazolam can be used to terminate SE. An initial bolus of 0.2 mg/kg should be given, followed by an infusion of 0.02 to 2 mg/kg/hr titrated to seizure termination on EEG monitoring. Pentobarbital has many adverse side effects, including vasodilation and myocardial depression that often necessitates vasopressor infusion, ileus and a relative immunosuppression; midazolam has fewer side effects. Its efficacy has not yet been compared with that of pentobarbital in clinical trials.

Other systemic complications to SE include rhabdomyolysis, hyperthermia, and severe acidosis. Vigorous hydration is essential. Forced diuresis with loop diuretics and alkalinization of urine is sometimes necessary. Acetaminophen may be helpful. Acidosis will spontaneously resolve once seizures are controlled and should not be treated with bicarbonate unless cardiac instability occur; hyperventilation can initially assist in normalization of pH. Because these complications resolve with termination of SE, seizure control should continue to be the main priority. Rarely, however, paralytic agents are used in refractory cases when side effects become life threatening and patient manipulation is required (e.g., intubation, neuroimaging, or venous access placement). It cannot be overstated that although paralytic agents will improve systemic symptoms, neurologically, the patient may have electrographic seizures and continue to incur neuronal damage. Continuous EEG monitoring is mandatory and active therapy to terminate seizures must continue.

Less conventional medications have also been used to terminate

SE. Propofol, etomidate, and lidocaine have been used successfully in the treatment of SE but have also been found to precipitate seizures in some patients; therefore their role in SE is not yet clear. The inhalational agents isoflurane and halothane, titrated to burst suppression on EEG, can stop seizures. Use in the ICU is difficult, however, because of the need for gas-scavenging equipment, and continuous observation is required.

Once seizures are under control, further workup for SE may be necessary. Patients with focal neurologic deficits should undergo head CT to rule out a precipitating lesion. In a patient with a fever, a lumbar puncture should be performed to evaluate for meningitis.

Subarachnoid Hemorrhage

SAH has an incidence of approximately 11 per 100,000. Nearly 10% to 25% of these patients will die within the first few days of hemorrhage. In one large study of 772 patients with SAH from aneurysm, although 75% of patients were alert or drowsy with no motor or speech deficits, only 58% were living independently without a major neurologic deficit 6 months later.

The most common cause for SAH is rupture of saccular aneurysms. They most commonly occur at anterior circulation bifurcations (i.e., the anterior communicating and the anterior cerebral arteries, the internal carotid, and the posterior communicating arteries) and the bifurcation of the middle cerebral artery. Twelve to 26% of patients have multiple aneurysms. Saccular aneurysms have a rupture rate between 1% per year, but it appears that the size of the aneurysm (>1 cm) may increase its risk of rupture. In one study, of 102 aneurysms <1 cm followed up prospectively, none ruptured in 824 patient-years of follow-up. Other causes of SAH include trauma, AVMs, and mycotic aneurysms.

A cataclysmic headache is the most common clinical presentation of SAH, although a mild headache may also herald an episode of bleeding. Nausea, vomiting, and focal neurologic deficits such as a third or sixth nerve palsy or a hemiparesis may be evident. The level of consciousness on presentation is associated with clinical outcome because patients with stupor or coma are less likely to do well. The Hunt and Hess scale (Table 20-2) has been used as a clinical indication of prognosis. Patients with grade I or II tend to do well, whereas patients with higher grades have a worsened prognosis. CT scan, however, may add prognostic information because pa-

TABLE 20-2. Hunt and Hess Scale for Clinical Grading of Patients with Subarachnoid Hemorrhage

Grade I	Asymptomatic or mild headache
Grade II	Moderate to severe headache, nuchal rigidity, no other neurologic deficit other than a cranial nerve palsy (e.g., third cranial nerve palsy)
Grade III	Confusion, lethargy, mild focal neurologic signs
Grade IV	Stupor or hemiparesis
Grade V	Coma, extensor posturing

tients with intraparenchymal or intraventricular hemorrhage appear to do worse. One small study showed that the chance of a good outcome was reduced from 89% to 44% in patients with a good clinical grade when bleeding into other structures was present.

A CT scan without contrast may be useful in initially detecting larger subarachnoid bleeds, but in patients with unexplained, sudden headache a lumbar puncture is more sensitive for detecting small SAHs. Intraarterial digital subtraction angiography remains the gold standard for diagnosis of an aneurysm. Currently, magnetic resonance angiography is approximately 85% accurate in diagnosing aneurysms >0.3 cm but may miss smaller aneurysms entirely.

COMPLICATIONS AND THERAPY

Rebleeding. Timing of aneurysm surgery has been the subject of great debate. Some feel that surgery should be delayed until the patient is clinically stable and potential cerebral swelling is diminished. Rebleeding, however, occurs in up to 30% in the first 2 weeks, with peak incidence in the first 24 hours. Mortality from rebleeding may be as high as 31%. Thus others have advocated early aneurysm clipping within 0 to 3 days to prevent rebleeding definitively. The International Cooperative Study on the Timing of Aneurysm Surgery (1980 to 1983) addressed this issue and failed to detect a significant advantage because less rebleeding after early surgery was offset by an increased risk for cerebral ischemia. However, a recent reanalysis in the North American centers suggested an advantage of early surgery over late surgery (11 to 32 days). Surgery during days 7 to 10 is associated with worsened outcome, likely because of vasospasm, which is discussed below.

Before surgery other maneuvers to attempt to decrease the risk of rebleeding include control of CPP by management of systemic blood pressure; profound drops in mean blood pressure also must be avoided. Adrenergic blocking agents such as labetalol are often used. Nitrates are avoided because they may cause cerebral vasodilation and potentially increase ICP. Patients are kept in quiet rooms to avoid excess stimulation. Analgesics are liberally administered, although they are titrated to avoid iatrogenic mental status changes, which would precipitate needless neurologic workup.

The use of antifibrinolytics such as epsilon-aminocaproic acid after SAH has been controversial. Review of most of the published studies, however, fail to demonstrate significant benefit from this therapy. One double-blinded, placebo-controlled study reduced bleeding from 24% to 9%, although the incidence of cerebral infarction was increased by 60% in the treated group. Hydrocephalus may also be more frequent in the treated group. Other studies have had similar results, and overall outcome is not significantly altered with antifibrinolytic therapy.

Hydrocephalus. Hydrocephalus occurs in 11% to 45% of post-SAH patients. Typically, communicating hydrocephalus results from diffuse obstruction of the resorptive arachnoid villi by blood. Noncommunicating hydrocephalus can also be seen when intraventricular hemorrhage results in large obstructive clots. It typically presents 4 to 20 days after SAH. Its most common clinical presentation is a subtle change in mental status, although Parinaud's syndrome, inability to move eyes upward and lack of pupillary constriction to accommodation, may be seen rarely. This diagnosis can be confirmed with a CT scan. Because hydrocephalus may be transient, repetitive lumbar punctures can sometimes obviate more invasive procedures. However, a ventriculostomy may be necessary and eventually ventriculoperitoneal shunting may be required. Sudden large drops in ICP by abrupt removal of CSF should be avoided in patients with unclipped cerebral aneurysms, which theoretically may cause an abrupt increase in CPP and increase in transmural pressure across the aneurysm, predisposing to rebleeding.

Cerebral Vasospasm. One of the most devastating complications of SAH is cerebral arterial vasospasm, which can cause delayed focal or diffuse ischemic neurologic deficits. It is uncertain why this follows SAH from saccular aneurysm rupture, but it occurs rarely after other causes of SAH, such as trauma. This may be due either to (1) the larger volume of blood in the subarachnoid space after aneurysmal bleeding, resulting in greater cytokine release and greater amounts of free radicals produced after the breakdown of heme products or (2) local mechanical pressure effects from the high-pressure arterial bleeding of the aneurysm or from the clot itself. Vasospasm occurs between 2 to 17 days after SAH, with peak incidence at days 7 through 12.

Angiographic vasospasm has been reported in up to 70% of patients after aneurysmal SAH. Twenty-eight percent have symptomatic vasospasm. Clinical findings primarily consist of diminished mental status followed by focal neurologic deficits. A head CT scan is important to distinguish between rebleeding or hydrocephalus as causes for neurologic decline. Although an angiogram remains the definitive diagnostic tool for vasospasm, transcranial Doppler imaging (TCD) has been used to determine the presence of arterial narrowing and consequent increase in mean velocities (>120 cm/sec). Unfortunately, TCD remains limited because the only vessels reliably insonated are the middle cerebral artery and the proximal anterior cerebral artery. Interrogation of the distal anterior cerebral artery, the posterior circulation, and smaller vessels, including small perforating arteries, is not possible. In one study that used a mean flow velocity of 120 cm/sec and above to indicate vasospasm, the sensitivity of TCD was 58.6% and the specificity was 100%.

After SAH decreased CBF and delayed cerebral ischemia and infarction are well documented. Therapy therefore is directed toward elevating and sustaining CBF. SAH patients should receive no less than 3 L intake per day. However, if symptomatic vasospasm occurs, CPP should be raised by increasing mean arterial pressure through plasma volume expansion with constant infusions of both normal saline solution and 5% albumin; this is "hypertensive, hypervolemic, hemodilutional therapy" (HHT or "triple H"). A pulmonary artery catheter is typically placed to monitor and optimize hemodynamics. In patients with secured aneurysms (i.e., after clipping) target pulmonary capillary wedge pressures (PCWPs) of 15 mm Hg and target systolic blood pressures of approximately 180 mm Hg are maintained with fluids and pressor agents, usually dopamine, if necessary. Hetastarch is avoided as a plasma expander in these patients because large volumes of colloid are often needed and repetitive, prolonged therapy with hetastarch has been associated with coagulopathy and subsequent intracranial hemorrhage.

In addition to fluid and hemodynamic management, the rheologic properties of blood are also optimized. Mannitol improves red blood cell deformability, and a 20% solution of mannitol at approximately 25 to 50 ml/hr is constantly infused. Serum osmolality should be monitored and kept <310 to 320 mOsm/L. Phlebotomy or blood transfusions are performed to maintain a hematocrit of 33% ± 13%, which has theoretically optimal viscosity and oxygen carrying capacity.

In some cases a continuous mannitol infusion causes an osmotic diuresis that makes maintenance of an optimal PCWP difficult. In such cases the mannitol infusion may need to be slowed or discontinued. Alternatively, desmopressin (DDAVP), 4 μg every 4 to 6 hours, may be given subcutaneously or intravenously in an attempt to prevent diuresis and to keep urine output <250 ml/hr. Careful electrolyte monitoring is necessary because SAH patients are also prone to salt wasting (see later discussion of hyponatremia).

The calcium channel blocker nimodipine is routinely used in the treatment of SAH. This agent has shown to improve neurologic outcome, although its mechanism is unproved. It was initially believed that this agent prevents constriction of vessels; however, clinical trials have shown no change in the incidence or severity of angiographic vasospasm. It is now postulated that improved outcome is related either to decrease in vasospasm in the microvasculature, which is not visualized by angiography, or to a modification of calcium influx into damaged cells, which limits the extent of neuronal injury. Nimodipine, 60 mg every 4 hours, should be administered enterally as soon after the ictus as possible, preferably before 96 hours. It is continued for 14 to 21 days. Patients with a Hunt and Hess grade of V do not appear to benefit from therapy but are usually treated anyway. Nicardipine is another dihydropyridine calcium channel blocker studied in SAH therapy; continuous intravenous infusion for 14 days after SAH has shown to decrease the incidence of vasospasm, but compared with placebo, nicardipine has not shown to improve clinical outcome at 3 months. Hypotension is seen in approximately 5% of patients treated with enteral nimodipine and in 28% to 33% of patients treated with intravenous nicardipine. Blood pressure needs to be monitored carefully; the hypotension is typically readily treatable with fluid administration. Pulmonary edema, presumably as a manifestation of high-output congestive heart failure, has also been associated with dihydropyridine therapy.

If medical management with HHT fails, other invasive therapies for vasospasm are available through interventional neuroradiology. These include percutaneous angioplasty (PTA) with soft, compliant silicone balloons, and direct local intraarterial injection of papaverine, a benzylisoquinoline alkaloid either prepared synthetically or obtained from opium, which has a direct spasmolytic effect on vascular and other smooth muscle. Sometimes these modalities are used in conjunction. Several studies suggest a 68% to 80% clinical improvement after PTA alone or with papaverine, although the effects of papaverine may last only a few days.

Seizures and Cerebral Edema.   Seizures occur in up to 7% of SAH patients, whereas cerebral edema complicates 10% to 13.6% of cases. Treatment of these conditions are discussed in earlier sections.

Spinal Cord Injury

The acute management of spinal cord injury (SCI) includes administration of methylprednisolone 30 mg/kg followed by a 24-hour infusion at 5.4 mg/kg/hr. In a multicenter placebo-controlled trial, the National Acute Spinal Cord Injury Study (NASCIS) showed that administration of methylprednisolone within 8 hours of injury improved neurologic recovery 6 weeks, 6 months, and 1 year after injury. Further analysis of this study showed that patients treated with methylprednisolone beyond the 8-hour window (i.e., greater than 8 hours posttrauma) recovered significantly less well at 6 months and 1 year than did placebo-treated patients.

Spinal cord–injured patients present several unique management problems. During the acute phase of injury 80% to 85% of deaths are caused by pulmonary disorders. SCI patients have an 80% to 100% incidence of deep venous thrombosis; this is discussed later. In addition, acute thermoregulatory problems occur because sweating and temperature-regulating functions below the level of the lesion are lost. This can result in persistent fevers; however, infection (i.e., pneumonia, urinary tract infection, sinusitis, and line infections) is common in these patients and must be ruled out before atelectasis or loss of thermoregulatory controls are invoked. Orthostasis and edema are commonly seen as a result of loss of vascular tone.

AUTONOMIC DYSREFLEXIA

Chronic problems that can occur in SCI patients include autonomic dysreflexia, also known as autonomic hyperreflexia. This phenomenon occurs in patients with complete spinal cord lesions at or above the level of the sympathetic efferents. It has been reported in approximately 80% of individuals with cord lesion at the T6 level and above. It may occur several years after SCI.

Autonomic dysreflexia can present as a medical emergency; the patient is hypertensive (systolic blood pressure as high as 240 to 300 mm Hg), with a throbbing headache and flushing and sweating above the level of the spinal cord lesion. Below the spinal cord level the patient is pale with vasoconstriction and pilomotor erection.

The pathophysiologic process involves the inability of the sympathetic and parasympathetic to communicate because of the cord lesion. In addition, the lesion must be above the sympathetic innervation of the splanchnic vascular bed. The patient has sensory irritation below the spinal cord lesion, most commonly, bladder distention, urinary tract infection, or fecal impaction; this sensory impulse is sent cephalad through the spinal cord, but the patient is not aware of it because of the cord lesion. The sensory impulse synapses with the intermediolateral column of the spinal cord below the cord lesion, which contains postganglionic sympathetic cell bodies; this results in a sympathetic response (vasoconstriction, piloerection) below the cord level. Because these impulses involve the splanchnic bed, which is a major reservoir for blood volume, resultant sympathetic vasoconstriction forces a large blood volume to the unconstricted vessels above the cord lesion, resulting in hypertension and headache. The aortic and carotid baroreceptors sense the hypertension and produce a parasympathetic response (i.e., vasodilation that cannot be transmitted below the level of the lesion); this results in nasal congestion and flushing and sweating above the level of the lesion.

Acute treatment involves relieving the irritating stimulus and treatment of the hypertension. A Foley catheter should be flushed or placed and urine checked for signs of infection. A rectal examination should be performed to evaluate for impaction or prostatitis. Epididymitis, decubiti, ingrown toenails, and pressure on a limb, including constricting bed clothes, leg-bag straps, or lying against a bed rail, have been reported to precipitate autonomic dysreflexia. Antihypertensive medications used acutely are vasodilators such as hydralazine and nitroprusside. As an alpha blocker, phentolamine has been recommended for acute treatment but is not always effective. Phenoxybenzamine, another alpha blocker, has been effective prophylactically in doses from 20 to 60 mg/day. Prevention of irritating factors that may precipitate events are the mainstay of therapy.

Anticholinergic agents such as propantheline and oxybutynin can prevent bladder spasms in patients prone to autonomic dysreflexia. An effective bowel regimen prevents constipation and impaction and dysreflexic episodes.

Neuromuscular Complications
CRITICAL ILLNESS POLYNEUROPATHY

In an intensive care setting neuromuscular strength is often not tested unless the patient is recovering and mobilized. In an intubated patient often the first indication of weakness is the failure to wean from the ventilator. Several metabolic abnormalities may contribute to this weakness, such as hypophosphatemia, hypomagnesemia, or hypocalcemia. Numerous medications may contribute to neuromuscular transmission defects (e.g., aminoglycoside or neuromuscular blocking agents). A necrotizing myopathy associated with critically ill patients has also been described. Disuse atrophy may play a role but is not usually responsible for profound neuromuscular weakness and has no electrophysiologic abnormalities. Critical illness polyneuropathy (CIP), described by Bolton in 1984, is probably a common and often overlooked entity in the ICU. CIP has been observed in patients critically ill for over 2 weeks with associated bacteremia or focal infection with systemic effects and with involvement of two or more organs. The patient appears to have lower motor neuron dysfunction with weakness, atrophy, and areflexia and may complain of paresthesias and numbness. The CSF profile typically is normal, although CSF protein rarely can be mildly elevated (<100 mg/dl). Electrophysiologic studies show axonal degeneration affecting both motor and sensory fibers. Electromyography (EMG) reveals fibrillation potentials and positive waves consistent with denervation.

CIP is a diagnosis of exclusion. Clinically, it most resembles the Guillain-Barré syndrome (GBS), although it differs by virtue of nearly normal CSF and its electrophysiologic characteristics. As opposed to GBS, CIP has few demyelinating features (i.e., latency and velocity of conduction) and F waves are not significantly affected, although there is evidence of significant axonal injury (i.e., decreased action potential amplitude). EMG shows denervation, which is seen in only about 10% of patients with GBS. Still these two entities may not be readily distinguishable and an etiologic workup may include search for heavy metal intoxication, *Campylobacter* gastroenteritis, and porphyria.

In a prospective study of 43 critically ill patients with sepsis and multiple organ failure, electrophysiologic abnormalities were found in 70% of patients; 30% had clinical signs of weakness, areflexia, and failure to wean from assisted ventilation. If patients survive their critical illness, most patients with CIP show both clinical and electrophysiologic improvement, with a surprisingly rapid recovery over several weeks. There is a 50% chance for complete recovery; although a small number, approximately 10% to 13%, may show no improvement and ultimately die. Current treatment is limited to physical therapy with range of motion, splints, and other measures to prevent contractures and deep venous thrombosis.

PROLONGED NEUROMUSCULAR BLOCKADE

There have been many case reports of prolonged paralysis after continuous infusion of neuromuscular blocking agents in critically ill patients. The majority of the patients reported have received vecuronium, although pancuronium and atracurium have also been implicated. The mechanism for this prolonged action is unknown. Renal failure, and occasionally hepatic failure, have been present with many cases, prompting theories that decreased clearance of vecuronium and its metabolites (notably, 3-desacetylvecuronium, which has 50% of the potency of parent compound) may play a role. It is unknown if atracurium has been associated with fewer cases of prolonged paralysis because it has been used with less frequency than vecuronium or because it undergoes ester hydrolysis and Hoffman degradation without neuromuscularly active metabolites. Clearance difficulties with vecuronium would explain short-term persistent paralysis (hours to a few days). However, persistent weakness over weeks is likely to be due to a different, unknown mechanism. Recovery time averages 9 weeks and ranges from 1.8 days to 6 months.

The concomitant use of steroids has been reported in 71% of cases of prolonged paralysis and may have contributed because steroids are known to cause myopathy. Vecuronium and pancuronium contain a steroid moiety. Because some patients show electrophysiologic and microscopic evidence of myopathic changes, it is postulated that these drugs exert some toxic effect on the muscle, which may worsen with additional steroid administration. However, steroid myopathy itself does not cause EMG abnormalities. Atracurium, on the other hand, is a benzylisoquinolinium-based muscle relaxant, although cases of prolonged paralysis have been reported with steroid use and atracurium infusion.

Currently, to minimize the potential of neuromuscular complications from paralytic agents, sedation should be optimized with benzodiazepines and opioids and use of prolonged pharmacologic neuromuscular junction (NMJ) blockade should be avoided whenever possible. However, when neuromuscular blockade is necessary and intermittent dosing, which may be preferable, is not adequate, many authors recommend use of neuromuscular monitoring during continuous infusion with a train-of-four (TOF) peripheral nerve stimulator to avoid excessive dosing with saturation of all receptors, indicated by a loss of all four twitches on TOF. A 90% blockade, which is essentially equivalent to one twitch, is assumed to be optimal. This technique will prevent prolonged NMJ blockade from overdosage. However, the hypothesis that TOF monitoring will decrease the complications of NMJ blockade remains unproved. Finally, because atracurium has been associated with fewer cases of prolonged paralysis, it may be the prudent choice for patients who require long periods (>24 hours) of paralysis to maintain adequate ventilation and oxygenation, especially in renal failure patients or patients requiring steroids. It should be noted, however, that laudanosine, a metabolite of atracurium, does produce seizures in some experimental animals in high levels (17 μg/ml). Laudanosine accumulates in patients with renal and hepatic dysfunction; thus atracurium should be used cautiously in this subset of patients, particularly in patients who may also have a known seizure disorder.

Brain Death

Each hospital should have policies and procedures regarding the determination of brain death. The Uniform Determination of Death Act and the clinical report of the medical consultants to the President's Commission for the Study of Ethical Problems in Medicine and Biomedical and Behavioral Research attempt to establish certain guidelines. For determining death, the patient must have sustained an irreversible cessation of circulatory and respiratory functions or, for brain death, irreversible cessation of all functions of the entire brain, including the brainstem. Most hospitals require two physicians to independently confirm brain death; usually one of the two physicians must be trained in the neurosciences, either neurology or neurosurgery.

The clinical examination yields the most important information. Once it is determined that the patient (1) has no toxic drug levels that could interfere with the examination, (2) is near normothermic (>32.3° C), (3) has no significant metabolic or endocrinologic disturbances (e.g., severe hypoglycemia), (4) has adequate cerebral perfusion pressure, and (5) has a sufficiently irreversible and sufficient cause for brain death, the neurologic examination should be performed.

The assessment includes mental status looking for unresponsiveness, pupillary response, corneal reflex, cervicoocular reflex (also called oculocephalic or doll's eyes response), vestibuloocular reflex (also called the oculovestibular response or cold water calorics) if the cervicoocular reflex is absent, and gag reflex. When these responses are lacking, an apnea test is performed. The patient is preoxygenated with 100% Fio_2 for 10 minutes with normocapnic ventilation. Then mechanical ventilation is stopped; modes that can be used include a T-piece with a tracheal cannula delivering a 10 L/min flow of oxygen or continuous positive airway pressure (CPAP) alone. The test is prematurely terminated if the patient becomes hemodynamically unstable or has evidence of oxygen desaturation. The patient is declared apneic if there is no ventilatory effort after the Pco_2 reaches 60 torr. Most institutions require observation of a patient for at least 6 hours before this determination is made. However, confirmatory tests, such as absent CBF on angiography or nuclear medicine scanning, can establish the irreversibility of the patient's condition and obviate the need for further observation. On motor examination, decerebrate or decorticate posturing or withdrawal to painful stimuli are not consistent with brain death. However, a stereotyped triple-flexion in response to a painful stimulus to the foot and other reflexes that are spinal cord mediated, will persist after brain death has occurred.

Irreversibility when making the diagnosis is critical. In the evaluation of the patient it must be determined that significant hypothermia or sedative or hypnotic medication overdose are not contributing factors. Paralytic agents will completely abolish the neurologic examination (except that pupillary responses will still be intact). Electrocerebral silence on EEG is problematic because it occurs transiently within 6 to 8 hours after circulatory arrest and will be present in cases of severe hypothermia (<27° C) or massive barbiturate overdose. Thus EEG should be performed 8 hours or more after the precipitating event. The EEG can be technically very difficult, requiring considerable technical expertise. Thus EEG is being used less frequently in the determination of brain death.

Criteria for declaring brain death in children are slightly different. Twenty-four hours of observation are typically required. Because children can tolerate hypothermia better than adults, longer periods of observation are especially necessary after cold drowning. In neonates the EEG is used with great caution because transient electrocerebral silence has occurred with good neurologic outcome. In addition, apparent EEG activity is sometimes seen in the absence of CBF.

Finally, although a patient must meet brain death criteria to become an organ donor, the failure to meet brain death criteria does not mean that the patient will recover as an aware individual. Studies on coma have enabled neuroscientists to predict outcome based on the patient's daily neurologic examination. Levy et al. evaluated nontraumatic hypoxic-ischemic coma and developed 1-year outcome estimates based on the examination up to 7 days postevent. For example, in comatose patients without eye opening by 7 days, 92% had no recovery or progressed to a vegetative state. Eight percent had severe disability, and no patient had moderate disability or good recovery. Such studies help clinicians make difficult decisions with families when a patient does not meet full criteria for brain death but has little chance for good recovery. In traumatic coma it remains more difficult to predict the final outcome, and caution should be used when making declarations for a patient's chance to recover from coma in this situation.

CARDIAC COMPLICATIONS

Intracranial pathologic processes such as stroke, SAH, seizures, and head trauma have been well documented to cause electrographic changes. These changes consist of both transient repolarization abnormalities and arrhythmias. Autonomic dysfunction with cardiac abnormalities such as ictal asystole has been implicated in sudden, explained deaths in patients with epilepsy. This may account for 5% to 17% of mortality in epilepsy patients. In patients with stroke, hypertensive encephalopathy, SAH, and increased ICP there have been reports of peaked P waves; decreased PR intervals; peaked, inverted, or notched T waves; ST segment elevation or depression; U waves; and prolonged QT intervals. Arrhythmias have included supraventricular tachycardias, sinus bradycardia, atrioventricular (AV) block, AV dissociation, nodal rhythms, and paroxysmal ventricular tachycardia.

When these cases of ECG abnormality were first reported, autopsies showed no pathologic cardiac changes, and it was initially hypothesized that the ECG changes were due to autonomic nervous system abnormalities arising from area 13 in the orbital-frontal cortex, without actual cardiac changes. Despite normal gross and light microscopic examinations, subsequent electron microscopy studies have shown that myofibrillar degeneration is present in the hearts of these patients. Myofibrillar degeneration (also known as contraction band necrosis or coagulative myocytolysis) describes a pattern of cardiac cell death where the cells die in a hypercontracted state with prominent contraction bands, which are dense eosinophilic transverse bands, and intervening granularity throughout the cytoplasm. This injury pattern was initially described in patients with chronically elevated catecholamine levels from pheochromocytoma. The pattern differs from that seen after ischemic myocardial injury (i.e., coagulative necrosis), where the cells die in a relaxed state without the presence of contraction bands. Thus the abnormalities on ECG after CNS insult reflect an injury pattern, and cardiac enzymes are elevated in most but not all patients. For unknown reasons the repolarization changes are best seen in the inferolateral and anterolateral chest leads.

The mechanism for damage is not entirely understood. Stimulation of the hypothalamus can lead to autonomic alterations, including cardiovascular changes, which are blocked by stellate ganglion interruption. Stimulation of the limbic cortex and the mesencephalic reticular formation can also cause myofibrillar degeneration. In response to sympathetic stimulation, a sudden cellular calcium influx with an efflux of potassium may occur, which would explain the lengthening QT, peaked T waves, and U waves. Arrhythmias result from the involvement of the cardiac conduction system because myofibrillar degeneration mostly occurs in the subendocardial region, which contains the conduction system.

This entity is important to recognize. Clearly, stroke patients with arteriosclerotic disease are at risk for both cardiac and cerebrovascular disease and may have ischemic myocardium; however, in patients with seizures, SAH, or head trauma without cardiac risk factors, ECG changes may be significant and need to be monitored.

Treatment does not include the usual reperfusion maneuvers associated with ischemic myocardial infarction (i.e., aspirin, heparin, or thrombolytics); however, close cardiac monitoring is essential. Use of agents such as calcium channel blockers or sympatholytics have not been explored.

RESPIRATORY COMPLICATIONS

Neurogenic Pulmonary Edema

Pulmonary edema typically results from high intravascular hydrostatic forces, such as cardiogenic pulmonary edema, or increased vascular permeability either from a high extravascular oncotic pressure or a breakdown of the pulmonary capillary integrity. After cerebral insults, an entity known as neurogenic pulmonary edema (NPE) occurs that cannot be attributed to a single mechanism but may be due to a combination of effects.

The study of subjects with acute hypothalamic lesions, head injury with increased ICP, or seizures shows that NPE is associated with elevated levels of norepinephrine and epinephrine, increased left atrial pressures, and severe systemic hypertension causing increased afterload with decreased cardiac output. This would suggest that after neurologic insult sympathetic stimulation results in a cardiogenic mechanism for NPE through increased pulmonary vascular pressures and increased hydrostatic transcapillary fluid flux. However, carefully controlled experiments show that NPE can occur even if left atrial pressure is kept normal. Other studies have shown the presence of sphincters in the pulmonary venules that appear to constrict after experimental head injury. This again would invoke a hydrostatic phenomenon as the mechanism for NPE.

Both human studies and animal studies have also shown that NPE is associated with a high protein content, which would suggest that vascular permeability is altered, because pulmonary edema from hydrostatic causes allows water efflux, with little protein extravasation. Thus it appears that both hydrostatic and permeability changes are present. Some have theorized that the high pulmonary vascular pressures damage endothelium and allow leakage of plasma and, occasionally, leakage of red blood cells.

Experimental lesions in the hypothalamus, bilateral nucleus tractus solitarius, and the ventral medulla can produce NPE. These areas regulate systemic arterial pressure and contain areas of afferent and efferent control of the pulmonary system. Spinal cord transection appears to prevent NPE in experimental animals. Similarly, unilateral lung denervation prevents NPE in the denervated lung.

Clinically, NPE can present in two distinct forms. The classic form appears early, within minutes to a few hours after acute CNS injury. Head trauma and seizures are the typical precipitating factors. Dyspnea is the first symptom; however, chest pain and mild hemoptysis may also be seen. Physical examination shows tachypnea, tachycardia, and rales. Laboratory results show hypoxemia, and a mild leukocytosis may be present. Chest radiography shows a bilateral alveolar filling process that typically resolves within 24 to 48 hours. The PCWPs and pulmonary artery pressures can be elevated or normal. A delayed form of NPE slowly progresses over 12 to 72 hours after CNS injury. The clinical manifestations are similar to the early form with the exception of the slower time course. The diagnosis of NPE is one of exclusion because the differential diagnosis often includes aspiration pneumonitis, pneumonia, atelectasis, or cardiogenic edema.

Treatment is supportive and often requires supplemental oxygen and positive pressure ventilation. PEEP may be necessary for adequate oxygenation; however, high levels of PEEP, as well as positive pressure ventilation alone, may increase CVP and decrease CPP and must be used with caution. Use of alpha- and beta-adrenergic blockade in experimental animals shows some promise. Dobutamine administration to augment cardiac output and reduce total peripheral vascular resistance has been advocated but has not been well studied.

Airway Management

In patients with closed head injury (CHI), those with a GCS ≤8 or with elevated ICP require endotracheal intubation. In addition, any uncooperative patient who will need significant sedation should also be intubated to maintain an airway and ensure adequate ventilation. Because up to 10% of patients with CHI also have cervical spine injury, cervical immobilization and intubation in the neutral position is essential until the neck can be fully evaluated. Nasotracheal intubation should be avoided in all patients with suspected basilar skull fractures and sinus injuries.

In addition to establishing an airway, preventing iatrogenic ICP elevations and maintenance of CPP are two essential goals during endotracheal intubation. Coughing significantly elevates ICP. Cough prevention with neuromuscular blocking agents appears to be more effective than with thiopental, lidocaine, or fentanyl. Barbiturates and lidocaine, however, are effective in attenuating ICP increases caused by tracheal stimulation when also given with a paralytic agent. Succinylcholine administration is controversial in the acutely head injured patients because it may transiently increase ICP because of increased carbon dioxide production or the effect of fasciculations. Coadministration of thiopental, lidocaine, or etomidate may minimize these changes. Defasciculation with another paralytic agent such as metocurine may also be effective. The use of rocuronium, a nondepolarizing, rapid-acting neuromuscular blocking agent may begin to play a greater role in rapid induction. Succinylcholine should be avoided in all patients who have been immobile for several days because of the risk of hyperkalemia that results from the depolarizing agent. Fatal cardiac arrhythmias can occur.

Hemodynamic parameters and ICP must be assessed before an appropriate hypnotic and dosage are chosen. Large drops in MAP can compromise CPP and should be avoided. In patients who are hypertensive, an antihypertensive agent or narcotic may be necessary to attenuate the hypertension associated with tracheal stimulation. Nitroprusside and nitroglycerin for blood pressure control should be avoided because they cause cerebral vasodilation and thereby elevate ICP. Anesthetic agents that should be avoided in this setting include halothane and ketamine because they increase ICP. Etomidate, which lowers CBF, may be useful in the hypovolemic patient to avoid drops in blood pressure, but the myoclonus associated with induction must be prevented with neuromuscular blocking agents.

Airway management in the convulsing patient is obviously easier if the seizures can first be controlled. In a patient who is having seizures for a short period, turning the head to the side may help prevent aspiration. In patients with SE or a prolonged postictal state and who are unresponsive, airway control with endotracheal intubation may become necessary. Intubation of a patient with tonic or clonic activity may be difficult. Termination of seizures may be achieved with benzodiazepines or high-dose barbiturates. If a paralytic agent is used to facilitate intubation, it will mask the clinical manifestations of seizures, but cerebral seizure activity and subsequent CNS damage will continue. For this reason a short-acting paralytic agent should be used, and administration of antiepileptic medications are essential. Continuous EEG monitoring to rule out sub-clinical seizures should be performed if more than one dose of a paralytic agent becomes necessary to maintain adequate ventilation.

In patients with cervical spine injury, maneuvers such as chin lift and jaw thrust can increase distraction and subluxation at the cervical injury site. Manual in-line traction can also increase distraction; therefore direct laryngoscopy should be performed with head and neck stabilization without traction in an emergency setting with a patient with neck injury. If the patient is awake and co-operative, fiberoptic laryngoscopy has a high success rate and may minimize neck movement. Awake intubation performed blindly may also be used, although nasotracheal intubation must be avoided in patients with suspected basilar skull fractures and should not be per-formed in an uncooperative patient who may become agitated and move because it may cause further cervical injury. Retrograde tra-cheal intubation has also been performed successfully in this sub-group of patients. In a patient with an anatomically difficult airway, cricothyroidotomy may be necessary. Finally, in patients who are stabilized in a halo or tongs, direct laryngoscopy is difficult, and of-ten fiberoptic or blind technique becomes necessary.

Respiratory Failure

Patients with neurologic disease present a unique subset of pa-tients requiring mechanical ventilation. In most postoperative set-tings patients primarily have a failure to adequately ventilate as a result of deep sedation from anesthesia or from pulmonary patho-logic processes; these patients can usually be extubated once they are awake and the pulmonary status improves. These problems also occur in neurosurgical patients; however, in this population central ventilatory drive may be impaired and cranial nerve dysfunction can diminish the ability of a patient to maintain or protect the airway.

The ninth and tenth cranial nerves are necessary for palatal sen-sation and movement, which are necessary for airway protection and the gag reflex. The twelfth cranial nerve provides tongue move-ment, and its impairment can also result in aspiration. However, it is less commonly recognized that at higher levels of ventilatory effort, upper airway muscles such as the adductors of the palate, dilators of the pharynx, and retractors of the tongue assist in preventing col-lapse of the upper airway; these muscles derive their innervation from the fifth, seventh, and ninth through twelfth cranial nerves.

Autonomic control of respiration is distributed throughout the neuroaxis. Bilateral frontal lesions result in Cheyne-Stokes respirations, which are characterized by seconds of hyperpnea alternating with apneic spells. Animal studies suggest this is due to an increased sensitivity to carbon dioxide and a decrease in forebrain ventilatory stimulus, causing apnea. Lesions throughout the brainstem result in abnormal patterns of breathing, including central reflex hyperpnea (a manifestation of NPE in some cases), apneusis, cluster breathing, and ataxic breathing—associated with low midbrain or pons, lower pons, high medullary, and lower medullary lesions, respectively.

Because diaphragmatic innervation is derived from C3 through C5, complete spinal cord lesions above the C3 level will result in complete respiratory failure and ventilatory dependence. However, in patients with lesions below this level but above the midthoracic levels, respiratory failure may also occur in the acute setting. This is a consequence of the action of the anterior intercostal muscles, innervated by the upper thoracic roots, to splint the chest wall outward while the diaphragm descends. Without this action the patient has a functional flail chest. After several weeks to months developing spasticity of these muscles alleviates this problem.

The first sign of respiratory failure in patients with intact respiratory drive is often tachypnea. Clinical evidence of respiratory failure should take precedence over laboratory values such as arterial blood gas results, although poor oxygenation may by itself be an indication for intubation. A rising P_{CO_2} is a late sign of inadequate ventilation, and intubation with mechanical ventilation should be initiated before it occurs. Other indications of impending respiratory failure include a forced vital capacity (FVC) <12 ml/kg and a peak negative inspiratory pressure (NIP) < -25 cm H_2O.

Successful ventilator weaning remains difficult to predict, especially in this population. Traditionally, minute ventilation <10 L, maximal inspiratory pressure < -15 cm H_2O, and vital capacity (VC) >12 to 15 ml/kg have been used as positive predictors of successful weaning trials but are often inaccurate. Two other indices that have been used are the ratio of frequency of breaths to tidal volume (f/V_T) and an integrative index of static compliance, respiratory rate, arterial oxygenation and maximum inspiratory pressure (CROP). Studies have shown that an f/V_T ratio of >105 and an NIP > -15 cm H_2O are good predictors of weaning failure. However, there are no indices that provide strong positive prediction of weaning outcome.

With current modes of ventilation, T-piece trials and CPAP are less frequently used for weaning of mechanical ventilation in neurologically impaired patients. The pressure support mode is often better tolerated by the patient, and progressively lowering the degree of pressure support assistance each day allows less taxing, less abrupt weaning capabilities. However, optimal weaning modes remain controversial.

INFECTIOUS COMPLICATIONS
Prophylactic Antibiotics

Attempts to determine the efficacy of antimicrobial prophylaxis in the neurosurgical setting regarding clean, nonimplant neurosurgical procedures, intracranial bolt placement, intraventricular catheters, and shunts, have been clouded with difficulties in study design and implementation. Because of the high morbidity and mortality of central nervous infections, however, it is common practice to give prophylactic antibiotics whenever the CNS is instrumented.

Studies of clean, nonimplant neurosurgical procedures have shown an incidence of infection in either control or placebo groups of 3.5% to 7.3%, whereas antibiotic treatment with gram-positive cocci coverage decreases infection to 0.5% to 1.8%. Subsequently, it is common practice to administer prophylactic antibiotics just before and several doses after surgery. Unfortunately, there is a paucity of well-designed clinical studies that clarify these issues, including dosages.

Temporary ventricular catheters have an 8% to 11% incidence of infection within 5 days. At 12 days the incidence rises to 40%. Thus the most effective method to diminish ventriculostomy infection is removal as soon as possible. If a ventriculostomy is needed for longer than 5 to 7 days, most often another is placed through a different burr hole. The second catheter has the same risks as though it were the first one placed. Daily antibiotic prophylactic therapy is also given while the catheter is in place. Risk factors leading to ventricular catheter infection include increased ICP and intraventricular hemorrhage. Once a CSF infection is detected, removal of the catheter is essential; direct ventricular instillation of an antibiotic is often undertaken but with few data to support its use.

Ventriculoatrial or ventriculoperitoneal shunts have a 3% to 27% incidence of infection. Seventy percent of these occur within the first 2 months after placement, whereas 90% occur within the first 6 months. This would suggest that inoculation occurs at surgery. True shunt infections involve internal colonization, usually by coagulase-negative staphylococci, which has a mucoid carbohydrate which allows binding to the catheter. True shunt infections differ from infections at the incisional site or at the intracutaneous portion (i.e., catheter tract infections), which commonly are due to *Staphylococcus aureus* or gram-negative bacilli. Once a diagnosis of infection is made, the shunt is externalized. Typical antibiotic practice during shunt placement includes preoperative dosing continued until the third postoperative day.

There have been no studies of ICP monitoring devices. With the fiberoptic systems available now, the risk for infection appears to be low. Despite this, prophylactic gram-positive antibiotic coverage is often given while the temporary monitor is in place.

Although vancomycin had been the drug of choice for antibiotic prophylaxis in many centers, the emergence of vancomycin-resistant enterococci has forced a shift to nafcillin, cefazolin, or ceftriaxone.

Meningitis

In the posttraumatic neurosurgical ICU population, meningitis complicates open, depressed skull fractures in 4% to 10% and basilar skull fractures in up to 22%. Postoperative meningitis must be considered whenever a patient who has undergone a procedure in proximity to the cranial or spinal dura mater is febrile and complains of headache or exhibits changes in mental status. Meningismus may be lacking in very young, elderly, or immunosuppressed patients, including those receiving corticosteroids. If a ventricular catheter is in place, CSF can be sent with relative ease. If not, a lumbar puncture should be performed with alacrity. If there is a possibility of an intracranial space-occupying mass (i.e., hematoma, abscess, or metastases), which is often the case for neurosurgical patients, broad-spectrum antibiotics (e.g., a third-generation cephalosporin such as ceftriaxone or cefotaxime) should be initiated while a CT scan is being arranged. Recent studies show that 33% of nosocomial meningitis are caused by gram-negative bacilli other than *Haemophilus influenzae*. This contrasts to 3% found in community-acquired episodes. If the patient has been hospitalized for a period of time, both gram-positive cocci and gram-negative bacilli, including *Pseudomonas* species should be covered (e.g., vancomycin, ceftazidime, and an aminoglycoside).

Interpretation of CSF results typically depends on a pleocytosis. The number of leukocytes of more than 5 per microliter is concerning, especially with neutrophilic predominance, but is usually >100 per microliter in 80% to 90% of cases. Protein content is >45 mg/dl in 90% of cases. Glucose content less than two thirds the serum level is seen in 45% to 50% of cases. In the neurosurgical population, especially those patients with recent SAH, cell counts and protein levels may be elevated as a result of a chemical meningitis from subarachnoid blood. In these patients a low glucose level can be helpful to determine whether a bacterial meningitis exists; however, because it is not a sensitive test, if uncertainty exists and there is any clinical suspicion, the patient should be treated empirically for bacterial meningitis.

The use of steroids in the treatment of meningitis is debated. In the pediatric population there is evidence to suggest that dexamethasone, by mediating the inflammatory cascade of cytokines, decreases sensorineural hearing loss and neurologic abnormalities after meningitis. In the adult population dexamethasone may decrease the mortality rate in *Streptococcus pneumoniae* meningitis. However, the increasing resistance of this organism to penicillin and third-generation cephalosporins is tempering enthusiasm for the use of steroids in adults with meningitis because these drugs may impair antibiotic penetration into the CNS by decreasing inflammation; this results in delayed sterilization of CSF. No recommendations in adults have been made, although in children the American Academy of Pediatrics recommends dexamethasone 0.6 mg/kg/day in four doses during the first 4 days of proved or strongly suspected bacterial meningitis.

GASTROINTESTINAL COMPLICATIONS
Bleeding Prophylaxis

Gastric mucosal abnormalities are seen in 70% to 100% of patients within 18 hours of admission into the intensive care unit; 2% to 10% of these have clinically significant bleeding. Patients with CNS injury or disease have an increased risk for gastrointestinal (GI) bleeding. Kamada reported a 30% incidence of GI bleeding in severely head-injured patients, and a 17% incidence in 433 patients with any degree of head injury. Other risk factors include prolonged mechanical ventilation, high-dose corticosteroid administration, sepsis syndrome, burn injury, major trauma or surgical procedures, hypotension, and renal and hepatic failure. One of the methods of stress prophylaxis is to neutralize the acidity of gastric acids (normal pH is <3.5) using antacids and H_2 blockers. A disadvantage of alkalinizing gastric pH is the proliferation of bacteria in the stomach, particularly gram-negative bacilli. Passive esophageal reflux and microaspiration of less acidic stomach contents may increase the risk of nosocomial pneumonia in mechanically ventilated patients. Treatment with sucralfate allows cytoprotection without effecting gastric pH.

Recent randomized controlled trials in a mixed population of ICU patients (i.e., surgical and medical) suggest that sucralfate may be as effective as H_2 blockers in preventing gastrointestinal bleeding and is associated with fewer nosocomial pneumonias (5% vs 21%). In one study in a medical ICU stress ulcer–related hemorrhage was seen equally in control patients and cimetidine- and sucralfate-treated patients. There was some suggestion, not statistically significant, that treated groups had a higher incidence of nosocomial pneumonia. However, it should be noted that enteral tube feedings, which are known to buffer stomach secretions, were given to a majority of control patients.

Currently, prophylaxis with sucralfate might be a reasonable first choice; however, it does require enteral access and can interact with other medications, including phenytoin, quinolones, and digoxin. If no enteral access is possible, intermittent infusions of H_2 blocker should be administered. Continuous infusions of H_2 blockers are superior to intermittent infusions in sustaining higher levels of gastric pH but not necessarily in decreasing risk of bleeding. Because of the possibility of increasing nosocomial pneumonia with alkaline stomach contents, bolus administration may be preferable. Of the H_2 blockers, cimetidine has the most adverse side effects and drug interactions. Famotidine and rantidine have fewer CNS complications. Famotidine is less frequently associated with thrombocytopenia.

NUTRITIONAL CONCERNS

Hyperglycemia at the time of induced cerebral ischemia has been shown to increase neurologic deficits in experimental animals.

In humans admission hyperglycemia appears to correlate with worsened neurologic outcome; however, it is not clear whether the hyperglycemia is causative or a reflection of the severity of neurologic damage. That is, it is possible that patients admitted with greater infarct size or worse medical conditions have a greater stress-related release of cortisol, growth hormone, and catecholamines, which results in insulin resistance. This, in turn, is reflected in higher admission glucose levels. It is postulated that hyperglycemic, ischemic animals do worse because elevation of cerebral glucose levels at the time of ischemia and relative hypoxia may increase the rate of anaerobic cerebral metabolism. The resultant cerebral lactic acidosis promotes free radical formation and subsequent neuronal damage. Cerebral acidosis may also cause local vasodilation and hyperemia, and promote cerebral edema. For this reason tight glucose control of neurologically injured patients has been advocated.

In the 1980s it was postulated that ketosis may play a role in treatment of neurologically damaged patients. Animal studies suggested that ketotic subjects had enhanced survival after hypoxia. Because ketones can supply as much as 60% of the energy requirements of the brain in fasting individuals, preexisting ketosis may reduce cerebral lactate formation. In addition, it may enhance hypoxic tolerance by maintaining the energy-producing capacity of the brain. For this reason, some investigators have advocated relative starvation if there is significant possibility of ischemia (e.g., in the postsubarachnoid population who have a risk of vasospasm). In addition, conventional alimentation formulas use glucose as the major nonprotein calorie source. Animal studies looking at other nonprotein sources of nutrition including glycerol, xylitol, sorbitol, and ketogenic energy substrates such as beta-hydroxybutyrate, acetate, and butyrate are in progress. Human studies are investigating medium-chain triglycerides in a similar role.

Despite this, because patients with head injury are hypermetabolic, early feeding of neurosurgical patients is as important as in any group found in an ICU. Moore and Jones have shown in patients with severe abdominal injury that septic complications are significantly reduced in patients with early (<18 hours) enteral feeding compared with control patients who were started on total parenteral nutrition (TPN), if they were not tolerating a diet by 5 days (4% vs 26%). Similarly, in one study of patients with head trauma early feeding with TPN (<48 hours) was associated with improvement in GCS in the first 18 days, although neurologic status at 1 year was only equivocally improved. Grahm et al. demonstrated that early (<36 hours) jejunal feeding decreased length of stay; late feeding initiated 4 to 5 days after head injury did not reduce the frequency of sepsis. In both studies early nutrition significantly reduced septic complications.

There are many theories as to why early nutrition may be beneficial in reducing septic complications. In animals enteral feedings appear to prevent atrophy of the GI tract and maintain the "gut barrier" that prevents bacterial translocation. Even if bacterial translocation does not occur in humans, disruption of the gut barrier may be responsible for release of cytokines and complement and initiate the systemic inflammatory response syndrome. Enteral feeding may also maintain the gut flora, and stimulate peristalsis and gut production of secretory immunoglobulin A (sIgA). sIgA presents antigens to the gut-associated lymphoid tissue. Parenteral glutamine also appears to maintain sIgA production. Finally, the reason that early parenteral nutrition is nearly as effective as early enteral nutrition in improving outcome may be related to the hypermetabolic response of injury. Early nutrition may attenuate protein catabolism and may decrease the stress response.

Thus, to improve neurologic outcome and to decrease septic complications, early nutrition, preferably enteral feedings, should be started within 36 to 48 hours of injury. However, serum glucose should be closely monitored and tightly controlled with insulin if necessary.

ENDOCRINOLOGIC COMPLICATIONS

Hypernatremia

Derangement in serum sodium level is a common occurrence in patients in an ICU. Hypernatremia typically reflects excessive free water loss from the skin, the kidney, the respiratory tract, or the gastrointestinal tract; in hypovolemic patients free water replacement is required (see below). In the neurosurgical unit neurogenic diabetes insipidus may occur with head trauma, primary brain tumors, metastatic brain tumors, and ruptured cerebral aneurysms. Approximately 15% to 20% patients with transsphenoidal resection of pituitary adenomas have neurogenic diabetes insipidus, but this condition resolves spontaneously 2 to 4 days after surgery. The diagnosis is dependent on a high serum sodium without diuretic use and a urine specific gravity of 1.005 for 2 hours with urine output 250 ml greater than fluid intake for over 1 hour or 1 liter urine output over 4 hours. DDAVP may be administered 2 to 4 units subcutaneously or intravenously every 6 to 8 hours titrated to urine output. Free water replacement may become necessary. Total body water (TBW) deficit is calculated by:

$$\text{TBW deficit} = \text{Desired TBW} - \text{Current TBW}$$

where

$$\text{Current TBW} = 0.6 \times \text{Current body weight (kg)}$$

$$\text{Desired TBW} = \frac{\text{Measured serum sodium} \times \text{current TBW}}{\text{Normal serum sodium}}.$$

When hypernatremia is present for over 24 hours, rapid correction may result in significant cerebral edema. Therefore it is prudent to correct half the TBW deficit over 24 hours and the second half over 2 to 4 days.

Hyponatremia

Hyponatremia is a common electrolyte abnormality in any ICU. Its evaluation requires measurement of serum osmolality to determine whether osmotically active compounds commonly found in neurosurgical patients (such as mannitol, glucose, or ethanol) may be responsible; in this case the serum is hyperosmolar as opposed to hypoosmolar. Next, an assessment of fluid status allows a differential diagnosis to be formulated. Congestive heart failure, cirrhosis, and nephrotic syndrome are associated with hypervolemic hypoosmolar hyponatremia. Hypovolemic hypoosmolar hyponatremia can be seen with dehydration caused by diarrhea, vomiting, renal losses (especially associated with diuretic use), adrenal insufficiency, and cerebral salt wasting (CSW). A euvolemic state is typically seen with hypothyroidism, and the syndrome of inappropriate antidiuretic hormone (SIADH).

CSW was first described by Peters in the 1950s. He speculated that hyponatremia after head injury was a result of corticotropin deficiency or CNS control of the kidney. In 1957 Schwartz described SIADH in patients with hyponatremia and hypoosmolality associated with bronchogenic carcinoma. Patients with CNS injury have elevated antidiuretic hormone. Also, nicotinic acetylcholine receptors on supraoptic neurons, neuropeptide Y, stress, and pain appear to stimulate antidiuretic hormone release. For this reason centrally stimulated SIADH has long been felt to be responsible for the hypoosmolar hyponatremia seen with CNS insults. Despite this, we now know that CSW is a distinct entity from SIADH. Clinically, CSW and SIADH appear to be similar; however, the most significant differences are plasma volume and clinical fluid status. In SIADH both plasma volume and clinical fluid status are normal to slightly increased; in contrast, patients with CSW are volume depleted. Thus it is important to distinguish between the two entities because fluid restriction is an important part of the therapy for SIADH. However, in one study of a group of patients with SAH and hyponatremia, probably from CSW, treatment with fluid restriction led to markedly worsened neurologic outcome with increased risk for cerebral infarction.

The mechanism of CSW is not completely understood. The most plausible theory involves atrial natriuretic peptide (ANP), which is known to be stimulated by atrial stimulation either by stretch or tachycardia but is also found in the anteroventral periventricular nucleus, which is adjacent to the anterior tip of the third ventricle. ANP acts as a vasodilator to decrease blood pressure and also decreases aldosterone production by direct action on the adrenal cortex. It predominantly acts on the kidney to increase urinary excretion of sodium and decrease renin production. Thus by several actions ANP lowers serum sodium. After SAH studies have shown that both antidiuretic hormone and ANP are elevated; however, over several days ADH returns to normal levels, but ANP continues to increase. The predominance of ANP over time likely leads to salt and water wasting, leaving the patient both salt and fluid depleted. Thus, in contrast to SIADH, replacement of sodium and administration of large amounts of fluid are essential to the management of patients with CSW. Addition of exogenous mineralocorticoid in the form of fludrocortisone may be helpful in this condition.

Rapid correction of significant hyponatremia (i.e., <120 mEq/L) should be avoided. Central pontine myelinolysis and extrapontine myelinolysis may occur 1 to 2 days after rapid correction. Clinically, the patient appears to be doing well and is awake and conversant after recovering from hyponatremia; however, 1 to 2 days later the patient is found obtunded with a quadriparesis that becomes spastic over time. Correction at a rate slower than 12 mEq/L/day or 0.5 mEq/L/hr decreases the incidence of this severely disabling or fatal complication. If hyponatremia is causing secondary life-threatening complications (e.g., seizures) correction at the same rate with loop diuretics, such as furosemide, and fluid replacement with normal saline solution should be adequate. "Hot salt" or 3% saline solution should be avoided as much as possible because it is often associated with overcorrecting hyponatremia. However, if the loop diuretic does not lower the urinary osmolality below 290 mOsm/L, 3% saline solution may be necessary.

Hypoadrenalism

It is not always recognized that patients with critical illness have an exaggerated cortisol response. Several studies have shown that baseline cortisol levels are much higher than those in healthy controls, often ranging from 40 to 50 mg/dl. These higher levels are not suppressible by dexamethasone infusion. In addition to elevated baseline corticotropin and cortisol concentrations, it also appears that cortisol-releasing hormone stimulation in critically ill patients results in significantly higher plasma corticotropin and serum cortisol levels than in controls.

Often in the workup of hyponatremia, thyroid and random cortisol levels are obtained. An elevated baseline cortisol level appears to be positively correlated with the degree of illness and with mortality rate. However, in the setting of hyponatremia and occasionally hypotension, hyperkalemia, and fever, a baseline cortisol level that would be adequate in a normal individual may reflect a relatively hypoadrenal state in a critically ill patient. There have been case reports of so-called occult hypoadrenalism in patients in an ICU with critical multisystem disease and hypotension with elevated cardiac output and low vascular resistance refractory to vasopressors. Despite cortisol levels that would appear to be adequate (i.e., ranging between 15.9 to 23.0 mg/dl), treatment with stress doses of hydrocortisone resulted in weaning of pressors within 24 hours. Although there have been no controlled studies, hypoadrenal shock may be a potential cause for refractory hypotension, fever, and electrolyte abnormalities in a critically ill patient. Hydrocortisone administration of 100 mg intravenously every 6 to 8 hours should be adequate therapy for such patients.

HEMATOLOGIC COMPLICATIONS
Coagulopathy

Disseminated intravascular coagulation (DIC) involves the pathologic activation of coagulation factors. As a result, clotting occurs and fibrinogen, platelets, and coagulation factors are consumed, leaving the patient with a curious mix of thrombosis with microangiopathic red blood cell destruction and a bleeding diathesis because clotting factors are used and destroyed. DIC has been associated with infection and the systemic inflammatory response syndrome and has a well-documented association with stroke and severe head injury. In one study of patients with closed head injury elevated prothrombin time (PT), partial thromboplastin time (PTT), or low platelet count was documented in 37.5% of patients on admission. In another large prospective study 8% of patients had laboratory evidence of DIC, and 32% of patients had some evidence of nonspecific coagulation abnormalities. Abnormal clotting studies have been associated with a higher risk of delayed neurologic insult as documented by CT scan (85% vs 31%).

The brain contains high levels of thromboplastin, which combines with factor VII to activate the extrinsic coagulation pathway. The diagnosis of DIC is made by laboratory tests, including decreased platelet count and fibrinogen level; PT and PTT are prolonged and fibrin degradation products, including D-dimer, are increased. In patients with a clinical bleeding diathesis, these laboratory tests should be obtained. Although platelet transfusions and administration of fresh frozen plasma (FFP) to correct laboratory abnormalities are often conversial in subclinical DIC, in neurosurgical patients potential intracerebral hemorrhage would be devastating. For this reason platelet transfusion and repletion of clotting factors with FFP should be performed if platelets are <50,000/μL and PT and PTT are elevated. Antifibrinolytic therapy (i.e., epsilon-aminocaproic acid), is not recommended, because systemic thrombosis may result. Heparin is used only when patients have evidence of systemic thrombosis and desperate measures are needed.

Venous Thromboembolic Disease

The incidence of deep venous thrombosis in patients after neurosurgical procedures has been reported between 18% and 50%. However, in patients with paralysis after SCI the incidence of deep venous thrombosis varies between 80% and 100%, depending on the method of detection. Invasive methods of investigation such as iodine 125–labeled fibrinogen scan and venography have the greatest sensitivity. The combination of clinical evidence of deep venous thrombosis with both positive impedance plethysmography and lower extremity Doppler ultrasound has a 100% sensitivity. The risk of deep venous thrombosis appears to be greatest during the first 12 weeks after SCI. In the nonparalyzed patient who is immobilized with spinal fracture but lacks the flaccid immobility of paralysis the incidence of deep venous thrombosis has been reported to be 0% to 8%. Significant pulmonary embolism occurs up to 3% to 8% of the general neurosurgical population and in 8% to 21% of patients with spinal injury.

Prophylaxis of thromboembolism continues to be a debated topic. Sequential compression devices, which contain an air-filled bladder that rhythmically compress the calf musculature, decreased the incidence of deep venous thrombosis from 78% to 40% in one small study by Green ($n = 15$). The addition of aspirin 325 mg twice daily and dipyridamole 75 mg three times daily decreased the incidence to 25%.

Anticoagulation with warfarin has been an effective prophylaxis for postsurgical orthopedic patients; however, trials of prophylactic warfarin anticoagulation in the neurosurgical population have posed significant bleeding risks and are not recommended.

Green compared fixed low-dose heparin of 5000 U twice daily with low-dose heparin adjusted to prolong the activated partial thromboplastin time (aPTT) to 1.5 times control values. Both were administered subcutaneously. Thromboembolism occurred in 31% with fixed-dose heparin compared with 7% with adjusted-dose heparin, a statistically significant difference. Patients with adjusted-dose heparin required a mean of 13,200 ± 2200 U of heparin per dose every 12 hours; 24% of these patients had significant bleeding complications, including GI, hemothorax, hematoma, or oozing from line site, which necessitated discontinuation of heparin.

Low-molecular-weight heparin (LMWH) may provide the safest, most effective means of thromboembolism prophylaxis. LMWH binds to antithrombin III in such a manner that it does not affect factor II and primarily has anti-X_a properties. As a result, it produces less frequent bleeding complications than heparin, and the aPTT does not reflect its activity; thus laboratory monitoring is superfluous. In pilot studies LMWH compares favorably with standard heparin in preventing thromboembolism and is associated with significantly fewer bleeding complications. One study treated patients with SCI with tinazeparin with a dose of 3500 anti-X_a U given subcutaneously once daily. Eighty-five percent of patients were free of thrombosis or bleeding after 8 weeks of treatment. Further multicenter trials are being proposed to confirm the efficacy and safety of these new agents.

Current recommendations regarding heparin anticoagulation after the diagnosis of deep venous thrombosis or pulmonary embolism are based on the desired safe loading doses that quickly are effectively therapeutic. Raschke described a weight-based nomogram with an 80 U/kg body weight bolus followed by an infusion of 13 U/kg/hr. The nomogram guided rate adjustments on subsequent PTTs. On this regimen only two of 62 patients (3%) have subtherapeutic anticoagulation after 24 hours. Five percent had subsequent thromboembolism and none had major bleeding complications.

Caval interruption with Greenfield filters has been used in patients with risks for anticoagulation therapy. Risks of these filters include distal migration and perforation of the vena cava. SCI patients often require "quad coughing" chest physical therapy for mobilization of pulmonary secretions. In one series of nine patients with Greenfield filters who also required quad coughing, four patients had distal migration of the filter, and three of the four had filter deformation. Two patients required laparotomy for bowel perforation. Thus caval interruption should be considered carefully in patients requiring quad coughing.

Suggested Readings

Balshi JD, Cantelmo NL, Menzoian JO: Complications of caval interruption by Greenfield filter in quadriplegics, *J Vasc Surg* 9:558, 1989.

Bleck TP: Seizures in the intensive care unit. In Parillo JE, Bone RC, editors: *Critical care medicine: principles of diagnosis and management,* St Louis, 1995, Mosby.

Bolton CF, Gilbert JJ, Hahn AF, et al: Polyneuropathy in critically ill patients, *J Neurol Neurosurg Psych* 47:1223, 1984.

Bracken MB, Holford TR: Effects of timing of methylprednisolone or naloxone administration on recovery of segmental and long-tract neurological function in NASCIS 2, *J Neurosurg* 79:500, 1993.

Cherian L, Peek K, Robertson CS, et al: Calorie sources and recovery from central nervous system ischemia, *Crit Care Med* 22:1841, 1994.

Gentleman D, Jennett B: Hazards of inter-hospital transfer of comatose head-injured patients, *Lancet* 2:853, 1981.

Grahm TW, Zadrozny DB, Harrington T: The benefits of early jejunal hyperalimentation in the head-injured patient, *Neurosurgery* 25:729, 1989.

Green D: Prevention of thromboembolism after spinal cord injury, *Semin Thromb Hemost* 17:347, 1991.

Haley EC, Kassell NF, Torner JC, et al: A randomized trial of two doses of nicardipine in aneurysmal subarachnoid hemorrhage, *J Neurosurg* 80:788, 1994.

Hansen-Flaschen J, Cowen J, Raps EC: Neuromuscular blockade in the intensive care unit: more than we bargained for, *Am Rev Respir Dis* 147:234, 1993.

Kamada T, Fusamoto H, Kawano S, et al: Gastrointestinal bleeding following head injury: a clinical study of 433 cases, *J Trauma* 17:44, 1977.

Kohi YM, Mendelow AD, Teasdale GM, et al: Extracranial insults and outcome in patients with acute head injury—relationship to the Glasgow Coma Scale, *Injury* 16:25, 1984.

Levy DE, Caronna JJ, Singer BH, et al: Predicting outcome from hypoxic-ischemic coma, *JAMA* 253:1420, 1985.

Miller JD, Butterworth JF, Gudeman SK, et al: Further experience with the management of severe head injury, *J Neurosurg* 54:289, 1981.

Moore EE, Jones TN: Benefits of immediate jejunostomy feeding after major abdominal trauma—a prospective, randomized study, *J Trauma* 26:874, 1986.

Origitano TC, Wascher TM, Reichman OH, et al: Sustained increased cerebral blood flow with prophylactic hypertensive hypervolemic hemodilution ("triple-H" therapy) after subarachnoid hemorrhage, *Neurosurgery* 27:729, 1990.

Pagni CA: Posttraumatic epilepsy. Incidence and prophylaxis, *Acta Neurochir Suppl* 50:38, 1990.

Povlishock JT: Pathobiology of traumatically induced axonal injury in animals and man, *Ann Emerg Med* 22:980, 1993.

Raschke RA, Reilly BM, Guidry JR, et al: The weight-based heparin dosing nomogram compared with a "standard care" nomogram: a randomized controlled trial, *Ann Intern Med* 119:874, 1993.

Samuels MA: Neurogenic heart disease: a unifying hypothesis, *Am J Cardiol* 60:15J, 1987.

Seelig JM, Becker DP, Miller JD, et al: Traumatic acute subdural hematoma: major mortality reduction in comatose patients treated within four hours, *N Engl J Med* 304:1511, 1981.

Simon RP: Neurogenic pulmonary edema, *Neurol Clin* 11:309, 1993.

Sloan MA, Haley EC, Kassell NJ, et al: Sensitivity and specificity of transcranial Doppler ultrasonography in the diagnosis of vasospasm following subarachnoid hemorrhage, *Neurology* 39:1514, 1989.

Temkin NR, Dikmen SS, Wilensky AJ, et al: A randomized, double-blind study of phenytoin for the prevention of post-traumatic seizures, *N Engl J Med* 323:497, 1990.

Witt NJ, Zochodne DN, Bolton CF, et al: Peripheral nerve function in sepsis and multiple organ failure, *Chest* 99:176, 1991.

INDEX